THE ROYAL MARSDEN HOSPITAL

Manual of Clinical Nursing Policies
and Procedures

Edited by
A Phylip Pritchard and Valerie-Anne Walker
Research Assistants, Department of Nursing Research

Contributors
Judith M Bibbings, RGN DipN, Sister, Recovery Unit
Derryn Borley, RGN RCNT, Assistant Director of Nursing Services
Monica Burchall, RGN, Sister, High Dependency Unit
Antionette Byrne, DipDiets CMS COPQ, Dietitian
Emma L Dilnutt, RGN RSCN RCNT, Clinical Nurse Specialist (Continuing
  Care)
Nest Howells, RGN DipN, Clinical Nurse Specialist (Stoma Care)
Sarah Hart, RGN Clinical Nurse Specialist (Control of Infection/Radiation
  Protection)
Jennifer M Hunt, BA MPhil RGN FRCN, Director of Nursing Services
Elizabeth M Janes, BSc RGN, Clinical Nurse Specialist (Nutrition)
Glynis A Markham, RGN RMN FETC, Assistant Director of Nursing Services
Cathryn Newton, BA RGN DipN, Sister Burdett Coutts and Eric Gibb Ward
Judith Pretty, RGN RCNT, Clinical Nurse Specialist (Head and Neck Unit)
Phylip A Pritchard, BA RGN RMN, Research Assistant, Nursing Research
  Department
Ray Rowden, RGN RMN ONC MBIM, Director of Nursing Services
Valerie D Speechley, RGN RCNT, Clinical Nurse Specialist (Intravenous
  Therapy)
Valerie-Anne Walker, BSc RGN, Research Assistant, Nursing Research
  Department
Richard J Wells, BA RGN RMN FETC Assistant Director of Nursing Services
Karen A Wright, RGN RCNT DipN FETC, Research Assistant, Nursing Research
  Department

THE ROYAL MARSDEN HOSPITAL

Manual of Clinical Nursing Policies and Procedures

Foreword by Robert Tiffany
Chief Nursing Officer

Introduction by Jennifer M Hunt
Director of Nursing Studies

Harper & Row, Publishers
London

Cambridge
Mexico City
New York
Philadelphia

San Francisco
São Paulo
Singapore
Sydney

First published 1984.
Reprinted 1985, 1986, 1987

Harper & Row Ltd
28 Tavistock Street
London WC2E 7PN

British Library Cataloguing in Publication Data
Royal Marsden Hospital
    Manual of clinical nursing policies and procedures.
    1. Nursing
    I. Title
    610.73   RT41

    ISBN 0-06-318288-2

Typeset by Gedset Cheltenham
Printed and bound by Butler & Tanner Ltd, Frome and London

CONTENTS

Foreword	xv
Acknowledgement	xvi
Introduction	xvii
1 ABDOMINAL PARACENTESIS	1
Reference material	1
Guidelines: Abdominal paracentesis	2
Nursing care plan	4
2 ASEPTIC TECHNIQUE	10
Reference material	10
3 BARRIER NURSING AND NURSING THE NEUTROPENIC PATIENT	12
Barrier nursing	12
Reference material	12
Guidelines: Barrier nursing	17
Nursing the Neutropenic Patient	21
Reference material	21
Guidelines: Nursing the neutropenic patient	23
4 BLADDER LAVAGE AND IRRIGATION	24
Reference material	24
Guidelines: Bladder lavage	28

Guidelines: Continuous bladder lavage 30
Bladder irrigation recording chart 32
Nursing care plan 33

5 BLOOD PRESSURE 35
Reference material 35
Guidelines: Blood pressure 40
Nursing care plan 41

6 BONE MARROW ASPIRATION 44
Reference material 44
Guidelines: Bone marrow aspiration 46
Nursing care plan 48

7 BOWEL CARE 49
General introduction 49
Reference material 49
Enemas 54
Reference material 55
Suppositories 56
Reference material 57
Rectal lavage 58
Reference material 59
Guidelines: Administration of enemas 62
Nursing care plan 64
Guidelines: Administration of suppositories 65
Guidelines: Administration of rectal lavage 67
Nursing care plan 70

8 CAESIUM-137 IMPLANTS AND APPLICATORS 72
Reference material 72

Guidelines: Care of patients with insertion of sealed
    radioactive sources   77
Guidelines: Care of patients with intraoral sources   78
Guidelines: Care of patients with gynaecological sources 79
Guidelines: Removal of the gynaecological caesium   79
Nursing care plan   81

9 CARDIOPULMONARY RESUSCITATION   83
Reference material   83
Guidelines: Cardiopulmonary resuscitation   87
Nursing care plan   90

10 CENTRAL VENOUS CATHETERIZATION   92
Reference material   92
Guidelines: Reading central venous pressure   98
Guidelines: Changing the dressing over a central
    venous catheter   100
Guidelines: Taking blood samples from a central
    venous catheter   103
Guidelines: Removal of catheters not skin tunnelled   105
Nursing care plan   108

**11 CYTOTOXIC DRUGS: HANDLING AND
ADMINISTRATION**   112
General introduction   112
Reference material   112
Intrapleural instillation of cytotoxic drugs   114
Reference material   114
Guidelines: Protection of nursing staff when
    handling cytotoxic drugs   116
Guidelines: Protection of the environment   119

Guidelines: Intravenous administration of cytotoxic
   drugs   120
Administration of cytotoxic drugs by other routes   121
Intramuscular and subcutaneous injection of
   cytotoxic drugs   122
Guidelines: Administration of intrapleural drugs   122
Guidelines: Intravesical instillations of cytotoxic
   drugs   123
Nursing care plan: Intravesical drug administration   126

12 DRUG ADMINISTRATION   128
Reference material   128
Guidelines: Oral drug administration   142
Guidelines: Administration of injections   145
Guidelines: Administration of rectal and vaginal
   preparations   153
Guidelines: Topical applications of drugs   154
Guidelines: Administration of drugs in other forms   154

13 ENTONOX ADMINISTRATION   156
Reference material   157
Guidelines: Entonox administration   159
Nursing care plan   160

14 EYE CARE   162
Reference material   162
Guidelines: Eye swabbing   169
Guidelines: Instillation of eye drops   171
Guidelines: Instillation of eye ointment   172

15 GASTRIC LAVAGE   176
Reference material   176

Guidelines: Gastric lavage   178

16 HEPATITIS B   182
Reference material   182
Guidelines: Hepatitis B   184

17 HUMIDIFICATION   189
Reference material   189
Guidelines: Humidification   191

18 INTRAPLEURAL DRAINAGE   192
Reference material   192
Guidelines: Management of underwater seal drainage   196
Guidelines: Changing drainage tubing and bottles   199
Guidelines: Removal of an intrapleural drain   200
Nursing care plan   202

19 INTRAVENOUS DRUG ADMINISTRATION   205
Reference material   205
Guidelines: Administration of drugs by continuous
  infusion   213
Guidelines: Administration of drugs by intermittent
  infusion   215
Guidelines: Administration of drugs by direct injection,
  bolus or push   219
Nursing care plan   222

20 IODINE-131 PROTOCOL   229
Reference material   229
Guidelines: Nursing the patient before the
  administration of iodine-131   234
Guidelines: Nursing the patient after administration
  of iodine-131   234

Guidelines: Emergency procedures   237

21 IRIDIUM-192 IMPLANTS   239
Reference material   239
Guidelines: Care of patients with insertions of
    sealed radioactive sources   241
Guidelines: Care of patients with intraoral sources   243

22 LAST OFFICES   244
Reference material   244
Guidelines: Last offices   244
Nursing care plan   247
Guidelines: Religious requirements for non-Christians   248

23 LIFTING   250
Reference material   250
Guidelines: Lifting   255

24 LIVER BIOPSY   257
Reference material   257
Guidelines: Liver biopsy   260
Nursing care plan   263

25 LUMBAR PUNCTURE   264
Reference material   264
Guidelines: Lumbar puncture   268
Nursing care plan   271

26 MOUTH CARE   273
Reference material   273
Guidelines: Mouth care   278
Nursing care plan   280

27 NASOGATRIC FEEDING 282

Reference material 282

Guidelines: Nasogastric intubation with Clinifeed tube 287

Guidelines: Nasogastric intubation with tubes other
than Clinifeed 289

Guidelines: Administration of a nasogastric feed 291

Nursing care plan 292

Appendix: Suggested management of a nasogastric
feeding regime 293

28 NEUROLOGICAL OBSERVATIONS 296

Reference material 296

Guidelines: Neurological observations 301

Nursing care plan 305

29 OXYGEN THERAPY 306

Reference material 306

Guidelines: Administration of oxygen therapy by
Venturi mask 313

Guidelines: Administration of oxygen by
MC mask 314

Guidelines: Administration of oxygen by nasal cannulae 315

Nursing care plan 316

30 PERITONEAL DIALYSIS 317

Reference material 317

Guidelines: Peritoneal dialysis 320

Nursing care plan 324

31 PRE - AND POSTOPERATIVE CARE 329

Reference material 330

Guidelines: Preoperative care 332

Guidelines: Postoperative care 334
Nursing care plan 335

32 PRESSURE SORES 339
Reference material 339
Guidelines: Treatment of pressure sores 349

33 PULSE 351
Reference material 351
Guidelines: Pulse 354
Nursing care plan 354

34 RESPIRATIONS 356
Reference material 356
Guidelines: Respirations 363
Nursing care plan 364

35 SCALP COOLING 367
Guidelines: Scalp cooling 368
Nursing care plan 370

36 SPECIMEN COLLECTION 371
Reference material 371
Guidelines: Specimen collection 374

37 STOMA CARE 381
Reference material 381
Guidelines: Stoma care 381
Guidelines: Collection of a speciment of urine from
    an ileal conduit or urostomy 395
Nursing care plan 396

38 SURGICAL WOUNDS AND DRAINS 399
Surgical wound management 399

Reference material   399
Surgical wound drains   401
Reference material   402
Guidelines: Clean wound without exudate   402
Guidelines: Clean wound with exudate   403
Guidelines: Dehiscent wound with minimal exudate   404
Guidelines: Dehiscent wound with copious exudate   405
Guidelines: Drain dressing (Redivac and
    closed drainage system)   406
Guidelines: Change of vacuum bottle (Redivac and
    closed drainage system)   407
Guidelines: Removal of drain (Redivac and closed
    drainage system)   407
Guidelines: Drain dressing (Penrose, Paul's tubing,
    corrugated and Norton Morgan drainage system)   408
Guidelines: Shortening of drain (Penrose, etc.,
    drainage system)   409
Guidelines: Removal of drain (Penrose, etc.,
    drainage dressing)   411

19 TEMPERATURE   412
Reference material   412
Guidelines: Temperature   415
Nursing care plan   416

40 TRACHEOSTOMY CARE   419
Reference material   419
Guidelines: Changing a tracheostomy dressing   423
Guidelines: Suction and tracheostomy patients   424
Guidelines: Changing a tracheostomy tube   426
Nursing care plan   428

41 TRACTION 430
Reference material 430
Guidelines: Skin traction 434
Nursing care plan 436

42 THE UNCONSCIOUS PATIENT 438
Reference material 439
Guidelines: The unconscious patient 440
Nursing care plan 444

43 URINARY CATHETERIZATION 446
Reference material 446
Guidelines: Urinary catheterization 449
Guidelines: Collection of catheter specimen of urine 454
Guidelines: Emptying a catheter bag 455
Nursing care plan 456

44 VENEPUNCTURE 459
Reference material 459
Guidelines: Venepuncture 464
Nursing care plan 468

45 VIOLENCE AND ITS MANAGEMENT 471
Reference material 471
Guidelines: Violence and its management 475

INDEX 482

FOREWORD

It gives me great pleasure to write the foreword to The Royal Marsden Hospital Manual of Clinical Nursing Policies and Procedures.

In this one volume my colleagues have compiled information that was previously only available from diverse sources, and have added to this material research data not hitherto easily available to nurses working outside research areas.

Delivering high quality care to different types of patient in varied clinical settings challenges the nurse to use many skills. The information contained in this manual will, I believe, greatly assist nurses to develop such essential skills on the basis of the relevant nursing principles involved.

I am sure that the reader will find this manual both interesting and useful — interesting because it provides information on the scientific bases of our nursing procedures and policies; useful because it gives precise detail on how to carry out procedures and identifies problems that patients may experience.

I am confident that this work will soon become an essential resource for individuals and organizations alike.

Robert Tiffany
Chief Nursing Officer
1984

ACKNOWLEDGEMENTS

We would like to express our gratitude to the contributors for their valuable work and remarkable tolerance of our editorial activities, members of the Nursing Practice Committee, those medical and paramedical colleagues in the hospital who have given us advice and support, and the library staff of the Royal College of Nursing.

We acknowledge our debt to our two typists, Jennifer Gilbert and Fiona Salmon, for their skilled work, useful suggestions and moral support.

We thank the members of staff at Harper & Row Ltd, notably Cathy Peck (Senior Editor), for their help and encouragement.

A P Pritchard
V-A Walker
1984

INTRODUCTION

This *Manual of Clinical Nursing Policies and Procedures* is very different from others that you may have used, because it gives the 'why' as well as the 'how' for each policy and procedure.

Our aim has been to make the manual research based, by using research findings wherever possible to determine the policies and procedures. Unfortunately we have found that in many areas there is little or no valid and reliable research; when this is so we have used what other information is available. In every case, however, we have tried to make sure that *the reasons* for what we ask you to do, are stated.

Every procedure has the following 2 sections:

1 Reference material
2 Procedure

Some procedures also have a third section: Nursing Care Plan.

REFERENCE MATERIAL

The reference material is a short review of the literature and other relevant material. Wherever possible research findings have been utilized. A reference list is included at the end so that you know where our information came from, and to assist you in looking up the topic if you need more detailed information.

PROCEDURE

The procedure gives you a list of the equipment needed, followed by a detailed, step-by-step account of the procedure, plus the rationale for the method proposed.

NURSING CARE PLAN

The nursing care plan gives a list of the problems which may occur, their possible causes and proposals for solving them. Items from this sheet can be used on the patient's own nursing care plan.

This is not a 'final' document. If you have more information to support or to challenge any of these policies and procedures, please let us know. We can then incorporate any changes in the second edition.

Jennifer M Hunt
Director of Nursing Services

1

ABDOMINAL PARACENTESIS

Definition

Abdominal paracentesis is used for the insertion of solutions into and the withdrawal of fluid from the peritoneal cavity.

Indications

Abdominal paracentesis is indicated under the following circumstances:

1　To obtain a specimen of fluid for analysis
2　To relieve pressure when abdominal fluid interferes with respiration or bladder function or is compressing the abdominal viscera and blood vessels
3　To insert substances such as radioactive gold colloid or cytotoxic drugs (e.g. bleomycin) into the peritoneal cavity
4　To achieve regression of serosae deposits responsible for fluid formation.

REFERENCE MATERIAL

Abdominal paracentesis is normally performed by a doctor assisted by a nurse. It is an invasive procedure performed at the patient's bedside.

The procedure is most frequently performed for diagnostic purposes. The removal of large amounts of peritoneal fluid is not routine because of the danger of inducing hypovolaemia, hypokalaemia and hyponatraemia. Immediately after removal of large amounts of peritoneal fluid, fluid moves from the vascular space and reaccumulates in the peritoneal cavity so that the problems that occurred before the procedure was performed reappear. In addition, ascitic fluid contains proteins, and body proteins in an already debilitated patient will be further depleted after abdominal paracentesis.

Anatomy and Physiology

The peritoneum is a semipermeable serous membrane consisting of two separate layers:

1 *Parietal layer*   This layer lines the walls of the abdominal cavity.
2 *Visceral layer*   This layer covers the organs contained within the abdominal cavity.

Those organs completely surrounded by peritoneum will be suspended from the posterior abdominal wall by a double fold of the membrane. It is in this way that a mesentery or fold of peritoneum by which the intestine is attached to the posterior abdominal wall is formed. It is between these two layers that the blood vessels reach the organs, for the abdominal aorta and its branches lie outside the peritoneal cavity.

The stomach, intestines (except for the duodenum and rectum), liver and spleen are almost completely surrounded by peritonuem. Duodenum, rectum and pancreas are covered only on their anterior surfaces.

The pelvic peritoneum is continuous with that of the rest of the abdominal cavity. It covers the front aspects of the rectum. In the male it passes forwards over the posterior and anterior surfaces of the bladder to become continuous with that on the anterior abdominal wall. In the female it passes from the rectum over the posterior and anterior surfaces of the uterus before reaching the bladder.

Functions of the Peritoneum

1 The peritoneum is a serous membrane which enables the abdominal contents to glide over each other without friction.
2 It forms partial or complete cover for the abdominal organs.
3 It forms ligaments and mesenteries which help keep the organs in position.
4 The mesenteries contain fat and act as a store for the body.
5 The mesenteries can move to engulf areas of inflammation and this prevents spread of infection.
6 It has the power to absorb fluids and exchange electrolytes.

References and Further Reading

Phipps W J et al. (1980) Shafer's Medical-Surgical Nursing, 7th edition, C V Mosby, p.550
Sears W G Winwood R S (1974) Anatomy and Physiology for Nurses, 5th edition, Edward Arnold, pp. 203-204
Wolff L (1979) Fundamental Nursing: the Humanities and the Sciences in Nursing, J B Lippincott, pp. 328-329

GUIDELINES: ABDOMINAL PARACENTESIS

Equipment

1 Sterile abdominal paracentesis set containing forceps, blade and holder, swabs, towels, suturing equipment, trocar and cannula, rubber tubing to attach to the cannula and guide fluid into the container.

2 Sterile dressing pack
3 Sterile receiver
4 Sterile gloves
5 Sterile specimen pots
6 Local anaesthetic
7 Needles and syringes
8 Antiseptic solution
9 Plaster dressing or plastic spray dressing
10 Large sterile drainage bag or container
11 Gate clamps

Procedure

Action	Rationale
1 Explain the procedure to the patient.	1 To obtain the patient's consent and cooperation.
2 Ask the patient to void his/her bladder.	2 If the bladder is full there is a chance of it being punctured when the trocar is introduced.
3 Ensure privacy.	
4 The patient should be sitting in an upright position or Fowler's position.	4 Normally the pressure in the peritoneal cavity is no greater than atmospheric pressure but, when fluid is present, pressure becomes greater than atmospheric pressure. This position will then aid gravity in the removal of fluid and the fluid will drain of its own accord until the pressure is equalized.
5 The procedure is performed by a doctor:	
a The abdomen is prepared aseptically and draped with sterile towels.	**a** To prevent local and/or systemic infection. The peritoneal cavity is normally sterile.
b Local anaesthetic is administered.	**b** To minimize pain during the procedure and thus ensure maximum cooperation from the patient.
c Once the anaesthetic has taken effect the doctor makes an incision approximately half way between the umbilicus and the symphysis pubis on the midline of the abdomen.	**c** To avoid puncturing the colon.
d The trocar and cannula are inserted via the incision and the rubber tubing is attached to the cannula.	

Action	Rationale
e The trocar is removed.	
6 If the cannula is to remain in position, sutures will be inserted and a supportive dry dressing applied and firmly taped in position.	6 To prevent trauma to the patient. To prevent local and/or systemic infection.
7 A closed drainage system is now attached to the cannula.	7 A sterile container with a non-return valve is necessary to maintain sterility.
8 Monitor the patient's vital signs and observe his/her peripheral circulation.	8 To monitor any reactions to the procedure. There may be major circulatory shifts of fluid which may precipitate a 'shock' syndrome. The sudden release of intra-abdominal pressure may cause vasolidation and a fall of blood pressure.
9 Apply a gate clamp to the tubing of the drainage system.	9 To exercise some control by maintaining a steady rate of flow. Approximately 1 litre can be removed safely before reducing the rate of flow.
10 Monitor the patient's fluid balance. Encourage a high protein and high calorie diet.	10 After removal of large amounts of peritoneal fluid, fluid moves from the vascular space and reaccumulates in the peritoneal cavity. Ascitic fluid contains protein in addition to sodium and potassium. Problems of dehydration and electrolyte imbalance may be present.

NURSING CARE PLAN

Problem	Cause	Suggested Action
1 Patient exhibits 'shock syndrome'	1 Major circulatory shift of fluid or sudden release of intra-abdominal pressure, vasolidation and subsequent lowering of blood pressure	1 Clamp the drainage tube with a gate clamp to prevent further fluid loss. Record the patient's vital signs. Refer to the medical staff for immediate intervention.
2 Cessation of drainage of ascitic fluid	2 **a** Abdomen is empty of ascitic fluid	2 **a** Check with the total output of ascitic fluid given on the patient's fluid balance chart.

Problem	Cause	Suggested Action
		Measure the patient's girth; compare this measurement with the preabdominal paracentesis measurement. Suggest to medical staff that the cannula should be removed. Discontinue the drainage system.
	b Patient's position is inhibiting drainage	**b** Change the patient's position, i.e. move the patient upright or on to his/her side to encourage flow by gravity.
	c The ascitic fluid has clotted in the drainage system	**c** 'Milk' the tubing. If this is unsucessful, change the drainage system asceptically.
3 Signs of local or systemic infection	3 Bacterial invasion at site of abdominal paracentesis cannula	3 Obtain a swab from the site of the cannula for cultural review. Apply a dry dressing. Refer to the medical staff.
4 Cannula becomes dislodged	4 Ineffective sutures, trauma or infection at site	4 Apply a dry dressing. Obtain a swab for culture. Inform the medical staff.

2

ASEPTIC TECHNIQUE

Definition

Aseptic technique is a method used to prevent contamination of wounds and other susceptible sites by ensuring that only sterile objects and fluids come into contact with these sites and that the risk of contamination is minimized.

Indications

Aseptic technique is intended to prevent infection of a wound or susceptible site due to

1 The size, position or nature of that wound or site, e.g. recent surgical incisions
2 Increased susceptibility of the host to infection, e.g. neutropenia or cachecia
3 Environmental factors, e.g. high humidity or other infected patients.

REFERENCE MATERIAL

The literature shows that a significant number of patients acquire some type of wound infection during their stay in hospital. Not only does this cause unnecessary suffering, it may also result in extended periods of hospitalization. Because aseptic procedures are used as a method of preventing wound infection, it is essential that they are both sound in theory and are carried out correctly.

Qualified nurses within any one hospital often demonstrate different aseptic techniques according to their training schools, practical experience, etc. It must be emphasized, however, that the success of the aseptic technique depends not on the type of procedure used but rather on how well the principles of asepsis are adhered to.

Principles of Asepsis

The aim of using an aseptic technique is to prevent the spread of infection by direct or indirect transmission. When dressing a wound, the most usual means of infection spread are as follows:

1 The hands of the staff involved
2 Inanimate objects, e.g. instruments and clothes
3 Dust particles or droplet nuclei suspended in the atmosphere.

Hand Washing

Hand washing greatly reduces the risk of infection transfer but studies have shown that this is rarely carried out in a satisfactory fashion. Fox (1974) showed that most nurses missed some part of their hands while washing and that right-handed people washed the left hand more thoroughly and vice versa. Areas where organisms may shelter include the wrists, under fingernails and under rings.

Transient bacteria can be almost completely removed from the hands by soap and water washing (Lowbury et al. 1974a). Conversely, soap and water do not reduce the number of resident bacteria by any significant amount. Resident skin flora, such as *Staphylococcus aureus*, are most effectively removed by rubbing the hands with an alcoholic solution of chlorhexidine, such as Hibisol. Lowbury et al. (1974b) showed that rinsing the hands with alcoholic chlorhexidine 0.5% removed more resident skin flora than washing the hands with a chlorhexidine 4% detergent wash, such as Hibiscrub.

It is suggested that a preparation such as Hibiscrub is used for cleaning physically dirty or contaminated hands while a preparation such as Hibisol should be used for disinfecting clean hands immediately prior to carrying out an aseptic technique. If a nurse has physically clean hands, he/she will not need to wash them during the aseptic procedure but should use a preparation such as Hibisol whenever disinfection is required, e.g. after opening the outer wrappers of dressings. This will also remove the need for the nurse to leave the bedside during the procedure to wash his/her hands at a basin, unless they become physically contaminated with blood, pus, excreta, etc. (assuming that adequate washing facilities are not available within the area where the procedure is being carried out).

It should be noted that preparations such as Hibiscrub may cause skin reactions in some people; in these cases soap and water may be used. Caution is required, however, if this method is adopted as the sludge or moist soap under the bar often becomes contaminated. A preparation such as Hibisol contains emollients that prevent drying of the skin.

Cleaning Inanimate Objects

The Sterile Field and Instruments All instruments, fluids and materials that come into contact with the wound must be sterile if the risk of contamination is to be reduced. The central sterile supplies department should normally provide all sterile instruments. In the event of supplies being short or in an emergency, it is acceptable to disinfect a clean instrument, such as a pair of scissors, by immersing it completely in alcoholic chlorhexidine 1 in 200 (70%) for 5-10 minutes.

Any equipment that becomes contaminated during the procedure must be discarded. On no account should it be returned to the sterile field.

The Dressing Trolley   The trolley should be washed thoroughly every day with detergent and water. It should not need cleaning between dressings unless a surface becomes physically contaminated since organisms cannot survive on cold, smooth, dry surfaces. The sterile field, usually made of thick waxed paper, will not allow the passage of organisms through it. Trolleys used for aseptic procedures must not be used for any other purpose.

Masks, Gowns and Aprons

The purpose of a mask is to protect the patient against organisms dispersed from the upper respiratory tracts of the staff. Masks used in operating theatres are usually of the 'deflector' type and are impervious to large droplets from the user's mouth. The use of paper masks on the ward, however, is not recommended, as their value is limited: 'Experimental studies and trials have shown that masks contribute little or nothing to the protection of patients in wards against infection and their routine use for aseptic ward procedures, including post operative dressings, is therefore unnecessary' (Lowbury et al. 1975).

It would seem that a greater reduction of droplet dispersion of organisms could be achieved by staff not talking unnecessarily during dressing procedures. Ideally, no staff with respiratory tract infections or sore throats should perform dressings. Nurses without infections who are likely to cough or sneeze while carrying out an aseptic procedure, e.g. sufferers from hayfever, should wear surgical masks to reduce the risk of droplet dispersion.

Nurses' clothing does become contaminated with organisms from the ward and from the nurses themselves. The front of the uniform is the area most likely to be contaminated, so it is advisable for nurses to wear protective clothing during aseptic procedures. This also prevents the transfer of bacteria from the uniforms to the patients.

Cotton material, because of its weave, allows bacteria to pass through it. It is therefore recommended that a disposable plastic apron, impermeable to bacteria, is worn during aseptic procedures. Aprons should be discarded after any dirty or infected dressing.

Airborne Contamination

The spread of infection is most likely to occur in a large open ward and ideally dressings should all be performed in a properly ventilated room. Many dressings, however, are carried out at the patient's bedside; in such cases ward cleaning should cease at least 30 minutes, and curtains should be drawn at least 10 minutes before a dressing is begun. To reduce opportunities for airborne contamination to a minimum, a wound should be exposed for the shortest time possible, dirty dressings being placed carefully in a bag, preferably plastic, which is sealed before disposal (Lowbury et al. 1975). Clean wounds should be dressed before contaminated wounds. Colostomies and infected wounds should be dressed last of all to minimize environmental contamination and cross-infection.

A potential source of infection can be water in which flowers or pot plants stand; these must be removed from the bedside before the screens are closed. Air movement should be kept to a minimum during the dressing. This means that adjacent windows should be closed and the movement of personnel within the area discouraged. The use of an alcohol-based hand wash solution at the bedside is advantageous as it reduces the air movement created by a nurse in leaving the cubicle to go to a sink; also it shortens the time that a wound is left exposed.

Selection of Hand Hygiene Preparations in General Use

Antiseptic Skin Cleansers

Hibiscrub   This is a cleansing solution containing chlorhexidine gluconate 4%. This solution should be used instead of soap as a preoperative scrub or disinfectant wash for hands and skin.

Betadine   This is a surgical scrub containing povidone iodine 7.5% in a nonionic detergent base. Betadine should be used as a preoperative or pre-procedural scrub for hands and skin.

Wide-spectrum Microbicides

Hibisol   This is a solution containing chlorhexidine gluconate 0.5% in isopropyl alcohol 70% with emollients. Hibisol may be used in undiluted form for hand and skin disinfection.

Manusept   This is an antibacterial hand rub containing triclosan 0.5% and isopropyl alcohol 70%. Manusept should be used for disinfection and for pre-operative and preprocedural hand preparation.

Chlorhexidine in Spirit Spray

Hibispray   This is a preparation of Hibitane in a spray containing chlor-hexidine gluconate 0.5% and isopropyl alcohol 70%. This spray may be used as a disinfectant on clean, dry surfaces.

References and Further Reading

Fox M K (1974) How good are hand washing practices? American Journal of Nursing 74: 1676-1678

Hayward M P (1980) An experimental study to determine the efficiency and effectiveness of a simplified dressing procedure, BSc thesis, Leeds Polytechnic

ICI (1981) ICI Antiseptics in Practice, ICI Pharmaceuticals Division

Lascelles I (1982) Wound dressing techniques, Nursing 2 (8): 217-219

Lowbury E J et al. (1974a) Disinfection of hands: removal of transient organisms, British Medical Journal 2: 230-233

Lowbury E J et al. (1974b) Preoperative disinfection of surgeons' hands: use of alcoholic solutions and effects of gloves on skin flora, British Medical Journal 4: 369-372

Lowbury E J et al. (1975) Control of Hospital Infection — a Practical Handbook, Chapman and Hall

GUIDELINES: ASEPTIC TECHNIQUE

Equipment

1   Sterile dressing pack containing gallipots or an indented plastic tray, wool balls, topical swabs, disposable forceps, dressing towel, sterile field, disposable bag
2   Fluids for cleaning and/or irrigation
3   Hypoallergenic tape
4   Appropriate hand hygiene preparation
5   Disposable plastic apron

Any other material required will be determined by the nature of the dressing: special features of a dressing should be referred to in the patient's nursing care plan.

Procedure

Action	Rationale
1 Explain the procedure to the patient.	1 To obtain the patient's consent and cooperation.
2 Screen the bed and position the patient comfortably so that the dressing is easily accessible without unduly exposing the patient.	2 To allow dust and airborne organisms to settle before the wound and the sterile field are exposed.
3 Wash your hands with an appropriate solution, such as soap and water or Hibiscrub.	
4 Put on a disposable plastic apron.	
5 Place all the equipment required for the dressing on the bottom shelf of a clean dressing trolley.	
6 Take the trolley to the patient's bedside, disturbing the screens as little as possible.	6 To minimize airborne contamination.
7 Open the outer cover of the sterile dressing pack and slide the contents on to the top shelf of the trolley.	

Action	**Rationale**
8 Open the sterile field using the corners of the paper only. Using the forceps in the pack, arrange the sterile field with the handles of instruments in one corner.	8 So that areas of potential contamination are kept to a minimum.
9 Attach a plastic disposal bag to the side of the trolley, below the level of the top shelf.	9 So that any contaminated material is below the level of the sterile field.
10 Open the other sterile packs, tipping their contents gently on to the centre of the sterile field. Pour lotions into gallipots or an indented plastic tray.	
11 Loosen the old dressing gently, touching only the hypoallergenic tape, etc., securing it.	11 So that the dressing can be lifted off easily with forceps.
12 Clean your hands with an alcohol-based hand wash solution, such as Hibisol.	12 Hands may have become contaminated by handling outer packets, etc.
13 Using forceps, or sterile disposable gloves if the dressing is large or bulky, remove the old dressing and discard it with the forceps, or gloves, into the plastic bag.	
14 Clean the wound as necessary, working from the inside to the outside of the area and dealing with the cleanest parts of the wounds first.	14 To minimize the risk of spread of infection from a 'dirty' to a 'clean' area.
15 Apply the new dressing with forceps and fix it in place with hypoallergenic tape, etc. There is no need to use forceps for securing the dressing as the wound is now covered.	
16 Make the patient comfortable and ensure that the dressing is secure.	16 The dressing may slip or feel uncomfortable as the patient changes position.
17 Fold up the sterile field, place it in the plastic disposal bag and seal the bag before moving the trolley.	17 To prevent environmental contamination.
18 Draw back the curtains.	
19 Dispose of waste in appropriate bags.	
20 Check that the trolley remains dry and physically clean.	

3

BARRIER NURSING
AND NURSING THE NEUTROPENIC PATIENT

BARRIER NURSING

Definition

Barrier nursing involves the use of practices aimed at controlling the spread of and destroying pathogenic organisms. These practices may require the setting up of mechanical barriers to contain pathogenic organisms within a specified area.

Indication

Barrier nursing is required under the following circumstances:

1 To prevent the spread of infection from patients with communicable diseases (i.e. contagious diseases such as glandular fever, or infectious diseases such as chicken pox)
2 To prevent the spread of infection from patients infected with organisms which are resistant to the usual range of antibiotics.

For the patient who acquires an infection in hospital the consequences can be considerable and may include the following:

1 Delayed or prevented recovery
2 Increased pain, discomfort and anxiety
3 Extended hospitalization, which has implications for the patient, the family and the hospital.

REFERENCE MATERIAL

Most precautions against transferring infection demand more effort, take more time and cost more than the comparable procedures in normal circumstances.

Sources of Infection

Self-infection

Self-infection results when tissue becomes infected from another site in the patient's body. The normal microbial flora of the human body consists largely of the organisms in the alimentary tract, upper respiratory tract and female genital tract and on the skin. This flora may include versatile pathogens (e.g. *Staphylococcus aureus*) that may cause disease in almost any tissue as well as others (e.g. micrococcus species and diptheroides) which are usually of very low pathogenicity; many organisms exist with capabilities between these extremes.

Cross-infection

Cross-infection may be caused by infection from patients, hospital staff or visitors who are suffering from the relevant disease (cases) or who are symptomless carriers. Food may also be a factor in cross-infection.

Routes and Reservoirs of Infection

1 Personal contact
2 Bedding
3 Equipment
4 Structual environment
5 Atmospheric air

Note: Water in flower vases usually contains a range of Gram-negative organisms, including *Escherichia, Klebsiella, Pseudemonas* and *Serratia* species, but the importance of this as a source of infection is uncertain.

Types of Isolation

Source Isolation (Barrier Isolation)

This form of isolation, i.e. physical isolation of the patient, is applied to patients who are infected and are hazardous to others. The need for isolation is determined by the ease with which the disease can be transmitted in hospital and, if it is transmittable, by its severity.

Protective Isolation (Reverse Barrier Nursing)

Patients whose susceptibility to infection is increased may require isolation for their own protection as an alternative to or as well as antibiotic treatment. The decision to use isolation is influenced by the individual circumstances and by the available facilities. Control of Infection Group, Northwick Park Hospital and Clinical Research Centre (1974) has outlined in detail the indications for protective isolation.

Design and Construction of Isolation Accommodation

The literature agrees that good isolation practice is more efficacious in a welldeisgned building. Easy, direct and short distance access to patients' supplies and facilities reduces the nursing load, thereby allowing more time to be devoted to the observation of the correct isolation procedures.

General Principles of Barrier Nursing

The main emphasis for successful barrier nursing procedures is on hand washing and protection of clothes. Several general principles need to be adhered to if effective barrier nursing is to occur.

Bacteriological Surveillance of Staff

Staff with symptoms or signs of communicable disease should be investigated for bacterial or viral infection. If pathogens are found, these members of staff should not come into contact with the patient being barrier nursed.

Hand Washing

Washing the skin quickly removes harmful organisms. Studies of hand washing by nurses and others, however, have shown that this procedure is not carried out efficiently. The use of disinfectants improves the cleaning process, although no method of chemical disinfection will produce a sterile hand. Soaps and detergent emulsions containing hexachlorophane build a protective barrier in the skin against Gram-positive organisms. A solution which is now widely used is one containing 4% chlorhexidine (Hibiscrub). A convenient and effective disinfectant for the hands is 70% alcohol with the addition of enough glycerine to prevent excessive drying of the skin. Washing in running water is essential. Basins should be deep enough to contain any splashing water and should be plugless. Taps should not be operated by hand but by elbow, knee or foot as appropriate.

Clothing and Gowns

Lidwell et al. (1974) have shown that disposable plastic gowns that cover the parts of the body that come into the closest contact with the patient reduce contact transfer substantially. More research is required to identify clothing that is a satisfactory obstacle to bacterial transfer.

Caps, Masks and Footwear

There is evidence that hair picks up bacteria readily from the environment. Because the head is moved directly above the patient it should be covered when a high degree of patient protection is necessary. If caps are to be used effectively they must cover all the hair.

Masks can be worn to protect the wearer or the patient. The wearer will only be protected if the mask fits the face closely.

Evidence that floors and footwear contribute to the risk of infection is, at present, inconclusive.

Bathing and Changing

There is no evidence to date that shower bathing has any useful effect in reducing the spread of microorganisms by an individual.

Terminal Disinfection

For diseases such as smallpox, anthrax, Lassa fever, Ebola fever and Marburg disease, formaldehyde is the agent of choice.

Food

Sterile water should be available if required. Complete food sterilization is not required except for the most stringent germ-free conditions. Bacterial contamination of food from central kitchens may be reduced by microwave irradiation combined with conventional heat.

Waste

Plastic bags have simplified and improved methods of disposal of waste, but care is needed to ensure that the bags are closed correctly. Separate routes for entry into and exit from the isolation area are the ideal. If this is not possible, correct bagging must be adhered to scrupulously. Any waste should be clearly labelled before leaving the isolation area. Bedpans and urinals should be bagged within the isolated area after use and then sent to be washed and sterilized.

Notification of Infection

If bacteriological analysis identifies an organism which necessitates barrier nursing, swift communication and action is needed to instigate this. Any problems may be discussed with the microbiologist or infection control clinical nurse specialist.

Isolation of the Patient

Effective barrier nursing practice is most easily achieved by isolating the patient in a single room with

1   An anteroom area for protective clothing
2   Hand washing facilities
3   Toilet facilities.

However, with good technique, an area in the ward away from especially vulnerable patients can be used.

Informing the Patient and Visitors

Careful explanation to the patient is essential so that he/she can cooperate fully with the restrictions. The nurse should be sensitive to the psychological implications of being labelled infectious and being confined in isolation. The patient's visitors must also be informed why the barrier nursing restrictions are necessary. Visitors may be allowed into the room, but only at the discretion of the bacteriologist. They must be taught to observe the correct procedures for entering and leaving the room. As children are more susceptible to infection than adults, any visit by a child should be discussed with the appropriate personnel.

Domestic Staff

The domestic manager must be informed as soon as barrier nursing is commenced. He or she will then provide the ward domestic with written instructions.

The ward domestic staff must clearly understand why barrier nursing is required and should be instructed on the correct procedure. The nursing staff must check that the ward domestics understand and are following their instructions correctly. If the patient is in a single room, a mop, cleaning fluid and disposable cloths should be kept in the room solely for this patient's use. If the patient is in a general ward, special care must be taken with the cleaning so that potentially infectious material is not transferred from the area around the infected patient to other patient areas. The infected patient's area must be cleaned last and separately.

Staff Allocation

A minimum number of staff should be involved with an infected case. The nurse concerned with the infected patient should not also attend to other susceptible patients. If barrier nursing is for an infectious disease, it is preferable that only personnel who have already had the disease should attend this patient.

The protection of staff against the risk of infection is one of the main functions of the occupational health department. This department offers an immunization and counselling service.

References and Further Reading

Bagshawe K D et al. (1978a) Isolating patients in hospital to control infection. Part I. Sources and routes of infection, British Medical Journal 2: 609-612

Bagshawe K D et al. (1978b) Isolating patients in hospital to control infection. Part II. Who should be isolated, and where? British Medical Journal 2: 684-686

Bagshawe K D et al. (1978c) Isolating patients in hospital to control infection. Part III. Design and construction of isolation accommodation, British Medical Journal 2: 744-748

Bagshawe K D et al. (1978d) Isolating patients in hospital to control infection. Part IV. Nursing procedures, British Medical Journal 2: 808-811

Bagshawe K D et al. (1978e) Isolating patients in hospital to control infection. Part V. An isolation system, British Medical Journal 2: 879-881

Control of Infection Group, Northwick Park Hospital and Clinical Research Centre (1974) Isolation system for general hospitals, British Medical Journal 1: 41-44

Infection Control Nurses' Association (1976). Stirling Conference of the Infection

Control Nurses' Association, Kimberley Clark

Lidwell O M et al. (1974) Transfer of micro-organisms between nurses and patients in a clean air environment, Journal of Applied Bacteriology 37(4): 649-656

GUIDELINES: BARRIER NURSING

Equipment

1 Isolation suite if possible
2 All items required to meet the patient's nursing needs during the period of isolation, such as crockery, linen, instruments to assess vital signs, etc.

Procedure

Action	Rationale
Preparation of the Isolation Room	
1 Place a barrier nursing sign outside the door.	1 To inform anyone intending to enter the room of the situation.
2 List requirements for personnel before entering and after leaving the isolation area.	
3 Remove all inessential furniture. The remaining furniture should be easy to clean and should not conceal or retain dirt or moisture either within or around it.	3 To minimize the risk of furniture harbouring microbial spores or growth colonies.
4 Stock the hand basin with a suitable antiseptic solution, e.g. Hibiscrub, and paper towels for staff use.	4 Facilities for hand washing within the infected area are essential for effective barrier nursing.
5 Place a suitable rubbish bag in the room on a foot-operated stand. This bag must be sealed before it is removed from the room, either by knotting (polythene bags) or by stapling the top (paper bags).	5 For containing contaminated rubbish within room.
6 Place a container for 'sharps' in the room.	6 To contain contaminated 'sharps' within the infected area.
7 When the 'sharps' container is full it must be kept in the room until collected for incineration. Advise the porter to wear gloves when handling such a container.	7 To protect hospital personnel.
8 Keep the patient's personal property to a minimum. Advise him/her to wear hospital clothing. All belongings taken into the room	8 The patient's belongings may become contaminated and cannot be taken home unless they are washable or cleanable. Anything

Action	**Rationale**
should be washable, cleanable or disposable.	else may have to be destroyed.
9 Provide the patient with his/her own thermometer and sphygmomanometer, water jug, glass and tray, and all items necessary for attending to personal hygiene.	9 Equipment used regularly by the patient should be kept within the infected area to prevent the spread of infection.
10 Keep dressing solutions, creams and lotions, etc., to a minimum and store them within the room.	10 All partially used materials must be discarded when barrier nursing ends (resterilization is not possible), therefore unnecessary waste should be avoided.
11 Set up a trolley outside the door to hold plastic gowns, gloves, an appropriate antiseptic solution and spare recording charts, e.g. for fluid balance.	

Entering the Room

1 Collect all equipment needed.	1 To avoid entering and leaving the infected area unnecessarily.
2 Roll up long sleeves to the elbow.	2 To protect clothing from contamination.
3 Put on a disposable plastic gown.	3 To protect clothing from contamination. Cotton gowns are ineffective against bacteria once wet.
4 Put on disposable gloves if you are intending to deal with contaminated material.	4 To reduce the risk of contaminating your hands.
5 Enter the room, shutting the door behind you.	

Attending to the Patient

1 *Meals* Meals should be served on disposable crockery and eaten with disposable cutlery if deemed necessary by the bacteriologist. Disposables and uneaten food should be discarded in the appropriate bag.	1 Contaminated crockery is a potential disease vector. Cleaning of same may be difficult and time consuming.
2 *Non-disposable crockery.* A personal water jug, glasses and tray should be kept at the bedside. These, and any other non-disposable crockery should be	2 Separation of contaminated crockery reduces the risk of the spread of infection in washing-up water.

Action	**Rationale**
washed separately from the rest of the ward's utensils.	
3 *Excreta* Ideally a toilet should be kept solely for this patient's use. If this is not available, a separate bedpan or urinal and commode should be left in the patient's room. Gloves must be worn by staff when dealing with excreta. Bedpans and urinals should be bagged in the isolation room, emptied and then washed in a bedpan washer, then dried and returned immediately to the patient's room.	3 To minimize the risk of infection being spread from excreta, e.g. via a toilet seat or a bedpan.
4 *Accidental spills* Any suspected contaminated fluids must be mopped up immediately and the area cleaned with a disinfectant	4 Damp areas encourage microbial growth and increase the risk of spread of infection.
5 *Bathing* An infected patient must be bathed last on the ward. Clean the bath after the previous patient *and* after the infected patient. If the patient has infected lesions, disinfectant may be added to the bath water, e.g. Steribath or Hibiscrub. Salt is not a disinfectant and has little antibacterial effect.	5 Leaving the bath dry after disinfection reduces the risk of microbes surviving and infecting others. Bacteria will not grow on clean, dry surfaces.
6 *Dressings* Gloves must be worn for doing all dressings. Waste materials and dirty dressings should be discarded in the appropriate bag.	6 Aseptic procedure minimizes the risk of cross-infection.
7 *Linen* Place linen in appropriate bags which should be tightly secured and placed directly into routine dirty linen bags, which must also be secured tightly. Linen bags should await laundry collection in the patient's room. Bags must not be stored outside the isolation room.	7 Storage of dirty linen within the room confines organisms to one infected area.
8 *Waste* Bags should be kept in the room for disposal of all the patient's rubbish. The bag's top should be sealed by knotting or	

Action	**Rationale**
stapling before it is removed from the room.	

Leaving the Room

1 Wash your hands with gloves on. Remove the gloves and discard them in the appropriate bag. Wash your hands again with an appropriate antiseptic solution.	1 Pathogenic contamination of gloves will be minimized before they are discarded.
2 Remove your gown and discard it in the appropriate bag. Wash your hands again with an appropriate antiseptic solution.	2 Hands may be contaminated by a dirty gown.
3 Leave the room, shutting the door behind you.	
4 Rinse your hands with an alcohol-based hand wash solution, such as Hibisol.	4 To remove pathogenic organisms acquired from such items as the door handle.

Transporting Infected Patients Outside the Barrier Nursing Area

1 Inform the department concerned of the diagnosis.	
2 Arrange for the patient to have the last appointment of the day.	2 The department concerned will then be empty of other patients; time can be allowed for special cleaning or disinfecting; hospital corridors, lifts, etc., are usually less busy at this time of day.
3 Provide the department concerned with the necessary gloves and aprons.	
4 Any porters involved must be instructed and given the necessary gloves, together with cleaning equipment for the trolley or chair.	4 Protection and reassurance of porters is necessary to allay fear, and to minimize the risk of infection being spread to them.
5 The nurse should escort the patient.	

Discharge of the Patient

1 Inform the bacteriologist when the patient is due for discharge.	1 The bacteriologist will advise on any special precautions.
2 The room should generally be stripped and aired. All textiles should be changed, and curtains sent to the laundry.	
3 Impervious surfaces, e.g. lockers, stools, blinds and thermometer	3 Wiping of surfaces is the most effective way of removing con-

Action	Rationale
holders, should be washed with soap and water.	taminants.Relatively inaccessible places, e.g. ceilings, may be omitted: these are not generally relevent to any infection risk.
4 The floor should be washed thoroughly.	

NURSING THE NEUTROPENIC PATIENT

Definition
One of the major side-effects of cytotoxic chemotherapy is neutropenia, a reduction in the number of neutrophils (granulocytes) as a percentage of the total white cell count. As the neutrophil count decreases, the incidence of infection increases. The longer the period of neutropenia, the higher the incidence of infection.

Indications
Barrier nursing of neutropenic patients is required

1   To protect the neutropenic or chronically immunosuppressed patient from hospital-acquired infection
2   To detect infection at an early stage and facilitate prompt treatment.

The procedure described below is intended to protect the patient whose period of neutropenia can reasonably be expected to be measured in days. It does not involve the special precautions of full protective isolation with protection from commensal infection in patients whose neutropenia is likely to be prolonged. Such patients should be nursed in a reverse barrier nursing unit. The present procedure should be used under the following circumstances:

1   Following high-dose cytotoxic chemotherapy with autologous bone marrow 'rescue'
2   Where there is idiosyncratic haematological sensitivity to cytotoxic agents, if the period of neutropenia is expected to be short.

REFERENCE MATERIAL
Bacterial, fungal and viral infections may all occur during a period of neutropenia.

Bacterial infections are commonly caused by Gram-negative organisms, such as *Pseudomonas* species, *Escherichia coli*, and *Klebsiella* species, normally found in the gastrointestinal tract, and *Staphylococcus epidermidis*, usually a skin contaminant.

The commonest fungal infection is *Candida albicans*, most usually in the oral cavity, but which may affect the oesophagus, bowel or vagina, and cause systemic infection, pneumonia and septicaemia.

Herpetic lesions may result from the herpes simplex virus, and herpes zoster is more common in patients who are immunosuppressed or neutropenic.

The main route of infection transmission is by contact transmission from hands and clothes. Airborne infectious microorganisms, notably staphylococi, may be inhaled or transferred to the patient through wounds, intravenous cannualae, etc. The patient may also infect himself directly from his own microorganisms.

Food chosen from the hospital menu is acceptable, but raw fruit salads and uncooked vegetables should be avoided to minimize or reduce endogenous infection.

Early detection of infection is vital. Four-hourly recordings of temperature, pulse and blood pressure will facilitate this.

The patient may carry out self-screening of the mouth, intravenous site and other areas of potential infection, if able, otherwise a nurse should do this and report any evidence of infection to allow prompt treatment with intravenous antibiotics.

Blood product therapy may be required during the neutropenic period.

Opinions vary as to the degree of protective care required, and to the ideal method; controlled trials are difficult to organize and to evaluate, and results are often conflicting. It is generally accepted, however, that the neutropenic patient who is given some protection will have fewer infections, fewer days of fever, and reduced morbidity and mortality compared with the unprotected patient.

The system chosen will depend on local resources. The success of the system relies heavily on the education and attitude of hospital staff, the patient, his/her relatives and friends who may wish to visit.

References and Further Reading

Bagshawe K D et al. (1978) Isolating patients in hospital to control infection. Part I. Sources and routes of infection, British Medical Journal 2: 609-612

Bates M (1980) Factors related to infection in cancer patients and implications for care, in Cancer Nursing Update, edited by R Tiffany, Balliére Tindall, pp. 81-85

Hodges D Griffiths G (1982) Prevention versus cure, Nursing Mirror 154 (7): 24-26

Jenner E A (1977) Intravenous infusion — a cause for concern? Nursing Times 73: 156-158

Lidwell O M et al. (1974) Transfer of micro-organisms between nurses and patients in a clean air environment, Journal of Applied Bacteriology 37 (4): 649-656

Remington J S Schimpff S C (1981) Please don't eat the salads, New England Journal of Medicine 304: 433-434

Smith B J (1983) The infection-prone child. 1. Aspects of microbiology, Nursing Times 79 (25): 56-60

Smith B J (1983) The infection-prone child. 3. Evaluation, Nursing Times 79 (27): 28-30

Stronge J L et al. (1980) Hospitals . . . should do the sick no harm. 11. Controlling infection by isolation, Part 2. Nursing Times 76: Supplement.

GUIDELINES: NURSING THE NEUTROPENIC PATIENT

Procedure

Action

Rationale

Preparation of the Room and Maintenance of General Cleanliness

1 A single room should be used if possible.

2 Bed linen should be changed frequently and blankets and cushions should be kept for the patient's exclusive use.

3 The room should be damp dusted and the floor mopped daily. Surfaces should not be left wet. Dressing and intravenous procedures should if possible be carried out before the room is cleaned.

4 Cleaning materials should be kept exclusively for the patient.

1 Reduces airborne transfer of microorganisms.

2 Indirect transfer of micro-organisms, particularly *Staphylococcus aureus*, is commonly associated with contaminated bed linen.

3 Damp dusting reduces transfer of airborne microorganisms. *Klebsiella* species are commonly found on moist surfaces.

Nursing Procedures

1 Hands should be washed thoroughly with a suitable anti-septic solution before attending to the patient.

2 A disposable plastic apron should be worn for all nursing procedures.

3 Four-hourly recordings of temperature, pulse and blood pressure should be maintained. Areas such as the mouth and intravenous sites should be inspected daily for evidence of infection.

1 Hands are regarded as the principle source of transfer of microorganisms. (For further information, see the procedure on aseptic technique, pages 10-11)

2 Staff clothing may be contami-nated with *Staphylococcus aureus* and Gram-negative organisms. A disposable plastic apron reduces the risk of transfer or organisms through the open-weave fabric of staff uniforms.

3 Detection of infection to allow prompt treatment. A neutropenic patient may have insuffucient circulating granulocytes to produce obvious signs of infection such as inflammation or pus. Hypotension may be the first sign of severe septicaemia.

Action	**Rationale**

Visitors

1 The patient should be asked to nominate close relatives and friends who may then, after education, visit freely. The patient or his representative should inform casual acquaintances or nonessential visitors that they should avoid visiting during the period of neutropenia.

2 The nominated visitors should stay away if they have obvious signs of infection.

1 The incidence of infection increases in proportion to the number of people visiting. Large numbers of visitors are difficult to screen and educate. Unlimited visiting by close relatives and friends diminishes the sense of isolation that the patient may experience.

2 To avoid transmission to the patient.

Diet

1 Educate the patient to choose only cooked food from the hospital menu and avoid raw fruit, salads and uncooked vegetables, whether on the menu or brought in by visitors.

1 To minimize or reduce endogenous infection.

4

BLADDER LAVAGE AND IRRIGATION

Definition

Lavage

Bladder lavage is the washing out of the bladder with sterile fluid.

Irrigation

Bladder irrigation is the continuous washing out of the bladder with sterile fluid.

Indications

Bladder lavage or irrigation is indicated for the following reasons:

Lavage

1   To clear an obstructed catheter
2   To remove potential sources of obstruction, e.g. blood clots or sediment from infection
3   To cleanse the bladder with urinary disinfectants when some types of urinary infections are present and to prevent the spread of such infection, e.g. to the kidney.

Irrigation

1   To prevent the formation and retention of blood clots, e.g. following prostatic surgery
2   On rare occasions to remove heavily contaminated material from a diseased urinary bladder.

REFERENCE MATERIAL

Solutions Used for Lavage and Irrigation

A small number of solutions is available for cleansing the bladder and the selection of a particular solution will depend on its therapeutic properties in relation to the patient's needs.

Normal saline is the agent most commonly recommended for lavage and irrigation and should be used in every case unless an alternative solution is prescribed. Normal saline is isotonic so it does not affect the body's fluid or electrolyte levels, therefore large volumes may be used as necessary. Three-litre bags of saline are available for irrigation purposes.

Studies on water and saline (Harper and Matz 1975, 1976) showed them to be the least erosive irrigating solutions when tested in rat bladders. The use of large volumes of sterile water is not recommended, however, as its absorption through the bladder wall may increase the blood volume to unacceptable levels.

The use of chlorhexidine gluconate as a bladder washout is not recommended unless it is specifically prescribed. The 0.02% solution provided for intravesical use is a disinfectant which is effective against vegetative bacteria, especially Gram-positive organisms. Its activity is reduced, however, by blood and other organic matter (Martindale 1977) and can cause haematuria and bladder erosion (Harper 1981).

Noxythiolin (Noxyflex) is occasionally prescribed as a bladder installation solution and is reported to be a more effective antibacterial and antifungal agent than chlorhexidine gluconate. A solution of 1% Noxyflex was found to be as effective as a 2.5% solution and caused less haematuria (MacFayden 1967). However, the significant amount of haematuria associated with the use of Noxyflex may restrict its use.

Cytotoxic Agents Given Intravesically

For the administration cytotoxic agents, see the separate procedure for cytotoxic drugs (pages 120-125)

Catheters Used for Lavage and Irrigation

A three-way urinary catheter must be used for irrigation in order that fluid may simultaneously be run into and drained out from the bladder. This catheter is routinely passed in theatre when irrigation is required, e.g. after prostatectomy. Occasionally bladder irrigation is started on the ward. If the patient has an ordinary catheter, this must be replaced with a three-way type (see Figure 4.1).

For bladder lavage it is not necessary to use a three-way catheter. There are three reasons for this:

1   Obstruction is more likely to occur when the drainage lumen is small, as in the three-way type.
2   The catheter may not drain if there is an obstruction. Such an obstruction is most likely to have occurred within the drainage lumen, and lavage via the side arm is unlikely to have much, if any, effect on the cause of the obstruction.
3   The risk of infection from the recatheterization with a three-way

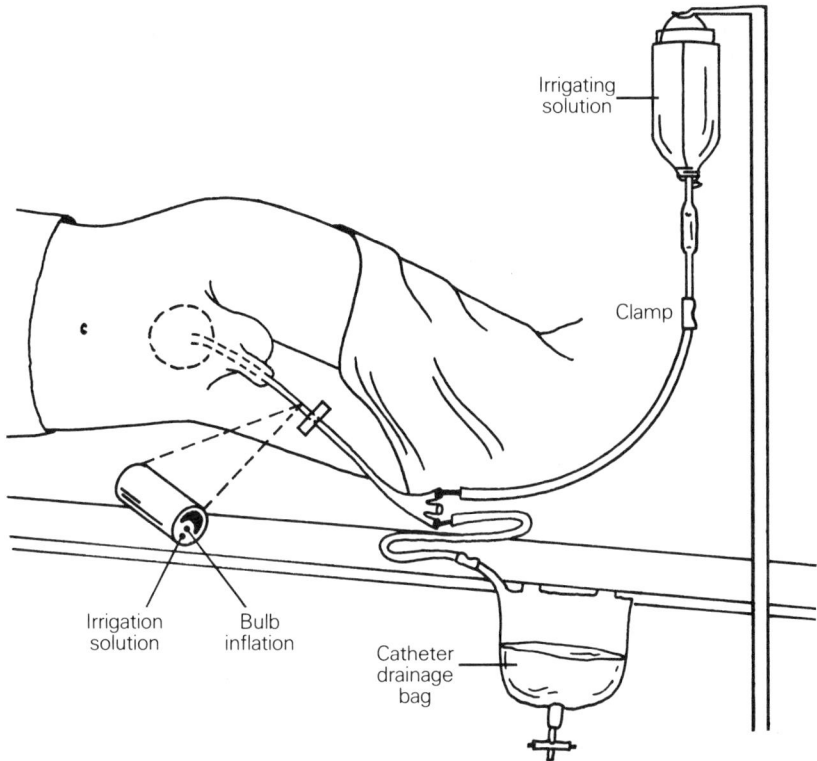

Figure 4.1 Closed urinary drainage system with provision for intermittent or continuous irrigation

catheter is much greater than the risk of infection from disconnecting a closed drainage system, provided that aseptic techniques are strictly adhered to.

It is recommended, however, that a three-way catheter is passed if frequent intravescial installations of drugs or antiseptic solutions are prescribed and the risk of catheter obstruction is not considered to be very great. In such cases the most important factor is minimizing the risk of introducing infection and maintaining a closed urinary drainage system, for which the three-way catheter allows.

References and Further Reading

Datta P K (1981) The post prostatectomy patient, Nursing Times 77:1759-1761

Harper W (1981) An appraisal of 12 solutions used for bladder irrigation or installation, British Journal of Urology 53: 433-438

Harper W Matz L (1975) The effect of chlorhexidine irrigation of the bladder in the rat, British Journal of Urology 47: 539-543

Harper W Matz L (1976) Further studies on effects of irrigating solutions on rat bladders, British Journal of Urology 48: 463-467

MacFayden I R (1976) Comparison of noxythiolin 'Noxyflex' and chlorhexidine

'Hibitaine' installation after intermittent catheterisation, Clinical Trials Journal 4: 654-656

Martindale W (1977) The Extra Pharmacopoeia, 27th edition, The Pharmaceutical Press

GUIDELINES: BLADDER LAVAGE

Equipment

1   Sterile dressing pack
2   Bladder syringe, 60 ml
3   Sterile jug
4   Antiseptic solution, such as Savlodil
5   Alcohol-based hand wash solution, such as Hibisol
6   Sterile gloves
7   Clamp
8   New catheter bag (for Foley-type catheter) or sterile spigot (for three-way catheter)
9   Sterile receiver
10   Sterile solution for lavage

Procedure

Action	Rationale
1 Explain the procedure to the patient.	1 To obtain the patient's consent and cooperation.
2 Screen the bed. Ensure that the patient is in a comfortable position allowing access to the catheter.	2 For the patient's privacy and to reduce the risk of cross-infection. Curtains are drawn at this stage so that dust and airborne organisms disturbed by the curtains do not settle on the sterile field.
3 Perform the procedure using an aseptic technique.	3 To prevent infection. (For further information see the procedure on aseptic technique pages 10-11)
4 Draw up solutions from vials, e.g. Noxyflex, using a 60 ml bladder syringe with needle adapter. Cap the syringe and place it in a sterile receiver.	4 It is easier to draw up solutions from vials in the clinical area than at the bedside.
5 Take the trolley to the bedside. Open the outer wrappings of packs and put them on the top shelf of the trolley.	
6 Prepare the sterile field. Pour the lavage solution into a sterile jug.	
7 Clean your hands with the appro-	7 To minimize the risk of infection.

Action	**Rationale**
priate antiseptic solution, such as Hibiscrub, and put on gloves.	
8 Clamp the catheter. Place a sterile paper towel under the junction of the catheter and the tubing of the drainage bag and disconnect them.	8 To prevent leakage when the catheter is disconnected. When the patient has a three-way catheter the drainage bag will not need disconnecting as the washout fluid is injected through the side arm of the catheter. This should be spigoted off after use and the fluid remaining in the bladder will drain into the catheter bag.
9 Clean your gloved hands with an alcohol-based hand wash solution, such as Hibisol. Using an aseptic technique, clean around the end of the catheter with sterile cotton wool and an antiseptic solution, such as Savlodil.	9 To remove surface organisms from gloves and catheter and thus reduce the risk of introducing infection into the catheter.
10 Draw up the irrigating fluid into the bladder syringe and insert the nozzle into the end of the catheter.	
11 Release the clamp on the catheter and gently inject the contents of the syringe into the bladder, trying not to inject air.	11 Rapid injection of fluid could be uncomfortable for the patient. Large volumes of air in the bladder cause distension and discomfort.
12 Remove the syringe and allow the bladder contents to drain by gravity into a receiver placed on a sterile towel.	
13 Repeat the last two steps (i.e. steps 11 and 12) of the procedure until the washout is complete or the returning fluid is clear.	
14 If the fluid does not return naturally, aspirate gently with the syringe.	14 Gentle suction is sometimes required to remove obstructive material from the catheter.
15 Connect a new catheter bag or sterile pigot if a three-way catheter is in place, and allow the remaining fluid to drain out.	15 A closed drainage system must be reestablished as soon as possible to reduce the risk of bacterial invasion through the catheter.
16 If the solution is to remain in the bladder, the catheter should be clamped when all the fluid has been injected and the clamp	

Action	**Rationale**
released after the desired period.	
17 Measure the volume of washout fluid returned and compare it with the volume of fluid injected. Record any discrepancies of volume in the appropriate documents.	17 To keep an accurate record of urinary output and to observe for catheter obstruction.
18 Make the patient comfortable, remove equipment and clean the trolley.	
19 Wash your hands.	19 To prevent cross-infection.

GUIDELINES: CONTINUOUS BLADDER IRRIGATION

Equipment

1   Sterile dressing pack
2   Antiseptic solution, such as Savlodil
3   Alcohol-based hand wash solution, such as Hibisol
4   Sterile gloves
5   Clamp
6   Sterile irrigation fluid
7   Disposable irrigation set
8   Infusion stand
9   Sterile jug

Procedure

Action	**Rationale**
Commencing Bladder Irrigation	
1 Explain the procedure to the patient.	1 To obtain the patient's consent and cooperation.
2 Screen the patient and ensure that the patient is in a comfortable position allowing access to the catheter.	2 For the patient's privacy and to reduce the risk of cross-infection. Curtains are drawn at this stage so that dust and airborne organisms disturbed by the curtains do not settle on the sterile trolley.
3 Perform the procedure using an aseptic technique.	3 To prevent infection. (For further information see the procedure on aseptic technique, pages 10-11.)
4 Open the outer wrappings of the pack and put it on the top shelf of the trolley.	
5 Insert the end of the irrigation	5 To prime the irrigation set so that

Action	**Rationale**
giving set into the fluid bag and hang the bag on the infusion stand. Allow fluid to run through the tubing so that air is expelled.	it is ready for use. Air is expelled in order to prevent discomfort from air in the patient's bladder.
6 Clamp the catheter.	
7 Prepare the sterile field.	
8 Clean your hands with an antiseptic solution, such as Hibiscrub. Put on gloves.	8 To minimize the risk of cross-infection.
9 Place a sterile paper towel under the irrigation inlet of the catheter and remove the spigot.	9 To prevent leakage of urine through the irrigation arm when the spigot is removed.
10 Discard the spigot.	
11 Clean your gloved hands with an alcohol-based hand wash solution, such as Hibisol. Using an aseptic technique, clean around the end of the irrigation arm with sterile cotton wool and an antiseptic solution such as Savlodil.	11 To remove surface organisms from gloves and catheter and to reduce the risk of introducing infection into the catheter.
12 Attach the irrigation giving set to the irrigation arm of the catheter. Keep the clamp of the irrigation giving set closed.	12 To prevent over-distention of the bladder, which can occur if fluid is run into the bladder before the drainage tube has been unclamped.
13 Release the clamp on the catheter tube and allow any accumulated urine to drain into the catheter bag. Empty the urine from the catheter bag into a sterile jug.	13 Urine drainage should be measured before commencing irrigation so that the fluid balance may be monitored more accurately.
14 Discard your gloves.	14 These will be contaminated, having handled the catheter bag.
15 Set irrigation at the required rate and ensure that fluid is draining into the catheter bag.	15 To check that the drainage system is patent and to prevent fluid accumulating in the bladder.
16 Make the patient comfortable, remove unncessary equipment and clean the trolley.	
17 Wash your hands.	17 To prevent cross-infection.

Care of the Patient during Irrigation

1 Adjust the rate of infusion according to the degree of haematuria. This will be greatest in the first 12 hours following surgery (average fluid input is 6-9 litres during the first 12 hours, falling to	1 To remove blood from the bladder before it clots and to minimize the risk of catheter obstruction and clot rentention.

Action	Rationale
3-6 litres during the next 12 hours). The aim is to obtain a drainage fluid which is rosé in colour.	
2 Check the volume in the drainage bag frequently when infusion is in progress, e.g. half-hourly or hourly.	2 To ensure that fluid is draining from the bladder and to detect blockages as soon as possible; also to prevent over-distention of the bladder and patient discomfort. Frequent checking means, in addition, that full catheter bags are noticed and can be emptied before they reach capacity.
3 Using rubber-tipped 'milking' tongs, 'milk' the catheter and drainage tube regularly, as required.	3 To remove unseen clots from within the drainage system and to maintain an efficient outlet.
4 Record the fluid balance chart accurately. The fluid balance of all patients having bladder irrigation must be monitored.	4 So that urine output is known and any related problems, e.g. renal dysfunction, may be detected quickly and easily.

BLADDER IRRIGATION RECORDING CHART

The bladder irrigation recording chart (see Figure 4.2) is designed to provide an accurate record of the patient's urinary output during the period of irrigation.

Procedure for the Use of the Chart

Record the time (column A) and the fluid volume in each bag of irrigating solution (column B) as it is put up.

When the irrigating fluid has all run from the first bag into the bladder, record the original volume in the bag in column C. Record the corresponding time in column A. Do not attempt to estimate the fluid volume run in while a bag is in progress as this will cause inaccuracies. If, however, a bag is discontinued, the volume run in can be calculated by measuring the volume left in the bag and deducting this from the original volume. This should be recorded in column C.

The catheter bag should be emptied as often as is necessary, the volume being recorded in column D and the corresponding time in column A. The catheter bag must also be emptied whenever the bag of irrigating fluid is empty, and the volume recorded in column D.

When each bag of fluid has run through, add up the total volume drained by the catheter in column D, and write this in red. Subtract from this the total volume run in (column C) to find the urine output. Write this in column E. Draw a line across the page to indicate that this calculation is complete and continue underneath for the next bag.

(A)	(B)	(C)	(D)	(E)	(F)
Date and time	Volume put up	Volume run in	Total volume	Urine	Urine running total

Figure 4.2 Bladder irrigation recording chart

NURSING CARE PLAN

Problem	Cause	Suggested Action
1 Fluid retained in the bladder when the catheter is in position	1 Fault in drainage apparatus, e.g.	
	a Blocked catheter	**a** 'Milk' the tubing. Wash out the bladder with normal saline.
	b Kinked tubing	**b** Straighten the tubing.
	c Overfull drainage bag	**c** Empty the drainage bag.
	d Catheter clamped off	**d** Unclamp the catheter.
2 Distended abdomen related to an overfull bladder during the irrigation procedure	2 **a** Irrigation fluid is infused at too rapid a rate	2 **a** Slow down the infusion rate.
	b Fault in drainage apparatus	**b** Check the patency of the drainage apparatus.

Problem	Cause	Suggested Action
3 Leakage of fluid from around the catheter	3 **a** Catheter slipping out of the bladder	3 **a** Insert the catheter further in and inflate the balloon more.
	b Catheter too large or unsuitable for the patient's anatomy	**b** If leakage is profuse or unacceptable for the patient's comfort, replace the catheter with one of smaller size.
4 Patient experiences pain during the lavage or irrigation procedure	4 **a** Volume of fluid in the bladder is too great for comfort	4 **a** Reduce the fluid volume within the bladder.
	b Solution is painful to raw areas in the bladder	**b** Inform the doctor. Administer analgesia as prescribed.

5

BLOOD PRESSURE

Definition

Blood pressure may be defined as the force which the blood exerts on the walls of the vessels in which it is contained. This may be represented as an equation:

blood pressure = cardiac output × peripheral resistance.

Indications

Blood pressure is measured for one of two reasons:

1   To establish a base-line in blood pressure
2   To monitor fluctuations in blood pressure.

REFERENCE MATERIAL

Blood flows from the heart, to arteries, to capillaries and to veins, as a result of differences in their internal pressure, pressure being least in the veins. These vascular pressures are controlled by the vasomotor centre in the medulla oblongata.

Normal blood pressure is maintained by reflex arcs derived from stretch receptors found in the wall of the proximal arterial tree, especially in the region of the aortic arch and carotid sinuses. When arterial pressure rises, there is increased stimulation of these nerve endings. The increased number of impulses along the vagus and glossopharyngeal nerves leads to reflex vagal slowing of the heart and reflex release of vasoconstrictor tone in the peripheral blood vessels. The resulting fall in cardiac output and the reduction of peripheral resistance tend to restore the blood pressure to the normal value. A fall in the arterial pressure decreases the stimulation of the arterial stretch receptors. The reflex tachycardia and vasoconstriction that ensue tend to raise the blood pressure to its normal value.

A fall in renal flow, due to a fall in arterial pressure, results in chemical changes which lead to stimulation of the suprarenal glands, leading in turn to salt and water retention. Such retention and vasoconstriction tend to raise arterial pressure.

Blood pressure varies, not only from moment to moment, but also with condition. It is lowest in neonates and increases with age, with weight gain and with stress and anxiety. Shock, myocardial infarction and haemorrhage are among the things that cause a fall in blood pressure as they reduce cardiac output and peripheral vessel resistance or they diminish venous return after fluid loss.

The conditions of hypertension (high blood pressure) and hypotension (low blood pressure) are defined by the following equations:

$$\text{hypertension} = \text{increased cardiac output} \times \frac{\text{greater total peripheral}}{\text{resistance}}$$

$$\text{hypotension} = \text{lessened cardiac output} \times \text{lesser total peripheral resistance.}$$

Normal Blood Pressure

Normal blood pressure is generally held to range from 100/60 to 140/90 mm Hg.

Systolic Pressure

The systolic pressure is the maximum pressure of the blood against the wall of the vessel following ventricular contraction and is taken as an indication of the integrity of the heart, arteries and arterioles.

Diastolic Pressure

The diastolic pressure is the minimum pressure of the blood against the wall of the vessel following closure of the aortic valve and is taken as a direct indication of blood vessel resistance.

Pulse Pressure

The pulse pressure is the difference between the systolic and diastolic readings.

Mean Arterial Pressure

The mean arterial pressure is the average pressure attempting to push blood through the circulatory system. This can be determined electronically or mathematically as well as by using an intra-arterial catheter and mercury manometer; e.g.

$$\text{mean arterial pressure (mathematically)} = \frac{1}{3}\frac{\text{systolic}}{\text{pressure}} + \frac{2}{3}\frac{\text{diastolic}}{\text{pressure}}$$

A blood pressure of 130/85 mm Hg gives a mean arterial pressure of 100 mm Hg.

Basal Blood Pressure

The basal blood pressure is the lowest blood pressure taken in a supine position after several days in hospital without treatment.

Factors Affecting Blood Pressure

1 Circulating blood volume
2 Elastic recoil of the arteries
3 Blood viscosity
4 Cardiac output
5 Neurogenic factors

Methods of Recording and Equipment

There are two main categories of method for recording the blood pressure: direct and indirect.

Direct methods are highly developed and of precise accuracy. The ideal direct method of measuring blood pressure involves the insertion of a minute pressure transducer unit into an artery for transmission of a waveform or digital display on a monitor. The most commonly used techniques involve placing a cannula in an artery and attaching a pressure-sensitive device to the external end.

The indirect method is the one most suitable for the nurse's purpose. All indirect methods are based upon the occluding technique devised by Riva-Rocci at the end of the last century and Korotkoff at the beginning of this century.

The Sphygmomanometer

The sphygmomanometer (see Figure 5.1) consists of a compression bag enclosed in an unyielding cuff, an inflating bulb, pump or other device by which the pressure is increased, a manometer from which the applied pressure is read, and a control valve to deflate the system.

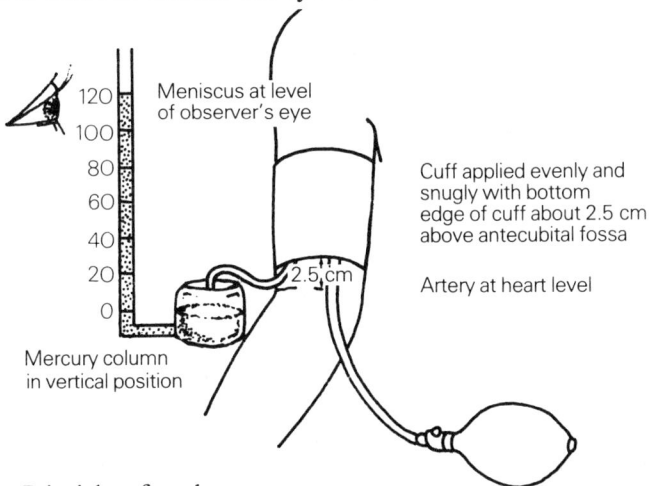

Figure 5.1 Principles of a sphygmomanometer

Manometer   Mercury sphygmomanometers are reliable, on the whole, and easily maintained. Care should be taken to avoid loss of mercury. Substantial errors may occur if the manometer is not kept vertical during the measurement. The air vent at the top of the manometer must be kept patent. Aneroid sphygmomanometers are generally less accurate than mercury ones.

Cuff   The cuff is an inelastic cloth that encircles the arm and encloses the inflatable rubber bladder. It is secured around the arm or leg by wrapping its tapering end to the encircling material, by Velcro surfaces or by hooks.

Inflatable Bladder   A bladder that is too short and/or too narrow will give falsely high pressures. One that is too wide and/or too long will give falsely low pressures. O'Brien and O'Malley (1979) recommended a bladder that is 20% greater than (1.2 times) the diameter of the extremity of the limb that is being used.

Control Valve, Pump and Rubber Tubing   The control valve is a common source of error. It should allow the passage of air without excessive pressure needing to be applied on the pump. When the valve is closed it should hold the mercury at a constant level and, when released, it should allow a controlled fall in the level of mercury. The rubber tubing should be long (approximately 80 cm) and with airtight connections that can easily be separated.

It is essential that the sphygmomanometer be kept in good working order. Conceicao et al. (1976) and North (1979) have shown that as many as 50% of the sphygmomanometers used in the hospitals they studied were inaccurate.

The Stethoscope

The stethoscope must be of a standard variety and in good working order.

Using the stethoscope, it is possible to identify a series of five phases as blood pressure falls from the systolic to the diastolic. These phases are known as Korotkoff's sounds (see Figure 5.2).

1   The appearance of faint, clear tapping sounds which gradually increase in intensity
2   The softening of sounds, which may become swishing
3   The return of sharper sounds which become crisper but never fully regain the intensity of the Phase 1 sounds
4   The distinct muffling sounds which become soft and blowing
5   The point at which all sound ceases.

The choice of Phase 4 or Phase 5 as the tone diastolic pressure is a controversial one, as can be seen from Burton (1967). It is recommended that both pressures should be recorded, e.g. 142/78/78 (if the levels are identical) or 142/82/78 (for different levels). If this practice is not followed, all nurses should agree on a predetermined diastolic end-point.

Blood pressure (mm Hg)

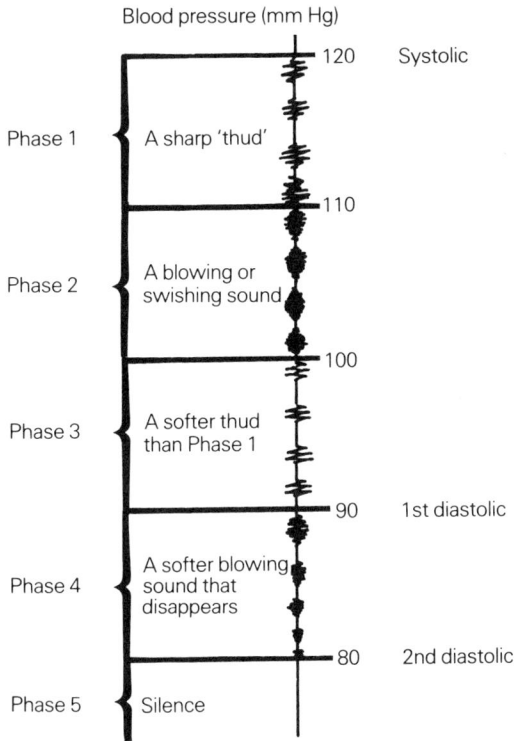

Figure 5.2 Korotkoff sounds

Some Additional Information

Much recent research has focused on the faulty techniques employed when nurses take blood pressures. Maxwell (1982) has shown that the number of obese patients diagnosed as hypertensive may be grossly overestimated due to the use of cuffs of the incorrect size. Thompson (1981) discussed, analysed and evaluated the methodology of blood pressure recording. Poor technique and observer bias as potential sources of error were also examined. He concluded that many nurses are often inadequately trained in blood pressure measurement and that, with increasing reliance on the nurse for recording vital signs, more attention needs to be paid to this area.

References and Further Reading

Bell G H et al. (1976) Textbook of Physiology and Biochemistry, Churchill Livingstone

Brunner L S Suddarth D S (1982) The Lippincott Manual of Medical-Surgical Nursing, Harper & Row, Volume 2, pp. 162-163, 170-171, 174

Burton A C (1967) The criterion for diastolic pressure and revolution and counter-revolution, Circulation 36: 805-809

Conceicao S et al. (1976) Defects in sphygmomanometers, British Medical Journal 2: 886-888

Jarvis C M (1980) Vital signs: a preview of problems, In Assessing Vital Functions Accurately, Intermed Communications, pp. 29-30

King E M et al. (1981) Illustrated Manual of Nursing Techniques, 2nd edition, J. B. Lippincott, pp. 470-471

Korotkoff M S (1905) On the subject of methods of measuring blood pressure, Bulletin of the Imperial Medical Academy of St Petersburg 11: 365-367

Maxwell M H (1982) Error in blood pressure measurement due to incorrect cuff size in obese patients, Lancet ii: 33-36

North L W (1979) Accuracy of sphygmomanometers, Association of Operating Room Nurses Journal 30: 996-1000

O'Brien E T O'Malley K (1979) ABC of blood pressure measurement: sphygmomanometer, British Medical Journal 2: 851-853

Thompson D R (1981) Recording patients' blood pressure: a review, Journal of Advanced Nursing 6 (4): 283-290

GUIDELINES: BLOOD PRESSURE

Equipment

1   Sphygmomanometer
2   Stethoscope

Procedure

Action	Rationale
1 Explain to the patient that his blood pressure is going to be taken.	1 To obtain the consent and co-operation of the patient.
2 Measure the blood pressure under the same conditions each time.	2 To ensure continuity and consistency in recording.
3 Ensure that the patient is in the desired position — lying, standing or sitting.	3 To obtain the required reading.
4 Use the correct size of blood pressure cuff.	4 To obtain the correct reading.
5 Apply the cuff of the sphygmomanometer to the arm above the antecubital fossa or to the leg above the popliteal fossa. The extremity should be positioned for maximum patient comfort and examiner accesibility. The leg should only be used if both arms are inaccessible.	5 The brachial and popliteal arteries are superficial in the antecubital and popliteal fossae.
6 Place the bell of the stethoscope over the artery.	6 When the bell of the stethoscope is placed over the artery, the sound

Action	Rationale
	will be heard with little distortion. The artery must be located by palpating with the fingertips.
7 Inflate the cuff to a point approximately 20-30 mm Hg above the last recorded reading or until the pulse can no longer be heard or palpated. Release the pressure valve on the cuff slowly.	7 Pressure exerted by the inflated cuff prevents blood from flowing through the artery. The systolic pressure is the point at which blood in the artery is first able to force its way through against the pressure exerted by the inflated cuff. It is found by slowly releasing the pressure valve. The point at which the first beat is heard is the systolic reading. The diastolic pressure is the point at which blood flows freely in the artery and is equivalent to the amount of pressure normally exerted on the wall of the arteries when the heart is at rest. While continuing to release the cuff pressure, a point is reached where the last distinct sound will be heard. The point at which the last beat is heard is the diastolic reading.
8 Record the systolic and diastolic pressures and compare the present reading with previous readings.	8 To monitor differences and detect trends. Any irregularities should be brought to the attention of the appropriate personnel.
9 Remove the equipment and clean it after use. The earpieces of the stethoscope should be wiped with a disinfectant solution that will not harm the ear.	9 To prevent the spread of infection.

NURSING CARE PLAN

Category	Frequency	Rationale
1 All new admissions	1 Once only, preferably when the patient has settled in	1 To provide a base-line.
2 Hypertensive patient	2 Four-hourly until condition is stable	2 To monitor the condition of the patient so that any necessary action can be taken.
3 Postoperative patient	3 Half-hourly, depend-	3 To detect postopera-

Category	Frequency	Rationale
	ing on the patient's condition, then 4-hourly until condition is stable	tive hypo- or hypertension.
4 Critically ill patient, e.g. unconscious patient	4 As often as determined by condition	4 To monitor blood pressure closely.
5 Pregnant client	5 Daily	5 To detect hypo- or hypertension.
6 Patient receiving a blood transfusion	6 When unit is put up. Observe the patient at 5 minute intervals for the first 15-20 minutes and take again 1 hour later if condition warrants it. If blood pressure fluctuates or the patient shows other signs of reaction, record again and as demanded by condition.	6 To record a base-line blood pressure and monitor any reaction to the transfusion.
7 Patient receiving intravenous infusion	7 Four-hourly.	7 To monitor circulatory overload.
8 Patient with local or systemic infection	8 Four-hourly until condition is stable	8 To detect any signs or symptoms of shock.
9 Patient receiving any drug known to cause fluctuations in blood pressure	9 Twice daily	9 To monitor reaction to the drug.
10 Patient with prolonged or profound neutropenia	10 Four-hourly until neutrophil count rises	10 To detect septicaemic shock that may not manifest itself in pyrexia or signs of local infection.
11 Patient not feeling well or nurse concerned about patient	11 Once. If outside the normal ranges, check again 2-3 hours later and take appropriate action.	11 To reassure the patient and nurse and to ensure that appropriate action is taken if blood pressure is remarkable.

Problem	Cause	Suggested Action
1 Falsely elevated blood pressure	1 **a** Using too narrow a cuff. The cuff bladder should be 20% wider that the diameter of the extremity in use.	1 **a** Use the correct size cuff.
	b Wrapping the cuff too loosely	**b** Wrap the cuff firmly but not tightly.
	c Deflating the cuff too slowly. Venous	**c** Release the pressure valve methodically.

Problem	Cause	Suggested Action
	congestion in the extremity will give a falsely high reading.	
	d Tilting the mercury column away from the vertical	**d** Maintain the sphygmomanometer in the vertical position.
	e Having the mercury column above eye level	**e** Place the sphygmomanometer at eye level.
	f Taking the blood pressure when the patient is upset, has just eaten, has just finished a cigarette or has been walking.	**f** Ensure that the patient has been relaxed for at least half an hour before taking the blood pressure.
2 Falsely low blood pressure	2 **a** Patient's arm above the level of his heart	2 **a** Ensure that the arm is below the level of the heart.
	b Having the mercury column below eye level	**b** Place the sphygmomanometer at eye level
	c Failure to notice an 'auscultatory gap', i.e. the sound, after fading out for about 10-15 mm Hg, returns	**c** Palpate the radial artery as the cuff is inflated.
	d Inability to hear feeble sounds	**d** Ask the patient to raise his arm before you inflate the cuff again. This decreases the venous pressure and should make the sounds louder. Then lower the arm, deflate the cuff, and listen. If the sounds are still feeble, chart the preparatory systolic pressure. Inform the medical staff.

6

BONE MARROW ASPIRATION

Definition

Bone marrow aspiration is the aspiration of sufficient bone marrow from the iliac crest or sternum, using a special needle, to enable laboratory testing.

Indications

Bone marrow aspiration is a procedure performed by trained medical staff to evaluate haematopoesis and so establish a diagnosis in certain haematological disorders, e.g. anaemia, leukaemia, myeloma, metastatic carcinoma. It is also performed to monitor both the course of the patient's disease and his/her response to therapy.

Contraindications

This procedure is contraindicated in those patients who are unable to co-operate, or who have a coagulation defect.

REFERENCE MATERIAL

Bone marrow aspiration was first introduced in Naples in 1909 by Pianese. By 1933 Custer had developed it into a routine technique. It is a quick and relatively simple method of obtaining a marrow specimen and can be performed either in the hospital ward or in an outpatient clinic.

Anatomy and Physiology

The bone contains two types of marrow:

1 Yellow marrow is a mainly fatty substance.
2 Red marrow is responsible for the production of red and white blood cells.

In certain diseases, such as leukaemia, the imature cells of the red marrow may proliferate and replace the yellow marrow.

Red marrow is found in the cavities of all bones during the first years of life. In adults it is found mainly in the flat bones, e.g. skull, vertebrae, clavicles,

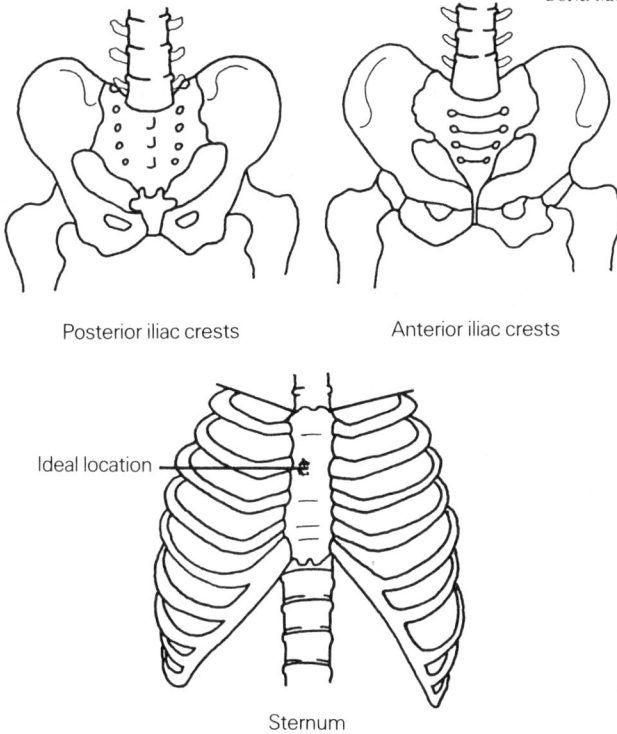

Posterior iliac crests   Anterior iliac crests

Ideal location

Sternum

Figure 6.1 Common sites for bone marrow examination, arranged in order of preference. Normally only aspirations, not biopsies, are done on the sternum because of its small size and proximity to vital organs

scapulae, sternum and iliac crests.

The preferred sites for marrow aspiration, in an adult, are the iliac crests and the sternum (see Figure 6.1). The iliac crests are often used for patients requiring frequent marrow aspirations as the use of the right and left crests can be alternated, both anterior and posterior surfaces may be used and there are no vital organs nearby that may be punctured during the procedure. The posterior iliac crest is often preferred as the procedure can then be performed outside the patient's field of vision, thus reducing his/her anxiety.

The actual aspiration of marrow from the bone cavity is painful despite the local anaesthetic which dulls the pain of the passage of the biopsy needle through the skin, subcutaneous layer and, to a large extent, the periosteum. To enable the patient to cope with the pain he/she should be warned about its inevitability beforehand but it should be emphasized that the pain will only be of short duration.

Very anxious patients and children may be prescribed a mild sedative, such as diazepam, to be given before the procedure begins. In some units the procedure is carried out under a light general anaesthetic.

Complications

Complications are extremely rare but include the following:

1 *Cardiac tamponade,* which can occur following sternal puncture
2 *Haemorrhage,* which occurs almost exclusively in those patients suffering from thrombocytopoenia. It may be avoided by applying adequate pressure to the puncture site for a few minutes following aspiration.

References and Further Reading

Abrahams P Webb P (1975) Clinical Anatomy of Practical Procedures, Pitman Medical pp. 111-114

Bevan J (1978) A Pictorial Handbook of Anatomy and Physiology, Mitchell Beasley, p. 34

Booth J A (1983) Handbook of Investigations, Harper & Row, pp. 49-51

Brunner L S Suddarth D S (1982) The Lippincott Manual of Medical-Surgical Nursing, Harper & Row, Volume 2, pp. 186-189

Frazer I Gough K R (1968) Bone marrow biopsy, In Biopsy Procedures in Clinical Medicine, edited by A E Read, John Wright & Sons, pp. 50-56

Markus S (1981) Taking the fear out of bone marrow examinations, Nursing (US) 11 (4): 64-67

Navarett D (1981) Assisting with bone marrow aspiration, in Mosby's Manual of Clinical Nursing Procedures, edited by J Hirsch and J Hancock, C V Mosby, pp. 226-228

Pagnana K D Pagnana T J (1982) Diagnostic Testing and Nursing Implications, C V Mosby, pp. 279-281

Skydell B Crowder A (1975) Diagnostic Procedures — A Reference for Health Practitioners and a Guide for Patient Counselling, Little, Brown, pp. 235-236

GUIDELINES: BONE MARROW ASPIRATION

Equipment

1 Antiseptic skin cleansing agent
2 Sterile dressing pack
3 Selection of syringes and needles
4 Local anaesthetic
5 Sterile gloves
6 Marrow aspiration needle and guard, e.g. Salah needle
7 Microscope slides and coverslips
8 Specimen bottles (plain and with heparin)
9 Plastic dressing or plastic dressing spray

Procedure

Action	Rationale
1 Explain the procedure to the patient.	1 To reinforce what the doctor has told him/her and thus ensure his/

Action	**Rationale**
	her cooperation.
2 Give medication as ordered, allowing sufficient time for it to have effect.	2 Usually this is only necessary for very anxious patients.
3 Help the patient into the correct position:	
a Supine	**a** For sternal puncture.
b Prone or on side	**b** For anterior or posterior iliac crest puncture.
4 Continue to observe the patient throughout the procedure. Assist the doctor as required. Reassure the conscious patient. Follow the appropriate procedure if the patient is anaesthetized.	
5 Procedure is performed by a doctor:	
a Skin is cleansed with antiseptic solution.	5 **a** To maintain asepsis throughout the procedure and thus minimize the risk of infection.
b Local anaesthetic is injected intradermally and through the various layers until the periosteum is infiltrated.	**b** To minimize pain during the procedure and to ensure the maximum degree of cooperation of the patient. Transitory pain will be felt both as the periosteum is punctured and when the marrow is aspirated.
c Once the local anaesthetic has taken effect the doctor inserts the marrow needle, with the guard on, into the anaesthetized area.	**c** The needle guard ensures the correct positioning of the needle in the marrow cavity and diminishes the risk, particularly in the sternal puncture, of inadvertently puncturing vital organs.
d If the patient has not been anaesthetized, the doctor warns the patient that he/she will feel a brief episode of sharp pain as the marrow is withdrawn. The needle is advanced into the bone marrow and the required amount of marrow is withdrawn.	**d** To allay anxiety and to ensure the patient's maximum cooperation
e The needle is removed from the puncture site.	
6 Once the doctor has removed the needle, apply pressure over the puncture site using a sterile topical swab until the bleeding stops.	6 To minimize bruising and to prevent haematoma formation. Prolonged pressure, 5-10 minutes, is required if the patient has a low

Action	Rationale
	platelet count (thrombocyto-poenia).
7 Once bleeding stops, cover the site with plaster or a plastic dressing. Ask the patient not to bath or wash the area for 24 hours.	
8 Make the patient comfortable. He/she may be mobile, as desired, depending on the level of sedation.	8 Some patients will have this procedure performed in the out-patient department and will be asked to wait in the clinic for a further 30 minutes to ensure that no further bleeding occurs.
9 Remove and dispose of equipment.	9 To prevent spread of infection.
10 Record necessary information in the appropriate documents and ensure that specimens are sent to the appropriate laboratory department, correctly labelled and with the necessary forms.	

NURSING CARE PLAN

Problem	Cause	Suggested Action
1 Pain experienced over the puncture site for 1-2 days following the procedure	1 Bruising of the tissues at the time of puncture or haematoma formation due to inadequate pressure on the puncture site following the procedure	1 Administer a mild analgesic as ordered by the doctor.
2 Haemorrhage from the puncture site following the procedure	2 Low platelet count or inadequate pressure on the puncture site following the procedure	2 Ensure that pressure is applied for a minimum of 5 minutes on the puncture site. Report excessive, uncontrollable bleeding to the appropriate personnel.
3 Haematoma formation over the puncture site	3 Haemorrhage following the procedure	3 Administer analgesics as ordered. If the haematoma is severe, report this to the doctor as aspiration may be required.

7

BOWEL CARE

GENERAL INTRODUCTION

It should be borne in mind that many patients are too embarrassed to talk about bowel function and will often delay reporting the problem until it has been present for a few days. Generally complaints will be either that the patient has diarrhoea or that he/she is constipated. Both diarrhoea and constipation should be seen as symptoms of some underlying disease or malfunction and managed accordingly.

The nurse's priority in either case is immediate resolution of the problem and re-education of the patient to avoid such problems in the future. In the management of diarrhoea, the nurse can ensure that the patient's diet is altered. Foods having a high fibre content can be avoided and fluid intake can be increased. Such measures as the provision of soft toilet paper, easy access to toilet facilities and a suitable barrier cream to prevent anal excoriation can be implemented and will be much appreciated by the patient. Constipation, however, demands the use of more elaborate nursing skills.

REFERENCE MATERIAL

Anatomy and Physiology

From the ileocaecal sphincter to the anus the colon is approximately 1.5 metres in length. Its main function is to eliminate the waste products of digestion by the propulsion of faeces towards the anus. In addition, it produces mucus to lubricate the faecal mass, thus aiding its expulsion. Other functions include the absorption of fluid and electrolytes, the storage of faeces and the synthesis of vitamins B and K by bacterial flora.

Faeces consist of any unabsorbed end products of digestion, bile pigments, cellulose, bacteria, epithelial cells, mucus and some inorganic material. They are semisolid in consistency and contain about 70% water.

The colon absorbs about 2 litres of water in 24 hours. If faeces are not expelled they will, therefore, gradually become hard due to dehydration and will be difficult to expel. If there is insufficient roughage (fibre) in the faeces, colonic stasis will lead to continued water absorption and the faeces will harden even further.

The movement of faeces through the colon towards the anus is by perstaltic action.

Faeces normally remain in the sigmoid colon until the stimulus to defaecate occurs. This stimulus varies in individuals according to habit. The stimulus can be controlled by conscious effort. After a few minutes the stimulus disappears and does not return for several hours. If these natural reflexes are inhibited on a regular basis they are eventually suppressed and reflex defaecation is inhibited. The result is that the individual becomes severely constipated. If the stimulus is responded to then faeces will move into the rectum.

The rectum is very sensitive to rises in pressure, even of 2-3 mm Hg, and distention will cause a perineal sensation with a consequent desire to defaecate.

A coordinated reflex empties the bowel from mid-transverse colon to the anus. During this phase the diaphragm, abdominal and levator ani muscles contract and the glottis closes. Waves of peristalsis occur in the distal colon and the anal sphincter relaxes, allowing the evacuation of faeces.

Constipation

Constipation is a symptom. Its management depends on its cause. Definitions and classifications differ but for most patients it means irregular, infrequent defaecation associated with the passage of hard faeces (see Figure 7.1). The patient usually complains of difficulty in defaecating with accompanying discomfort or pain.

Traditionally, the treatment of constipation has been left to the nurse (Milton-Thompson 1971). As the patient often presents in hospital with an acute problem of constipation, nurses will need to formulate a short term plan to evacuate the bowel as completely and as quickly as possible. For this reason enemas, suppositories and laxatives have remained the treatments of choice. Very often little thought is given either to the cause of the problem or to a more long term plan. Duffin et al. (1981) have shown that a total of 3428 enemas were given on the geriatric wards of a district general hospital over a 6-month period. There were 1120 admissions in this period which gave an overall average of three enemas per patient. The same study found that although the enemas frequently produced a good bowel evacuation, they also embarrassed the patient and produced symptoms ranging from nausea and abdominal pain to faecal incontinence. Hurst (1970) felt that enemas were probably only of use where there was a mechanical delay between the splenic flexure and anus. Dorgu (1971) felt that the main benefit of enemas was that they acted within minutes of their administration and were useful in acute conditions of impaction before drug therapy could be effective.

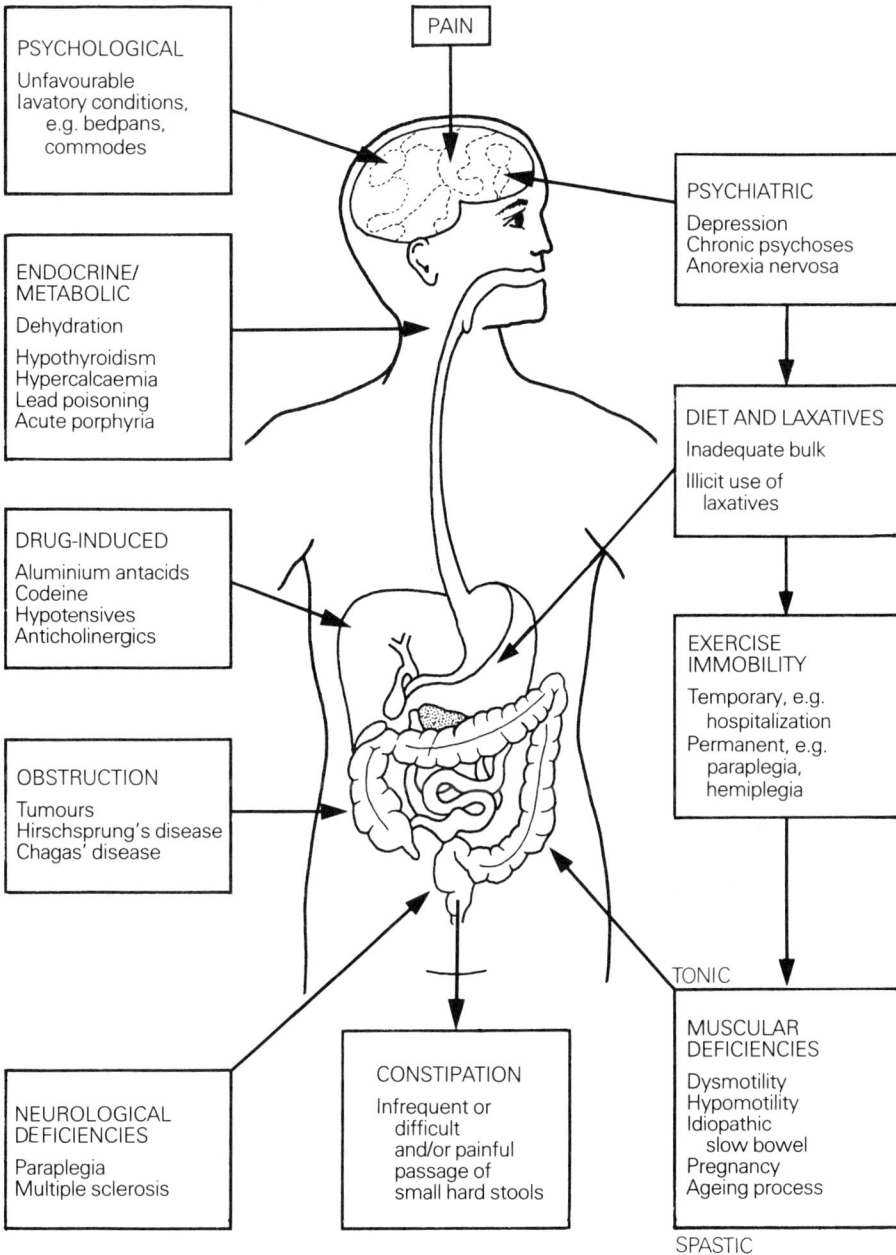

Figure 7.1 Classification of constipation — combined sources

Assessment of the problem

The myth of daily bowel evacuation being essential to healthy living has persisted through the centuries. This myth has resulted in laxative abuse becoming one of the commonest types of drug abuse in the Western world.

On the use and abuse of purgatives Hurst (1970) showed that £10 000 000 was expended in 1921 on patent medicines, the majority of which contained purgatives. In the 1960s, a survey of Londoners showed that over 30% were treating themselves with laxatives (Rutter and Maxwell 1976).

However, the indications for their use are fairly limited. The nurse should always stress the importance of diet and exercise to the patient before recommending other ways of evacuating the bowel.

Defining constipation is undoubtedly a problem while the notion of essential daily evacuations persists. The first objective should be for the nurse to assess what is 'normal' for that patient. A bowel action every third day may be quite adequate for some people; for others three times a day will be the norm. This does not mean that the first person is constipated or that the second has diarrhoea.

Many factors may affect normal bowel functioning. Among those pertinent to hospital admission are the following:

1   Change in diet
2   Lack of exercise
3   X-ray investigation of the bowel involving the use of barium.
4   The use of drugs, particularly analgesics.

Purgatives are often required to overcome these effects.

The nurse should always make a rectal examination to establish whether the patient is constipated and to what degree. Wilson and Muir (1975) in their trial on geriatric faecal incontinence found that there was little correlation between a nurse's subjective assessment of whether a patient was constipated and the actual evidence gained from a rectal examination.

Wherever possible the most natural means of bowel evacuation should be employed. This will mean, after initial solution of the problem by the use of purgatives, re-educating the patient about dieting and exercise.

The use of the bedpan should always be avoided if possible. If the patient can get out of bed, a commode is preferable as the amount of energy expended is considerably less than that required for balancing on a bedpan. Lewin (1976) quoted from research by an American team investigating the straining forces of bowel evacuation by objective methods. They showed that straining was increased three to six times when a patient used the bedpan and that its use requires a 50% greater consumption of oxygen than a commode by the bedside.

In all cases manual evacuation of the rectum should be avoided. It is a distressing, often painful and potentially dangerous procedure for the patient. It may be necessary to sedate the patient before carrying out the procedure. It is recommended by Pirrie (1980) that it should be performed by medical staff only.

Laxatives

The use of purgatives should be avoided and certainly they ought not to be used unless prescribed by a doctor. Purgatives alter the natural functioning of the alimentary tract and often a period of no bowel evacuations will follow their use. This usually causes the patient to take more laxatives and a cycle of dependence ensues (Mortimer 1970).

Table 7.1 Types of laxatives

Type of laxative	Example	Brand names and sources
Bulk producers	Dietary fibre	Bran, wholemeal bread
	Mucilaginous	Metamucil, Isogel,
	polysaccharides	Normacol
	Methylcellulose	Celevac
Stool softeners	Synthetic surface active agents	Dioctyl
Lubricants	Liquid paraffin	Agarol, Petrolagar
	Mineral oil, hydrocarbon mixtures	
Osmotic agents	Sodium, potassium and magnesium salts	Magnesium sulphate, Epsom salts, milk of magnesia
Chemical stimulants	Anthracene compounds	Senna, Senokot, Dorbanex
	Polyphenolic compounds Castor oil	Bisacodyl, Dulcolax
	Bile salts	Cholic acid, Taxol, Veracolate

Stool softeners lower the surface tension of the faeces and allow penetration by water. They act within 24-48 hours. Liquid paraffin is a stool softener as well as a lubricant, but its use should be avoided as droplets of oil may be accidentally inhaled, especially by the very young or the elderly, and cause lipoid pneumonia or even pulmonary tumours which may imitate carcinoma (Milton-Thompson 1871). Repetitive use of liquid paraffin and the mineral oils also interferes with the absorption of fat-soluble vitamins and may increase the risks of alimentary tract malignancies (Jones 1979).

Osmotic agents retain water in the small bowel and increase the flow of fluid into the colon. This increased volume will cause peristalsis and consequent expulsion of faeces. Osmotic agents work within 3-6 hours. Magnesium salts are contraindicated for patients suffering from chronic renal failure as magnesium poisoning may result (Milton-Thompson 1971). Sodium-containing laxatives should not be used for patients with cardiac problems or inflammatory bowel disease (Corman et al. 1975).

Chemical stimulants cause irritation of mucosa, nerves or smooth muscle. Most of the stimulants act within 2-8 hours. The amount of abdominal cramping produced and the time taken for them to work varies from drug to drug. These drugs can produce electrolyte imbalance, histological changes (melanosis coli) and damage to the mysenteric plexi. Eventually permanent damage to the motility of the colon can occur, leading the patient to take increasing doses of the drug (Rutter and Maxwell 1976).

Recently more favour has been shown towards the bulk laxatives, particularly those, such as bran, which can be incorporated into the diet. Bulk laxatives work by increasing the mass of the faeces. They do this by attracting water. This in turn promotes peristalsis and reduces the time taken by the faeces to move through the colon. An increased fluid intake is required when bulk laxatives are used, particularly in the elderly, to prevent intestinal obstruction occurring. Another problem initally is that bulk laxatives tend to distend the abdomen, often making the patient feel full and uncomfortable. Sometimes this leads to temporary anorexia. Harris (1980) discussed fully the merits of introducing bran into the diet, especially of the elderly, and the consequent drastic reduction in the number of enemas administered. She also showed that the cost of using bran compared to other laxatives, even other bulk laxatives, was very much lower. It is often forgotten that bran also reduces glucose absorption from the small intestine and increases the time taken for the blood sugar level to reach its maximum.This could be beneficial when treating patients with maturity onset diabetes, although caution is needed if they are receiving oral hypoglycaemics.

ENEMAS

Definition

An enema is the introduction into the rectum or lower colon of a stream of fluid for the purpose of producing a bowel action or instilling medication.

Indications

Enemas may be prescribed for the following reasons:

1 To clean the lower bowel prior to surgery or childbirth, prior to X-ray examination of the bowel using contrast medium, prior to endoscopy examination or in cases of severe constipation
2 To introduce medication into the system
3 To soothe and treat irritated bowel mucosa

4   To decrease body temperature (due to contact with the proximal vascular system)
5   To stop local haemorrhage
6   To decrease cerebral oedema

Contraindications

Enemas are contraindicated under the following circumstances:

1   Cases of paralytic ileus
2   Cases of colonic obstruction
3   The administration of tap water or soap and water enemas which may cause circulatory overload, water intoxication, mucosal damage and necrosis, hyperkalaemia and cardiac arrythmias
4   The administration of large amounts of fluid high into the colon which may cause perforation and haemorrhage
5   Following gastrointestinal or gynaecological surgery, where suture lines may be ruptured (unless medical consent has been given).

REFERENCE MATERIAL

Types of enemas

Evacuant Enemas

An evacuant enema is a solution introduced into the rectum or lower colon with the intention of its being expelled, along with faecal matter and flatus, within a few minutes. The following solutions are commonly used:

1   Phosphate enemas with standard or long rectal tubes in single dose disposable packs
2   Dioctyl sodium sulphosuccinate 0.1%, sorbitol 25% in single dose disposable packs
3   Sodium citrate 450 mg, sodium alkylsulphoacetate 45 mg, sorbic acid 5 mg in single dose disposable packs
4   Sodium citrate 450 mg, sodium laurylsulphoacetate 45 mg, glycerol 625 mg with citric acid, potassium sorbate and sorbitol in single dose disposable packs
5   Sodium citrate 450 mg, sodium laurylsulphate 75 mg, sorbic acid 5 mg, in a viscous solution in single dose disposable packs
6   Oxyphenisatin (Veripaque) in powder for reconstitution
7   Tap water.

Enemas containing dioctyl sulphosuccinate lubricate and soften impacted faeces. Phosphate enemas are useful in bowel clearance prior to X-ray examination and surgery.

Tap water may be dangerous when administered as an enema to a child or to those with poor cardiac function as excessive absorption could lead to circulatory overload (Milton-Thompson 1971).

Green soap was formerly very popular as an evacuant enema, especially prior to childbirth. Its use has now, however, fallen into disfavour due to numerous adverse reports of mucosal damage, necrosis, extensive sloughing of mucosa, severe haemorrhage, anaphylactic shock and death (Lewis 1965; Smith 1967; Pike et al. 1971; Edgell and Johnson 1973). The limiting factors in soap are alkalis, potash and phenol. In Hirschprung's disease, deaths following soap enema have occurred when a potassium-based soap was used. Hyperkalaemia resulted, causing cardiac arrythmias (Lewin 1976). Soap is probably a simple irritant; the higher the concentration the greater the mucosal inflammation.

Retention Enemas

A retention enema is a solution introduced into the rectum or lower colon with the intention of its being retained for a specified period of time. Two types of retention enema are in common use:

1   Arachis oil (may be obtained in a single dose disposable pack)
2   Olive oil.

Enemas containing oil will soften and lubricate impacted faeces. Rentention enemas given to administer medications will be prescribed by the doctor. The product must be checked with the prescription by two nurses before its administration.

SUPPOSITORIES

Definition

A suppository is a solid or semisolid pellet introduced into the anal canal for medicinal purposes.

Indications

The use of suppositories is indicated under the following circumstances:

1   To empty the bowel prior to certain types of surgery
2   To empty the bowel to relieve acute constipation or where other treatments for constipation have failed
3   To empty the bowel prior to endoscopic examination
4   To introduce medication into the system
5   To soothe and treat haemorrhoids or anal pruritus.

Contraindications

The use of suppositories is contraindicated when one or more of the following pertain:

1 Chronic constipation, which would require repetitive use
2 Cases of paralytic ileus
3 Cases of colonic obstruction
4 Following gastrointestinal or gynaecological operations, unless on the specific instructions of the doctor.

REFERENCE MATERIAL

Many elderly people find repeated enemas both unpleasant and uncomfortable and in cases of severe stasis and impaction whole gut irrigation or colonic lavage may be preferable (Currie 1979). Hunt (1974) states that the advantages of colonic lavage are that it clears the colon more effectively when visual observation of the interior of the colon is necessary and in cases of disordered action with constipation. However, the disadvantages include the risk of bowel perforation and the inadvertant washing away of the protective mucus which the bowel secretes. Its use is contraindicated in cases of diverticular disease and colitis.

Suppositories may be favoured as they are both easier to administer (see Figure 7.2) and generally cause the patient less discomfort.

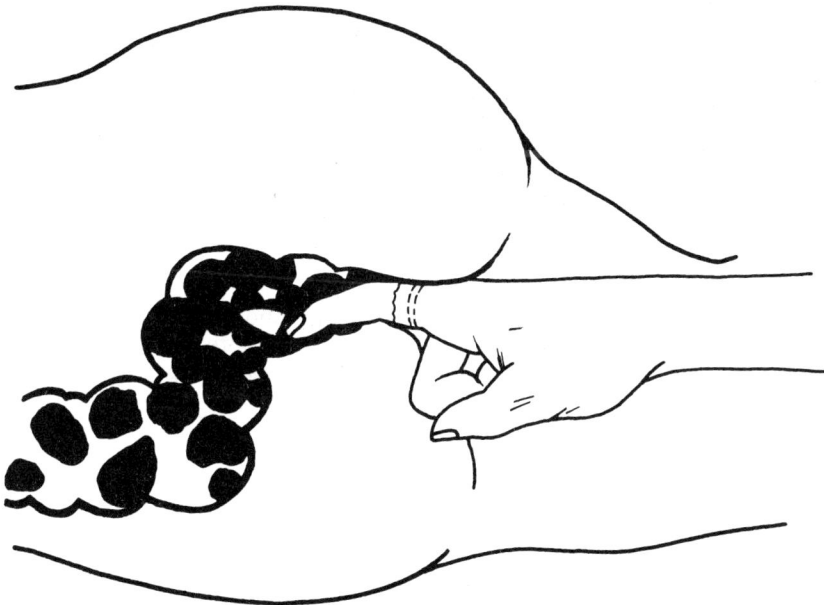

Figure 7.2 Administration of suppositories

Administration of Suppositories

The use of suppositories dates back to about 460 BC. Hippocrates recommended the use of cylindrical suppositories of honey smeared with ox gall (see Hurst 1970). Several types are now commercially available.

Lubricant suppositories, e.g. glycerine, should be inserted directly into the faeces and allowed to dissolve to enable softening of the faecal mass (see Figure 7.2). However, stimulant types, such as bisacodyl, must come into contact with the mucous membrane of the rectum if they are to be effective. Other types, such as sodium bicarbonate and anhydrous sodium acid phosphate (Beogex), exert their influence by releasing carbon dioxide, causing rectal distention when they contact water or mucous membrane.

Walker (1982) has shown that if a suppository is being used to obtain a systemic action it should be inserted blunt end forward to minimize rectal discomfort or irritation and maximize the retention period. For local action to promote defaecation it should be inserted in the conventional manner (Figure 7.3)

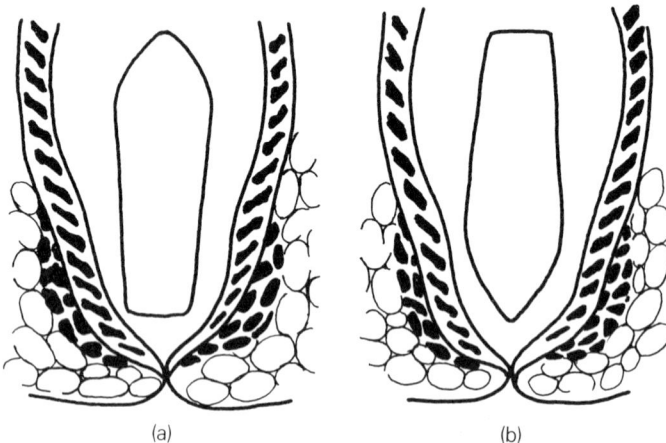

(a)   (b)

Figure 7.3a   A suppository administered in the conventional manner to have a local action and promote defecation.   **b** A suppository administered blunt end forward to minimize local discomfort and maximize systemic therapy

RECTAL LAVAGE

Definition

Rectal lavage is the washing out of the rectum using large volumes of nonsterile fluid.

Indications

Rectal lavage is performed for the following purposes:

1   To clear the lower bowel prior to investigation by barium enema and thus enable good images to be obtained
2   To assist in clearing the lower bowel prior to major abdominal surgery and thus decrease the risk of infection and aid satisfactory healing
3   To clear the lower bowel of residual faecal matter following previous surgery, e.g. formation of colostomy.

Contraindications

Rectal lavage is contraindicated in patients who have a history of any one of the following:

1   Severe or prolapsed haemorrhoids
2   Anal fissure
3   Inflammatory bowel disease
4   Large tumour in the rectum or sigmoid colon
5   Post-radiation proctitis
6   Internal fistulae
7   Previous extensive deep X-ray therapy to the pelvis
8   Recent bowel surgery
9   Congestive cardiac failure
10 Impaired renal function.

In the first eight of the contraindications listed above, the reason for employing caution is because of the damage that could be inflicted by the mechanical aspects of rectal lavage. When the bowel has already been traumatized there is a greater potential risk of causing irritation or, in extreme cases, perforation, while inserting the catheter and running large volumes of fluid in and out of the rectum.

With the last two contraindications the potential risk lies with the possibility of large amounts of fluid and/or electrolytes becoming absorbed through the bowel. (Generally speaking, with the amounts and type of fluid used and the relatively short time that it stays in the bowel, it should not present a major problem.)

REFERENCE MATERIAL

Choice of Fluid

Several solutions can be used to clear the bowel.

Soap Solutions

Soap solutions can be made from either 'hard' soap, i.e. from olive oil and sodium hydroxide, or 'soft' soap, which is a combination of potassium and vegetable products. Soft soaps are more irritating than hard soaps and the usual dilution is 5 ml of soap in 1000 ml or more of water. Soap solutions stimulate peristalsis by chemical irritation and intestinal distention. However, they can also cause a whole range of symptoms, which extends from simple hyperaemia to gangrene and the occasional fatality. Lewis (1965) in his survey of five Seattle hospitals reported 'definite undesirable and unnecessary morbidity' related to the use of soap solutions. He further reported that the strengths of solutions used were arbitrary and haphazard, often far exceeding the recommended concentration.

Soap solutions are unsuitable for use prior to bowel surgery or rectal examination because of their effect on the mucosa, and Lewis's investigations leave much doubt as to whether they are of any real value. (See the material on soap enemas above.)

Hypertonic Solutions

Hypertonic solutions, e.g. sodium phosphate and sodium biphosphate in solution, act by drawing water from the intestinal cells by osmosis. This increases the fluid in the faecal mass, causing first distention then contraction and defaecation.

For patients who have a large amount of faecal matter to evacuate, small volumes of these solutions are very effective. Hypertonic solutions should not be given to patients whose capacity to utilize sodium is affected as some sodium may be absorbed. These are available as commercially prepared enemas but are not suitable for administration in large volumes.

Tap Water

Rectal lavage is a procedure that is normally used in combination with other methods of clearing the bowel, e.g. oral aperients and dietary restrictions. In this situation, it can be anticipated that there will be very little residue remaining in the lower bowel. What is needed, therefore, is a simple, nonsterile solution that can be used with relative safety in large volumes to wash out the residual faecal matter. The solution which fulfils these criteria ideally is tap water.

Rectal lavage using tap water is not without risk as large volumes of this hypotonic solution can upset the patient's electrolyte balance. Water is drawn by osmosis into the intestinal cells and water intoxication can result with symptoms of weakness, sweating, pallor, vomiting, coughing and dizziness. However, this is a relatively rare complication and generally tap water is very well tolerated.

The other advantages of tap water are as follows:
1   It is cheap and easily available.
2   It can be easily warmed to the correct temperature.
3   It is nonirritant to the bowel mucosa.
4   It does not cause excessive peristalsis with resulting cramps and colic.

Caution should be exercised when giving tap water lavage to infants or patients with altered kidney or cardiac reserve, but otherwise tap water is the solution of choice.

Isotonic Saline

For patients with compromised electrolyte status an isotonic saline solution can be substituted. This is prepared by adding two teaspoonsful of salt to 1 litre of plain water. Its effect on the bowel is similar to that of water in that it stimulates peristaltic action by distending the intestinal walls. With isotonic saline, however, there is less danger of electrolyte imbalance.

Choice of Catheter

Several manufacturers produce rectal catheters. The criteria for selection should be as follows:

1   The catheter should be of an adequate length. Most are approximately 30 cm.
2   The lumen should be large enough to allow the free drainage of particulate matter, i.e. a minimum Charrière gauge of 24.
3   The tip of the catheter should be open ended or have large opposed eyelets to minimize the possibility of blockage.
4   The catheter should be made from a soft flexible material; rubber or plastic are suitable.

References and Further Reading

British Medical Association The Pharmaceutical Society of Great Britain (1982) British National Formulary, 3rd edition, British Medical Association, etc., pp. 43-49
Cooper P (1976) The treatment of constipation, Midwife, Health Visitor and Community Nurse 12: 165
Corman M et al. (1975) Cathartics, American Journal of Nursing 75: 273-279
Currie J E J (1979) Whole gut irrigation, Nursing Times 75: 1570-1571
Dorgu R E O (1971) Bowel Function — Disorders and Management, Butterworth
Duffin H M et al. (1981) Are enemas necessary? Nursing Times 77: 1940-1941
Edgell R W Johnson W D (1973) Postpartum hypotension and erythema: an adverse reaction to soap enema, American Journal of Obstetrics and Gynecology 117: 1146-1147
Harris W (1980) Bran or aperients? Nursing Times 76: 811-813
Hunt T (1974) Colonic irrigation, Nursing Mirror 139 (1): 76-77
Hurst Sir A (1970) Selected Writings of Sir Arthur Hurst (1879-1944), Spottiswoode, Ballantyne
Jones E (1979) Constipation: keeping a true perspective, Nursing Mirror 149 (13): Supplement, p.x
King E M et al. (1981) Illustrated Manual of Nursing Techniques, 2nd edition, J B Lippincott, pp. 222-229, 331
Lewin D (1976) Care of the constipated patient, Nursing Times 72: 444-446
Lewis A E (1965) Dangers inherent in soap enemas, Pacific Medicine and Surgery 73: 131-133
Milton-Thompson G J (1971) Constipation, Nursing Mirror 132 (2 April): 30-33
Mortimer P M (1970) A worrying problem — constipation, Health Visitor 43: 47-48
Pike B F et al. (1971) Soap colitis, New England Journal of Medicine 285 (4): 217-218

Pirrie J (1980) Constipation in the elderly, Nursing 1st series, no. 17: 753-754

Rutter K Maxwell D (1976) Constipation and laxative abuse, British Medical Journal 2: 997-1000

Smith D (1967) Severe anaphylactic reaction after a soap enema, British Medical Journal 215 (4): 215

Thompson M Bottomley H (1980) Normal and abnormal bowel function, Nursing lst series, no. 17: 721-722

Walker R (1982) Suppository insertion, World Medicine 18: 58

Wislon A Muir T (1975) Geriatric faecal incontinence, Nursing Mirror 140 (16): 50-52

GUIDELINES: ADMINISTRATION OF ENEMAS

Equipment

1   Disposable incontinence pad
2   Disposable gloves
3   Topical swabs
4   Lubricating jelly
5   Rectal tube and funnel (if not using a commercially prepared pack)
6   Solution required or commercially prepared enema pack (check prescription with another nurse before adminstering a medicinal enema, e.g. Predsol retention enema)
7   Bath thermometer

Procedure

Action	Rationale
1 Explain the procedure to the patient.	1 To obtain the patient's consent and cooperation.
2 Ensure privacy.	2 To avoid unnecessary embarrassment to the patient.
3 Ensure that a bedpan, commode or toilet is readily available.	3 In case the patient feels the need to expel the enema before the procedure is completed.
4 Warm the enema to the required temperature, testing with a bath thermometer. A temperature of 40.5-43.3 °C is recommended for adults. Oil retention enemas should be warmed to 37.8 °C.	4 Heat is an effective stimulant of the nerve plexi in the intestinal mucosa. An enema temperature of body temperature or just above will not damage the intestinal mucosa. The temperature of the environment, the rate of fluid administration and the length of the tubing will all have an effect on the temperature of the fluid on reaching the rectum.
5 Assist the patient to lie in the required position, i.e. on the left	5 This allows ease of passage into the rectum by following the

Action	**Rationale**
side, with knees well flexed, the upper higher than the lower one, and with the buttocks near the edge of the bed.	natural anatomy of the colon. In this position gravity will aid the flow of the solution into the colon. Flexing the knees ensures a more comfortable passage of the enema nozzle or rectal tube.
6 Place a disposable incontinence pad beneath the patient's hips and buttocks.	6 To reduce potential infection caused by soiled linen. To avoid embarrassing the patient if the fluid is ejected prematurely following administration.
7 Wash your hands and put on disposable gloves.	7 To reduce cross-infection.
8 Place some lubricating jelly on a topical swab and lubricate the nozzle of the enema or the rectal tube.	8 To prevent trauma to the anal and rectal mucosa by reducing surface friction.
9 Expel excessive air and introduce the nozzle or tube slowly into the anal canal while separating the buttocks.	9 The introduction of air into the colon causes distention of its walls, resulting in unnecessary discomfort to the patient and increases peristalsis. The slow introduction of the lubricated tube will minimize spasm of the intestinal wall.
(A small amount of air may be introduced if bowel evacuation is desired.)	(Evacuation will be more effectively induced due to the increased peristalsis.)
10 Slowly introduce the tube or nozzle to a depth of 10-12.5 cm.	10 This will bypass the anal canal (2.5-4 cm in length) and ensure that the tube or nozzle is in the rectum.
11 If a retention enema is used, introduce the fluid slowly and leave the patient in bed with the foot of the bed elevated by 45°.	11 To avoid peristalsis. The slower the rate at which the fluid is introduced the less pressure is exerted on the intestinal wall. Elevating the foot of the bed aids in retention of the enema by force of gravity.
12 If an evacuant enema is used, introduce the fluid slowly until the pack is empty or the solution is completely finished.	12 The faster the rate of flow of the fluid the greater the pressure on the rectal walls. Distention and irritation of the bowel wall will produce a strong persistalsis which is sufficient to empty the lower bowel.

Action	Rationale
13 If using a funnel and rectal tube, adjust the height of the funnel according to the rate of flow desired.	13 The forces of gravity will cause the solution to flow from the funnel into the rectum. The greater the elevation of the funnel, the faster the flow of the fluid.
14 Clamp the tubing before all the fluid has run in.	14 To avoid air entering the rectum and causing further discomfort.
15 Slowly withdraw the tube or nozzle.	15 To avoid reflex emptying of the rectum.
16 Dry the patient's perineal area with a gauze swab.	16 To promote patient comfort and avoid excoriation and infection.
17 Ask the patient to **a** Retain the enema **b** Hold the enema for 10-15 minutes before evacuating the bowel	17 To enhance the evacuant effect.
18 Ensure that the patient has access to the nurse call system, is near to the bedpan, commode or toilet, and has adequate toilet paper.	
19 Remove and dispose of equipment.	19 To avoid infection.
20 Wash your hands.	
21 Record in the appropriate documents that the enema has been given, its effects on the patient and its results (colour, consistency, content and amount of faeces produced).	21 To monitor the patient's bowel function.

NURSING CARE PLAN

Problem	Cause	Suggested Action
1 Unable to insert the nozzle of enema pack or rectal tube into the anal canal	1 **a** Tube not adequately lubricated. **b** Patient in an incorrect position.	1 **a** Apply more lubricating jelly. **b** Ask the patient to draw his/her knees up further towards his/her chest.
	c Patient apprehensive and embarrassed about the situation.	**c** Ensure adequate privacy and give frequent explanations to the patient about the procedure.
	d Patient unable to relax his/her anal sphincter	**d** Ask the patient to take deep breaths and 'bear down' as if defaecating.

Problem	Cause	Suggested Action
2 Unable to advance the tube or nozzle into the anal canal.	2 Spasm of the canal walls.	2 Insert the tube or nozzle more slowly, thus minimizing spasm.
3 Unable to advance the tube or nozzle into the rectum.	3 **a** Blockage by faeces. **b** Blockage by tumour	3 **a** Allow a little solution to flow and then insert the tube further. **b** If resistance is still met, stop the procedure and inform a doctor.
4 Patient complains of cramping or the desire to evacuate the enema before the end if the procedure.	4 Distention and irritation of the intestinal wall, which produces a strong peristalsis sufficient to empty the lower bowel.	4 Temporarily stop the insertion of fluid by clamping the tubing or lowering the funnel until the patient says the feeling has subsided.
5 Patient unable to open his/her bowels after an evacuant enema and the fluid has not returned.	5 Reduced neuro-muscular reponse in the bowel wall.	5 Insert a rectal tube and try to siphon the fluid off. Measure and record the amount. If this is not successful, perform rectal lavage. (For further information see the procedure on rectal lavage, pages 67-70. Measure and record the amount returned.

GUIDELINES: ADMINISTRATION OF SUPPOSITORIES

Equipment

1 Disposable incontinence pad
2 Disposable glove
3 Topical swabs or tissues
4 Lubricating jelly
5 Suppository(ies) as required (check prescription with another nurse before administering a medicinal suppository, e.g. aminophylline)

Procedure

Action	Rationale
1 Explain the procedure to the patient.	1 To obtain the patient's consent and cooperation.

Action	Rationale
N.B. If you are administering a medicated suppository, it is best to do so after the patient has emptied his/her bowels.	To ensure that the active ingredients are not impeded from being absorbed by the rectal mucosa or that the suppository is not expelled before its active ingredients have been released.
2 Ensure privacy.	2 To avoid unnecessary embarrassment to the patient.
3 Ensure that a bedpan, commode or the toilet is readily available.	3 In case of premature ejection of the suppositories or rapid bowel evacuation following their administration.
4 Assist the patient to lie in the required position, i.e. on the left side, with his/her knees flexed, the upper higher than the lower one, with the buttocks near the edge of the bed.	4 This allows ease of passage of the suppository into the rectum by following the natural anatomy of the colon. Flexing the knees will reduce discomfort as the suppository is passed through the anal sphincter.
5 Place a disposable incontinence pad beneath the patient's hips and buttocks.	5 To avoid unnecessary soiling of linen, leading to potential infection and embarrassment to the patient if the suppositories are prematurely ejected or there is rapid bowel evacuation following their administration.
6 Wash your hands and put on gloves.	6 To reduce cross-infection.
7 Place some lubricating jelly on the topical swab and lubricate the *blunt* end of the suppository if it is being used to obtain systemic action. Separate the patient's buttocks and insert the suppository, blunt end first, advancing it for about 2-4 cm. Repeat this procedure if a second suppository is to be inserted.	7 Lubricating reduces surface friction and thus eases insertion of the suppository and avoids anal mucosal trauma. Research has shown that the suppository is more readily retained if inserted blunt end first. (For further information see the reference material section above.) The anal canal is approximately 2-4 cm long. Inserting the suppository beyond this ensures that it will be retained.
8 Once suppository(ies) have been inserted, clean any excess lubricating jelly from the patient's perineal area.	8 To ensure the patient's comfort and avoid anal excoriation that may then lead to infection.
9 Ask the patient to retain the suppository(ies) if it is of an	9 This will allow the suppository to melt and release its active ingredients.

Action	Rationale
evacuant type. If it is medicated, ask the patient to retain the suppository for 20 minutes, or until he/she is no longer able to do so.	
10 Remove and dispose of equipment.	10 To avoid infection.
11 Record that the suppository(ies) have been given, the effect on the patient and the result (amount, colour, consistency and content) in the appropriate documents.	11 To monitor the patient's bowel function.

GUIDELINES: ADMINISTRATION OF RECTAL LAVAGE

Equipment

1 Rectal lavage pack containing a large funnel, rubber tubing, a straight connector, a 1 litre jug, and a rectal catheter (Charrière gauge 24)
2 Nosterile topical swabs
3 Lubricating jelly
4 Disposable gloves
5 Disposable incontinence pad
6 Plastic sheet and draw sheet
7 Large nonsterile jug
8 Bucket
9 Gate clip or clamp
10 Toilet paper or tissues
11 Disposable plastic apron
12 Large disposable bag
13 Measured volume of warm tap water (37-40 °C)

Procedure

Action	Rationale
1 Explain the procedure to the patient.	1 To obtain the patient's consent and cooperation.
2 Prepare the area where lavage is to be performed, i.e. the patient's bed or a couch in the room where rectal lavage is to take place. Protect the bed or couch with a plastic sheet and draw sheet. Place a disposable incontinence pad on the floor.	2 To prevent nondisposable equipment becoming contaminated with faecal matter, thus minimizing the risk of cross-infection.

Action	**Rationale**
3 Wash and dry your hands, clean the trolley and prepare the equipment for the procedure by opening the pack and laying out the contents on the top of the shelf.	3 Although this is not an aseptic procedure, care must be taken to avoid unnecessary contamination.
4 Attach a large disposable bag to the trolley.	4 To provide a suitable receptacle for safe disposal of potentially large amounts of contaminated waste.
5 Fill a large nonsterile jug with a measured volume of warm (37-40 °C) tap water. Check the temperature with a lotion thermometer. Place the filled jug on the lower shelf of the trolley. Put a bucket for receiving effluent by the side of the bed or couch.	5 As the bowel is not sterile, there is no need to use sterile fluid. A large volume needs to be available for use, although the total amount used will vary with each patient. If the solution is too warm, the intestinal mucosa may be damaged; if too cold, unnecessary cramping may occur.
6 Assist the patient to lie in the required position, i.e. on the left side, with his/her knees well flexed, the upper higher than the lower one, and with the buttocks near the edge of the bed. Tilt the bed slightly if possible.	6 This position allows ease of access for insertion of the catheter into the rectum, follows the natural anatomy of the colon and aids gravity in promoting the flow of fluid into the sigmoid and descending colon. Tilting the bed also aids the flow.
7 Check that the patient's clothing is tucked out of the way and that both the patient and the bed are adequately protected. Ensure that the patent is as comfortable as possible before continuing with the procedure.	7 As the procedure can be lengthy and is potentially messy, the patient needs to be as relaxed and well protected as possible to aid successful completion.
8 Wash your hands and put on disposable gloves and a disposable plastic apron.	8 To reduce cross-infection.
9 Connect up the funnel, tubing and rectal catheter, using a straight connector between the latter two items. Fix a gate clamp or clip in position approximately 15 cms from the end of the rectal catheter.	9 To allow the tubing and the catheter to be primed and filled with fluid, thus preventing the entry into the rectum and discomfort to the patient.
10 Using nonsterile topical swab lubricate the last 15 cm of the rectal catheter with a generous	10 To aid insertion and minimize patient discomfort and trauma to

Action	**Rationale**
amount of jelly.	the rectal mucosa.
11 Fill a small jug with 1 litre from the measured volume of warm tap water.	11 A small jug is more manageable and allows measurement of the amount of fluid used each time.
12 Prime the catheter and tubing.	
13 Gently insert 7.5-10 cm of the catheter into the rectum.	13 The rectum is approximately 12.5 cm long and the anal canal 2.5 cm. Inserting the catheter 7.5-10 cm ensures that the rectum will be adequately filled with the minimum trauma to the patient.
14 Encourage the patient to take deep breaths.	14 Deep breathing relaxes the anal sphincter.
15 Check that the patient is comfortable.	
16 Fill the funnel with approximately 400 ml of fluid from the jug.	15 The rectum will hold 200-400 ml without causing trauma.
17 Hold the funnel about 30 cm above the rectum, release the clamp and allow the fluid to run into the rectum, holding the catheter in position.	17 Aqueous solution exerts a pressure of 0.225 kgf for every 30 cm of elevation. The pressure should not exceed 0.45 kgf as this may cause cramping or even rupture of the intestinal wall.
18 Before the funnel is completely empty, invert it over the bucket to allow the lavage fluid and faecal material to drain out.	18 To prevent unnecessary amounts of air entering the rectum and causing the patient discomfort.
19 Refill the funnel with another measure of fluid, keeping the tubing pinched or clamped and the funnel at patient level until it is filled.	
20 Repeat the last two procedures until **a** The effluent runs clear **b** A maximum volume of 6 litres has been used.	**b** If the bowel is not clear after this volume, other methods need to be employed.
21 Note how much fluid was used during the procedure.	21 To ensure that not more than 6 litres is used.
22 At the end of the procedure **a** Measure the amount of efffluent obtained and compare it with the volume run in.	**a** To ensure that the patient has not absorbed fluid in such a quantity that will carry the risk of fluid overload.

Action	Rationale
b Clear away and dispose of equipment.	**b** To avoid infection.
c Ensure that the patient is clean and dry.	
23 Settle the patient into bed, on an incontinence pad and with a bedpan or commode at hand.	23 To reduce potential infection caused by soiled linen.

NURSING CARE PLAN

Problem	Cause	Suggested Action
1 Fluid will not run in freely	1 **a** Catheter is pressed against the bowel wall	1 **a** Gently manoeuvre the catheter around in the rectum.
	b Catheter is blocked with faecal material	**b** Remove the catheter and unblock. Reinsert and recommence procedure.
	c Insufficient gravity flow	**c** Raise the funnel slightly, but never over 60 cm above the mattress.
2 Leakage of fluid around the catheter	2 **a** Poor positioning of the catheter or displacement following insertion.	2 **a** Check that the catheter is 7-10 cm into the rectum. Hold it gently in position.
	b Poor tone of the anal sphincter muscles	**b** Ask the patient to try and tighten muscles as fluid is run in. Elevate the foot of the bed to aid flow.
3 Discomfort and/or cramping when the fluid is run in	3 **a** Fluid is too cold	3 **a** Check the temperature of the fluid and warm it if necessary.
	b Pressure of the fluid entering the rectum is too high	**b** Lower the funnel to stop fluid from running until the spasm passes, but leave the catheter in to relieve distention.
	c Extreme tension and anxiety	**c** When the spasm has passed, gradually raise the funnel and allow fluid to enter very slowly. Encourage deep breathing through the mouth to relax the abdominal muscles and decrease colonic pressures.

Action		Rationale
4 Severe pain accompanied by perspiration, pallor and tachycardia	4 **a** Perforation of the rectum **b** Perforation of the gut around the site of a large tumour due to increased peristalsis	4 **a** Stop the procedure immediately. **b** Check the patient's vital signs. Inform a doctor. Do not allow the patient to eat or drink until seen by a doctor.
5 Blood is returned in the effluent	5 **a** Insertion of the catheter has caused internal haemorrhoids to bleed **b** Trauma to rectal mucosa	5 **a** Stop the procedure and inform a doctor. Record the appropriate amount of blood that has been passed and observe further bowel motions.
6 Large discrepency between the amount of fluid run in and the effluent obtained	6 **a** Excessive leakage on to pads during the procedure **b** Patient has retained a certain amount of fluid that may be passed later **c** Patient has absorbed the excess fluid	6 **a** Try to estimate the amount of fluid on pads, etc. **b** Measure carefully all subsequent bowel actions. **c** Check the patient's vital signs. Record further intake and output carefully. Inform a doctor.
7 Sudden onset of pallor, perspiration, vomiting, coughing and dizziness	7 Water intoxication due to excessive absorption of water from the rectum	7 Stop the procedure immediately. Inform a doctor. Check the patient's vital signs.

8

CAESIUM-137 IMPLANTS AND APPLICATORS

Definition

Casium-137 is a radioisotope that can be used in the form of implants or in applicators.

The half-life of caesium-137 is 30 years. It emits gamma and beta radiation, the latter being screened out by the plastic casing around the source. Caesium has largely replaced iridium as a source in brachytherapy.

Indications

Caesium implants are now used instead of radium for interstitial, intracavity or superficial therapy, especially in the treatment of carcinoma of the cervix.

REFERENCE MATERIAL

Oral Implants

Caesium-137 may be used in a needle-like implant that can be positioned directly into the tissue surrounding the tumour. This is a fairly common treatment for early lesions of the cheek, lip and anterior two-thirds of the tongue. If bone involvement is suspected, e.g. in the mandible, alternative treatment will be given.

Preparation of the Patient

Dental assessment of the patient is usually carried out prior to oral brachytherapy so that caries, mouth infections and dental extractions may be dealt with in case of the oral blood supply being impaired by the treatment. The patient is usually admitted 24 hours prior to the implant, during which time the nature of the procedure and the implications of having a radioactive source should be explained to the patient. Ideally, the patient should be nursed in a cubicle or in a bed away from other patients to reduce the amount of radiation exposure to other people.

Insertion of Needles

The sources (see Figure 8.1) are inserted in theatre under a general anaesthetic. They are inserted individually in a predetermined pattern so that the implant covers the whole growth with a safety margin of at least 1 cm. Each needle is positioned by pushers so that its eye, through which silk is threaded, is just visable beneath the mucosal surface. Each silk is then stitched to the tongue with a single suture. When all the needles have been inserted, the silks are counted and gathered together. They are threaded through a piece of rubber to prevent friction and trauma to the mouth. The silks are strapped to the cheek to prevent any needle being swallowed should it work loose. Small beads are attached to the ends of the threads to facilitate counting the needles. X-rays are always taken to check the positions of the needles and to enable estimation of the dose distribution.

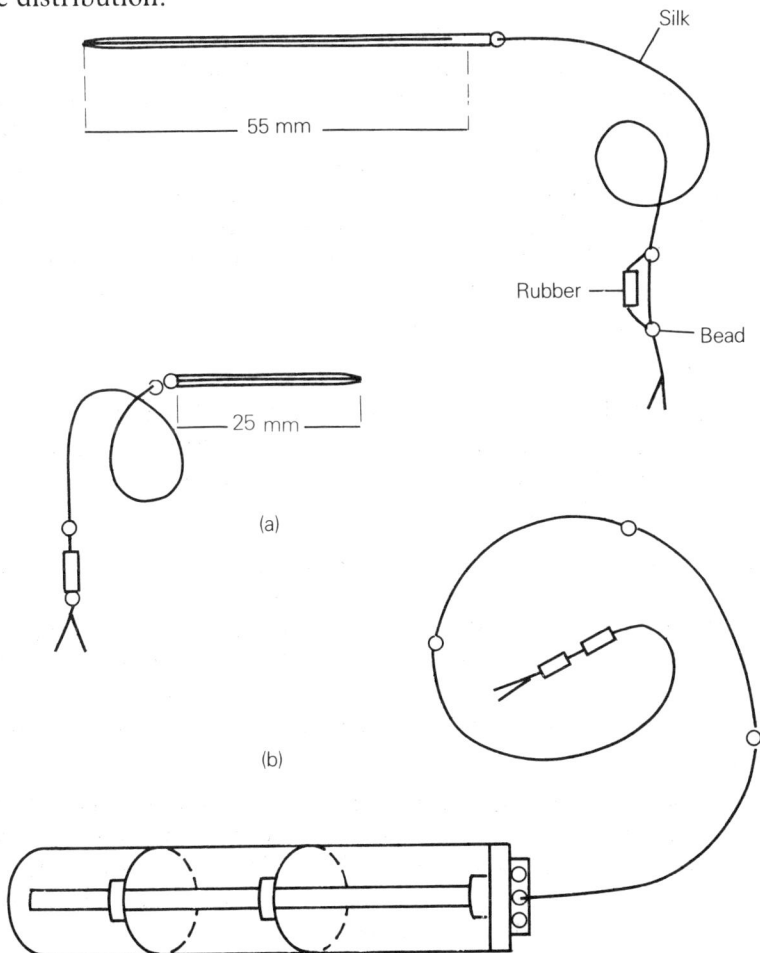

Figure 8.1a Caesium needles **b** A Dobbie applicator

Removal of Implants

The staff of the physics department are normally responsible for calculating how long a radioactive implant is to stay in place. This is usually about 6 days, depending on the size of the tumour. Removal is carried out in theatre by the radiotherapist.

Discharge of the Patient

The patient is usually discharged the day after the removal of the implant. The patient should be warned about the brisk local reaction which he/she may experience due to rapid cell breakdown induced by the radiation. In order to minimize the risk of infection or soreness the patient should be taught how to care for the treated area, e.g. frequent oral toilet.

Gynaecological Applicators

Caesium-137 may be used in applicators that are placed against the tissue and held in position by packing. The commonest malignancies treated by use of radioactive applicators are tumours of the female genital tract. Intracavity applicators are used which deliver a high dose to the region of the cervix, the paracervical tissue, the upper part of the vagina and the uterine body. The applicators are inserted under a general anaesthetic, and the position of the applicator is checked by X-ray before the patient returns to the ward. A urinary catheter is also inserted in theatre to reduce the risk of the sources becoming dislodged by the patient when micturating.

Types of Applicator

There are several different types of applicator available and choice is usually determined by the site of the tumour, the anatomy of the patient and the preference of the treatment centre. The most commonly used types of applicator are described below (see Figure 8.2).

Stockholm Applicator   This is used for carcinoma of the body of the uterus or cervix. Usually a uterine tube and two vaginal packets are inserted. Occasionally, if the vaginal vault is small, one packet is omitted or replaced by a vaginal tube. The radioactive material is held in place with a flavine sealed gauze pack. It is usually left in for 22 hours. Tubes and packets have strings attached for removal and colour-coded beads indicate which should be removed first.

Modified Stockholm Applicator   This is used for carcinoma of the body of the uterus and cervix. It consists of a uterine tube and a square box which connect together by a point and a hole. The vagina is then packed with gauze saturated with proflavine. They are usually left in for 20 hours. The box should be removed first. The uterine tube is plain.

Fletcher Applicator   This is used for carcinoma of the corpus or cervix, but

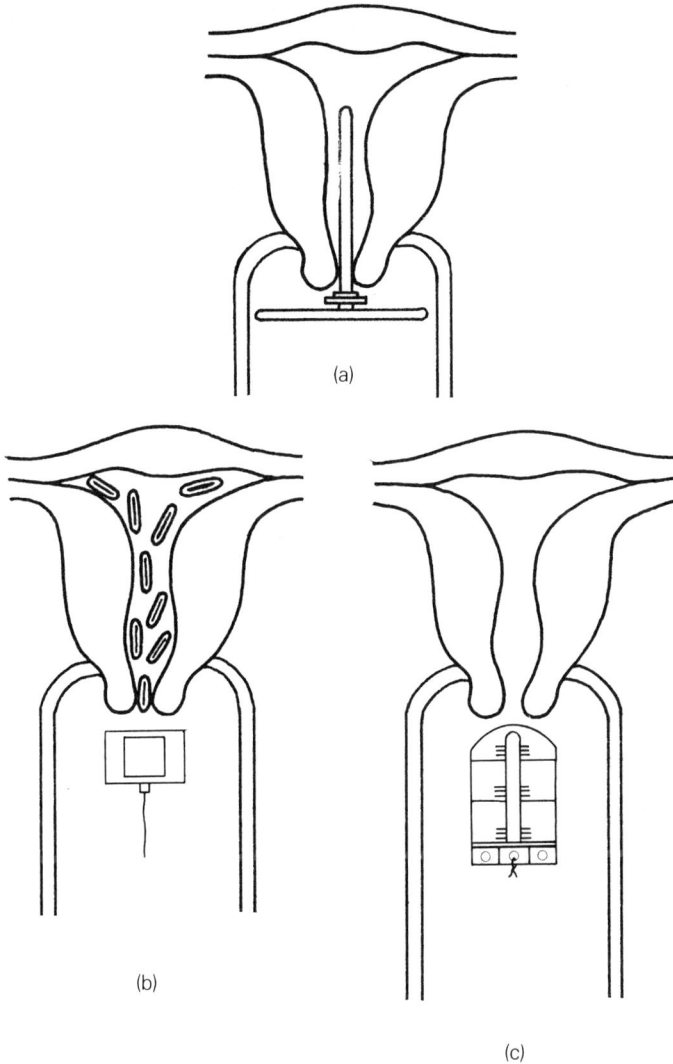

Figure 8.2 Gynaecological caesium applicators. **a** Modified Stockholm applicator.
b Heyman's capsules and packet. **c** Dobbie applicator

the patient needs to have a fairly capacious vaginal vault. Hollow applicators, a
uterine tube and two vaginal ovoids are inserted in theatre and loaded with the
radioactive sources later, on the ward, by the radiotherapist. The apparatus is
held in place with a flavine pack. Long ends project through the vulva so that
afterloading can be done. These insertions are usually left in for 60-72 hours.
No strings are needed as the apparatus itself projects from the vulva.

Curietron Afterloading Applicator This is used for carcinoma of the corpus or cervix, but patients need to have a fairly capacious and symmetrical vault. Hollow metal applicators, consisting of two vaginal ovoids and a uterine tube, are inserted in the theatre and are loaded with radioactive 'Curietron' sources later, on the ward, by the radiotherapist. The apparatus is held in place with approximately 90 cm of ribbon gauze flavine pack. The long ends of the applicators project through the vulva so that afterloading can be carried out. The patient may need to be nursed with a sorbo pad or pillow under the dorsal area to keep the projecting ends off the bed.

These insertions last 60-72 hours. Patients usually have two insertions but may sometimes be given a single preoperative insertion or a single insertion following external irradiation.

Heyman's Capsules These are used for carinoma of the corpus where there is enlargement of the uterus and and expanded uterine cavity. They consist of small metal capsules, each of which contains a small, radioactive source. As many capsules as possible are placed into the uterus. Usually two vaginal packets are used as well. They are held in place by a flavine gauze pack and are left in for about 12-18 hours. Each capsule has a flexible wire attached, strapped to the thigh, for removal, and a numbered tag to indicate the order of removal.

Dobbie Applicator This is used to irradiate the whole vagina. A perspex cylindrical applicator, with radioactive sources in the centre, is inserted into the vagina and sutured in place to the vulva. It is usually left in for about 18 hours. Strings are attached to the applicator for removal.

Modified Dobbie Applicator This is a polyacetal (Delrin) cylindrical applicator with a long hollow through the middle. A uterine tube is loaded and slipped into the long hollow. The applicator is inserted into the vagina and sutured in place. It is usually left in position for about 18 hours, but this will depend on the rectal dose of radiation. Strings are attached to aid removal.

Preparation of the Patient

The patient is usually admitted 12-48 hours prior to the procedure so that any preanaesthetic investigations may be performed. An enema or suppositories are usually given to reduce the chance of the patient having a bowel action while the sources are in place. This could dislodge the sources. Some patients, however, have diarrhoea on admission due to previous radiotherapy and will need regular medication, such as codeine phosphate, both before and during the application of the sources. It is arguable whether the vulval area needs to be shaved. The patient should be bathed before any premedication is administered. A full explanation should be given to the patient along with information about the implications of having a radioactive source inside her.

References and Further Reading

Amersham International Ltd (1981) Radioisotope Sources for Brachytherapy, Amersham International

Royal Marsden Hospital (1968) Rules for the Protection of Nursing Staff Exposed to Ionising Radiation, revised edition, Royal Marsden Hospital

Tiffany R (1979) Cancer Nursing Radiotherapy, Faber & Faber

GUIDELINES: CARE OF PATIENTS WITH INSERTIONS OF SEALED RADIOACTIVE SOURCES

Action	Rationale
1 When transferring patients from theatre to ward, the nurse and porter should remain at the head and foot of the bed and at least 120 cm from the centre of the bed in the event of any delay in the transfer. If the source is intraoral, the nurse should stand at the foot of the bed.	1 To minimize the risk of exposure to radiation.
2 A yellow radiation hazard board should accompany the patient back from theatre. This must remain at the bottom of the bed or outside the cubicle until the source is removed.	2 To warn everybody that the patient has a radioactive source.
3 Nursing staff must calculate the time allowed with the patient in any 24-hour period. This time should be written on the yellow hazard notice on the bed or cubicle door.	3 To minimize exposure to radiation.
4 A Geiger counter should be available on the ward.	4 To monitor radioactivity if a dislodged source is suspected, e.g. in the bed linen.
5 One nurse should be delegated responsibility for the nursing care of the patient. The time spent with the patient should be shared between all of the staff on duty and time spent in nursing procedures must be kept to a minimum.	5 To minimize the risk of over-exposure to radiation.
6 Every nurse must wear a radiation badge above the level of the lead shield.	6 To record the extent of exposure to radiation.
7 All bed linen and waste materials removed from the patient area should be monitored before being removed from the ward.	7 To prevent loss of an accidentally dislodged source.

8 If a source becomes dislodged, use the long-handled forceps provided to put the source into a lead pot. Care should be taken not to damage the source. It must never be handled directly with the fingers.

8 To minimize the dose of radiation received.

9 Visitors must remain at least 120 cm away from the patient. The visit should not last longer than the time shown on the warning notice. No children or pregnant women are allowed to visit.

9 To minimize the risk of over-exposure to radiation.

GUIDELINES: CARE OF PATIENTS WITH INTRAORAL SOURCES

Action	**Rationale**
1 Encourage frequent mouth care. The patient should void the solution into a bowl, not into a handbasin.	1 To reduce the risk of infection. To prevent the loss of a dislodged source.
2 Provide a soft, pureed or liquid diet.	2 To reduce the risk of the patient dislodging the source with his/her tongue. Eating is often difficult when implants are present.
3 Avoid spicy, hot food. Discourage the patient from smoking and from drinking spirits.	3 To prevent exacerbation of local reaction or soreness.
4 Encourage the ingestion of carbonated drinks.	4 To alleviate dryness.
5 Provide crushed ice for the patient to suck or soluble aspirin as a mouthwash.	5 To minimize oral pain and discomfort.
6 Give steroids as prescribed.	6 To prevent and/or minimize swelling.
7 Provide writing equipment for the patient.	7 To reduce the need for oral communication. This is liable to increase soreness and alter the distribution of the sources.
8 Provide paper tissues and a bowl for saliva.	8 The patient may have difficulty in swallowing due to soreness and oedema.
9 The sources should be checked at regular intervals, e.g. at the beginning of a span of duty.	9 To make sure that the sources have not become dislodged.
10 The patient must be confined to the cubicle or space around the bed. Washing must be carried out	10 To minimize the risk of radiation exposure to other people on the ward.

Action	**Rationale**
in the bed area, but the general toilet facilites should be used provided that the patient remains at a distance from other people.	

GUIDELINES: CARE OF PATIENTS WITH GYNAECOLOGICAL SOURCES

Action	**Rationale**
1 The patient must remain in bed in a recumbent or semirecumbent position while the applicators are in place.	1 To prevent the applicators becoming dislodged or changing their position with relation to the internal organs.
2 Rolling from side to side is permitted and should be encouraged if the patient is at risk of developing a pressure sore.	2 To promote comfort and to relieve prolonged pressure on any one area.
3 On return from theatre, the sanitary towel should be checked for discharge. Disposable pants may be worn. Check that the catheter is correctly positioned to allow drainage.	3 To secure the position of the sanitary towel. To ensure that urine is draining freely.
4 Observe for any blood or other discharge from the vagina. Check the temperature and pulse every 2 hours. Administer prescribed analgesics antiemetics and antidiarrhoeal agents.	4 To monitor haemorrhage, shock and other postoperative complications. 5 For the patient's comfort.
6 Encourage fluid intake as soon as the patient is allowed to drink.	6 To ensure adequate hydration. To reduce the risk of urinary tract infection.
7 If the source is to be in for longer than 24 hours: **a** Encourage a fluid intake of 50-100% a day over and above the patient's normal intake. **b** A low residue diet may be taken.	**a** To ensure adequate hydration. To reduce the risk of urinary tract infection. **b** To prevent the stimulation of a bowel action.

GUIDELINES: REMOVAL OF GYNAECOLOGICAL CAESIUM

The removal of applicators is usually performed by nursing staff. Only nurses holding a certificate of competence, or nurses supervised by a suitably qualified nurse, should perform this procedure.

Equipment

1 Sterile gynaecological pack containing large receiver, green towel, paper towel, long dissecting forceps, sanitary towel, cotton wool balls
2 Equipment for the administration of Entonox
3 Douche set and sodium bicarbonate solution
4 Solutions of choice for swabbing, e.g. Savlodil, normal saline
5 Sterile gloves
6 Sterile scissors or stitch cutter
7 Clean draw sheet
8 Geiger counter
9 Bedpan

Procedure

Action	Rationale
1 Explain the procedure to the patient.	1 To obtain the patient's consent and cooperation.
2 Check the date and time for removal on the form that was received from the physics department when sources were inserted.	2 The accurate timing of the removal is essential for the administration of the correct therapeutic dose of radiation.
3 Check that any preremoval drugs (e.g. sedatives, analgesics) have been administered.	
4 Check, with another nurse, the exact time of removal and the number of applicators.	4 To reduce the risk of error.
5 Ensure that:	
a The lead shield is suitably positioned beside the patient.	a To shield the nurse from exposure to radiation.
b The lead pot is also suitably positioned with the lid removed.	b So that sources can be placed in the pot immediately after removal.
6 Begin the administration of Entonox at least 2 minutes before commencing the procedure.	6 To allow time for the effects of the gas to be felt. (For further information see the procedure on Entonox administration, pages 159-160.)
7 Prepare a trolley, put on gloves and open the pack before going to the bedside.	7 This is a clinically clean, not an aseptic procedure. To reduce the time spent in close proximity to the source.
8 Working from behind the lead shield, assist the patient into the dorsal position with knees apart. Remove the sanitary towel.	8 To obtain access to the sources.

Action	**Rationale**
9 Remove any sutures, if present. Remove the vaginal packing.	
10 Remove the caesium sources in reverse order of insertion. Contact the radiotherapist immediately if difficulty is encountered in removing a source. Place the removed sources in a lead pot immediately and cover with the lid.	To contain radioactivity.
11 Remove the lead pot to a designated area, e.g. an isotope sluice or safe. Ensure that the lid of the pot or the sluice door is locked.	11 To remove the radioactive source from the ward area. To prevent unauthorized access to the source.
12 Monitor the patient's level of radioactivity.	12 To ensure that no sources remain inside the patient.
13 Remove the urinary catheter.	
14 Douche the patient with sodium bicarbonate solution and/or swab the vulva and perineal area with a solution such as Savlodil or normal saline. Ensure that the patient has a clean sanitary towel in position and is made comfortable.	14 To promote patient hygiene and comfort.
15 Monitor the bed linen, paper bags, vaginal packing and other waste material. (Two nurses should monitor the patient independently.)	15 To ensure that no source has been lost or remains inside the patient.
16 The patient should remain in bed until the physics department staff are satisfied that all sources are accounted for.	16 To ensure that all sources have been accounted for before the patient moves around.
17 Remove the radiation warning notice.	

NURSING CARE PLAN

Problem	**Cause**	**Suggested Action**
1 Patient has a bowel action		1 Inform the radiotherapist.
2 Patient removes caesium source herself	2 Confusion, e.g. post-anaesthetic	2 Using long-handled forceps place the source in the lead container or safe. Inform the radiotherapist and the physics department.

Problem	Cause	Suggested Action
3 Pyrexia	3 **a** Pelvic cellulitis or abcess **b** Reaction to the proflavine pack **c** Urinary infection **d** Physiological reaction to the breakdown of the tumour **e** Chest infection **f** Peritonitis due to perforation of the uterus	3 If the patient's temperature remains over 37.5 °C for two consecutive readings, inform the radiotherapist. The caesium may have to be removed if the pyrexia persists.

9

CARDIOPULMONARY RESUSCITATION

Definition

Cardiac arrest may be defined as the abrupt cessation of cardiac function. The heart may be in one of two states during cardiac arrest, either asystole or ventricular fibrillation.

Indications

Indications of cardiac arrest are as follows:

1   Sudden loss of consciousness
2   Absence of radial, femoral and carotid pulses
3   Cessation of respirations
4   Dilatation of the pupils
5   Marked cyanosis.

REFERENCE MATERIAL

Principles

The primary objectives of cardiopulmonary resuscitation are twofold:

1   To restore effective circulation and ventilation
2   To prevent irreversible cerebral damage due to anoxia. When the heart fails to maintain the cerebral circulation for approximately 4 minutes, the brain may suffer irreversible damage.

Resuscitation consists of meeting the following needs (ABC sequence):

1   A(irway) is met by maintaining an open, clear airway.
2   B(reathing) is met by maintaining artificial ventilation.
3   C(irculation) is met by maintaining external cardiac massage.

Causes

1   *Cerebral*   Cerebral causes are due to depression of the respiratory

centre, e.g. overdose of depressant drugs, hypothermia, trauma, hypotension, lesions of the central nervous system.

2 *Respiratory* Respiratory causes are due to respiratory obstruction, e.g. foreign bodies, pulmonary embolism, pneumothorax, haemothorax, drowning.

3 *Cardiac* Cardiac causes are due to coronary occlusion, pericardial tamponade, cardiac myopathy, and electrocution.

4 *Hepatic* Liver disfunction may cause electrolyte imbalance, e.g. hyper- or hypokalaemia.

Treatment

Treatment of cardiac arrest is carried out in three stages:

1 Cardiopulmonary resuscitation
2 Correction of acid-base balance
3 Assessment and correction of electrolyte balance.

Drugs

A range of drugs is used in the treatment of cardiac arrest:

1 *Sodium bicarbonate 8.4%* To correct acidosis associated with cardiopulmonary arrest.

2 *Adrenaline 1:10 000* To increase exitability and tone of the myocardium.

3 *Calcium chloride 10%* To increase the contractability of the myocardial muscle.

4 *Isoprenaline 0.002%* To maintain cardiac output by stimulating the ventricles to contract with greater power.

5 *Atropine sulphate* To increase the heart rate by blocking the slowing effect of vagal activity.

6 *Aminophylline* To reduce pulmonary oedema, left ventricular fibrillation and bronchospasm. To a lesser extent it causes coronary artery dilatation, increases urinary output and the rate and power of cardiac contraction.

7 *Lignocaine* To lower the excessive excitability of cardiac contraction.

8 *Frusemide* To increase diuresis and reduce pulmonary oedema.

Aftercare

1 Monitor pulse, blood pressure and urinary output.
2 Connect up oscilloscope.
3 Give oxygen therapy.
4 Transfer to special units (coronary care).

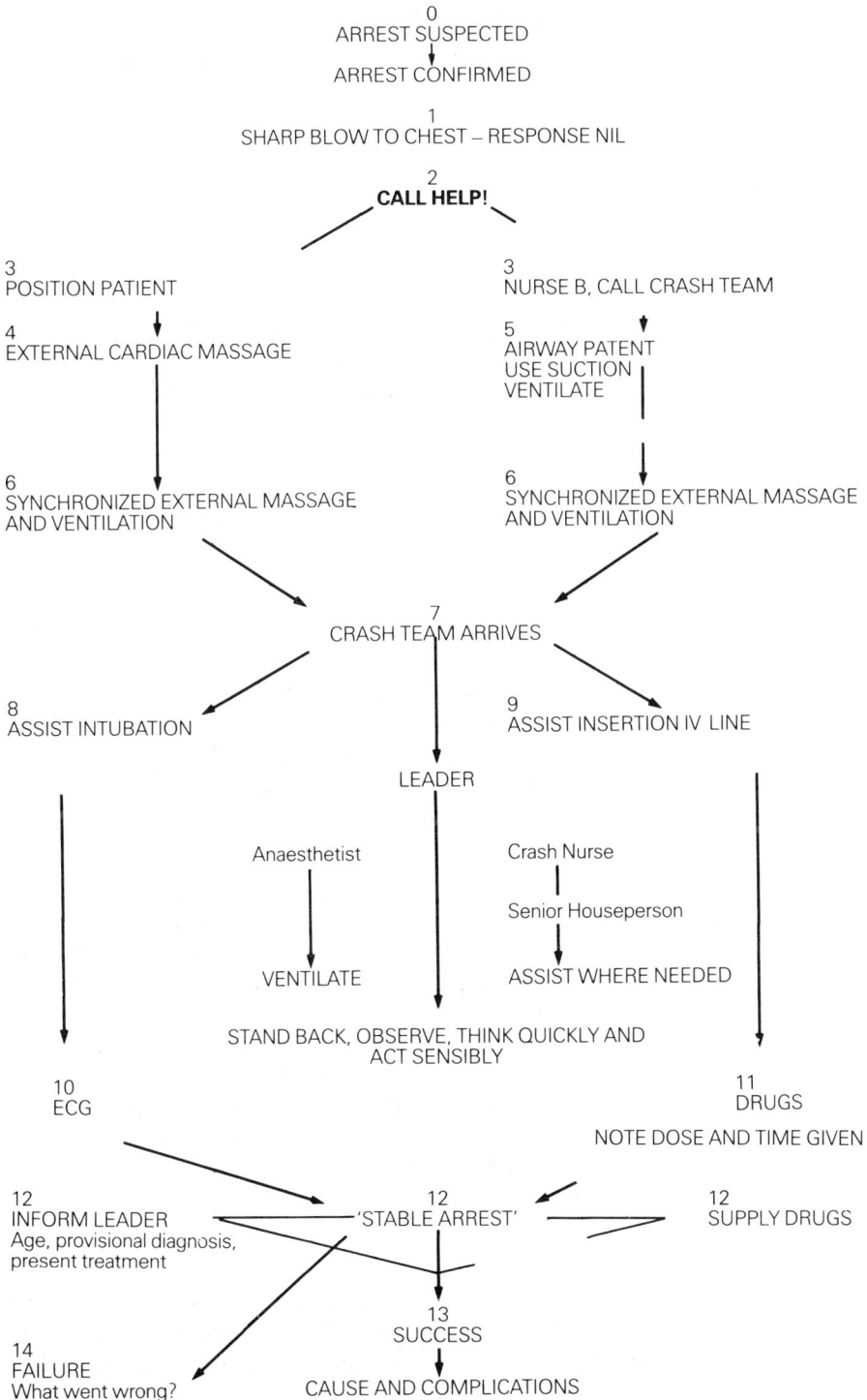

Figure 9.1 Flow chart to illustrate the management of cardiopulmonary resuscitation

Intravenous Infusion and Intubation

If the procedure is performed by a doctor, the nurse's responsibilities are as follows:

1   To check what equipment the doctor needs to use and to prepare it for use
2   To assist as required
3   To clear away equipment.

Defibrillation

The carrying out of defibrillation by nurses is more common in the United States than it is in the United Kingdom, although those nurses working in special units in this country are accepting responsibility for this procedure. A useful outline of the principles and the equipment may be found in Matheny (1981).

The Resuscitation Team

Wilson and Aarvold (1975) recommend that four or five personnel are adequate:

1   A senior physician to diagnose and direct the treatment
2   An anaesthetist, anaesthetic nurse or a nurse trained to perform endotracheal intubation
3   One or two nurses to perform external cardiac massage
4   One nurse to administer prescribed drugs and intravenous infusion.

These authors also warn of the dangers engendered when personnel not directly involved gather around the area where the arrest has occurred.

Statistics

It has been estimated by Thompson (1982) that 80-90% survival can be anticipated on the coronary care unit in patients with primary ventricular fibrillation. Survival rates on the ward are approximately 20% lower. Survival rates in the community are nil. Peatfield et al. (1977), in a study based on the Central Middlesex Hospital, found that of 1063 arrests in the hospital over a 10-year period, 345 patients were successfully resuscitated but 252 of these died later in hospital, giving 93 survivors. The number of cardiac arrest calls varied between 77 and 134 per year and the percentage surviving to discharge varied from 4 to 13.8%. Survival rates for males and females were equal. (The study was based on arrests in the general areas of the hospital, excluding the coronary and intensive care units.)

Ethics

The criteria used to assess the suitability of a patient for resuscitation are controversial. Factors that need to be considered are the patient's age, the nature and extent of the principal and/or secondary diseases, the quality of life experienced by the patient prior to admission and that to be expected after discharge. All personnel in the clinical team must be aware of the resuscitation status of each individual patient.

References and Further Reading

Brunner L S Suddarth D S (1982) The Lippincott Manual of Medical-Surgical Nursing, Harper & Row, Volume 2, pp. 23-28
Cochrane G M (1978) Saving life after cardiac arrest, Nursing Mirrror 147 (2): 17-20
Matheny L G (1981) Defibrillation: when and how to use it, Nursing (US) 11 (6): 69-72
Peatfield R C et al. (1977) Survival after cardiac arrest in hospital, Lancet i: 1223-1225
Thompson D R (1982) Cardiac Surgery, Ballière-Tindall, pp. 183-185
Wilson P Aarvold J A (1975) The organization and operational nursing management of cardiac arrest, International Journal of Nursing Studies 12: 23-32

GUIDELINES: CARDIOPULMONARY RESUSCITATION

Equipment

All items should be kept together and a checklist of these items should be drawn up. The list should be checked at least once a week and immediately after use.

1 Airway
2 Ambu bag with valve and mask
3 Oxygen tubing
4 Tongue forceps
5 Mouth gag
6 High capacity clearance catheters for aspriating the buccal cavity
7 Laryngoscope with spare bulbs and batteries
8 Intubating forceps
9 Endotracheal tubes
10 Topical swabs
11 Lubricating jelly
12 Syringe
13 Artery forceps
14 Endotrachael suction catheters
15 Hypoallergenic tape
16 Scissors
17 Catheter mount and swivel connector
18 Plaster
19 Tracheostomy set
20 Tracheostomy tubes
21 Emergency cardiac drugs
22 Intravenous infusion giving sets
23 Intravenous infusion cannulae
24 Syringes and needles
25 Swabs saturated with isopropyl alchohol 70%

26   Intravenous infusion stands
27   Cardiac needle
28   Oscilloscope
29   Electrode pads
30   Defibrillator
31   Lubricating jelly suitable for defibrillation paddles

Procedure

Action	Rationale
1 Note the time of the arrest, if witnessed.	1 Lack of cerebral circulation for approximately 3—5 minutes will result in irreversible brain damage.
2 Give the patient a short, sharp blow to the chest.	2 This may restore a cardiac rhythm which will give an adequate cardiac output.
3 Summon help. If a second nurse is available, he/she should call the emergency resuscitation team, bring equipment needed for cardiopulmonary resuscitation, prepare the environment and screen off the area.	3 Cardiopulmonary resuscitation is more effective when carried out by two people. Two nurses carrying out efficient cardiac massage and assisted ventilation can support the patient for 20 minutes plus. Medical intervention is required immediately.
4 Lie the patient in a supine position on a firm, non-metallic surface.	4 To allow for effective compression of the sternum against the spine during cardiac massage and to safeguard patients and personnel if defibrillation is required.
5 Ensure a clear airway by removing debris, secretions, vomit and prostheses from the buccal cavity. Hyperextend the neck by tilting the chin upwards and backwards.	5 Maintains a clear airway by moving the tongue away from the pharyngeal wall.
6 Insert the airway.	
7 Compress the lower third of the sternum with the heel of one hand. Place the palm of the other hand over the back of this hand. Keep your arms straight and elbows locked.	7 The heart is situated between this area of the sternum and the spine. Pressure will massage the heart and maintain circulation. The brain is more susceptible to ischaemia than anoxia and external cardiac massage should commence prior to ventilation, if both cannot be instituted simultaneously.
8 Place the mask of the Ambu bag over the patient's mouth and nose.	8 To inflate the lungs. To ensure an airtight seal.

Action	**Rationale**
9 Depress the bag in a rhythmical fashion.	9 To ensure a constant, steady supply of oxygen.
10 Attach the Ambu bag to an oxygen source as soon as possible. A minimum of 4 litres per minute at 100% should be delivered.	10 Brain damage begins to occur once the blood's small store of oxygen is used up. There is a lack of sufficient oxygen in atmospheric air (approximately 21%).
11 Inflate the lungs and compress the heart in the ratio 1 : 4. Cardiac massage must continue until the patient is able to maintain his/her own blood pressure.	11 To maintain circulation and oxygenation at an acceptable rate (a pulse of 60 beats per minute and respirations of 15 per minute).
12 When the resuscitation team arrives, one nurse should be responsible for recording information in the appropriate documents.	12 To ensure accurate information about the nature and course of the emergency.
13 Remove the head of the bed if the patient is in bed.	13 To allow easy access to the patient's head. To assist in the intubation procedure.

At this stage the resuscitation team becomes responsible for the management of the emergency. All other personnel not directly involved should return to their duties.

Intubation

14 Continue to ventilate and oxygenate the patient before intubation begins.	14 Cardiac arrhythmias due to hypoxia are decreased.
15 Attach the patient to an oscilloscope by applying electrode pads.	15 Accurate recording of cardiac rhythms will enable appropriate treatment to be initiated.
16 Before handing equipment to the medical staff check that: **a** The suction equipment is operational. **b** The endotrachael tube is lubricated. **c** The endotracheal tube cuff inflates and deflates. **d** The catheter mount and the swivel connector are attached.	
17 Recommence ventilation and oxygenation immediately intubation is completed.	

Action	Rationale

Intravenous Line

Such a line will allow for the restoration of acid-base and electrolyte imbalance, the adminstration of drugs and the replacement of body fluids.

	Action		Rationale
18	Asepsis must be maintained throughout.	18	To prevent local and/or systemic infection.
19	The correct rate of infusion is required.	19	To ensure maximum drug and/or solution effectiveness.
20	Accurate recording of the administration of solutions infused and drugs added is essential.	20	To provide a point of reference in the event of any queries.

Defibrillation

Used to terminate ventricular fibrillation.

NURSING CARE PLAN

Problem	Action	Rationale
1 Only one nurse available immediately	1 **a** Shout for help and keep shouting. **b** Inflate the lungs and compress the heart in the ratio 2 : 15.	1 **a** To make it obvious that help is needed. **b** This will give a pulse of 80 beats per minute.
2 Absence of chest expansion	2 **a** Check that the airway is clear and that the head is in the correct position. **b** If an Ambu bag is used, check that the valve is working, i.e. that the flaps open and close. **c** Check that the mouthpiece of the Ambu bag is covering the nose and the mouth.	2 **a** To provide and maintain a clear airway so that forceful ventillation may occur. **c** To provide an airtight seal.
3 Patient is a child	3 **a** Omit precordial thump. Use only two fingers over the lower sternum to compress the heart. **b** An increased rate of compression is also necessary.	3 **a** Undue pressure will fracture a child's ribs, with potential rupture of the lungs leading to haemopneumothorax. **b** Children normally have a pulse rate of 20-40 beats per minute more than an adult.

Problem	Action	Rationale
	c Ensure that appropriate equipment of paediatric size is available, e.g. airway and Ambu bag.	**c** Adult-size equipment would cause trauma and be inadequate for this purpose.
	d If equipment is unavailable, use mouth to mouth-nose method, i.e. cover child's mouth and nose and inflate lungs.	**d** To ensure an airtight seal and adequate oxygenation.
4 Patient has a radioactive source implanted	4 See procedures on iodine-131 and iridium-192 (pages 234-238 and 241-243).	

10

CENTRAL VENOUS CATHETERIZATION

Definition
Central venous catheterization is the catheterization of a large vein leading to the superior or inferior vena cava.

Indications
This procedure is indicated in the following circumstances:

1 To monitor central venous pressure in seriously ill patients
2 For the administration of large amounts of intravenous fluid or blood, e.g. in cases of shock or major surgery
3 To provide long term access for
   a Hydration or electrolyte maintenance
   b Repeated administration of drugs, such as cytotoxic and antibiotic therapy
   c Repeated transfusion of blood or blood products
   d Repeated specimen collection
4 For total parenteral nutrition.

REFERENCE MATERIAL

Insertion of the Catheter
Common Sites of Insertion
The catheter may be inserted at any of the sites listed below (see Figure 10.1):

1 Subclavian vein
2 Cephalic vein at axilla
3 Jugular vein — internal or external
4 Antecubital fossa.

If the site chosen is the antecubital fossa, a long line catheter will be used as this has to pass through the cephalic, the basilic or the brachial vein.

Internal jugular vein

External jugular vein

Subclavian vein

Axillary vein

Incision

Cephalic vein

Skin insertion

Brachial vein

Basilic vein

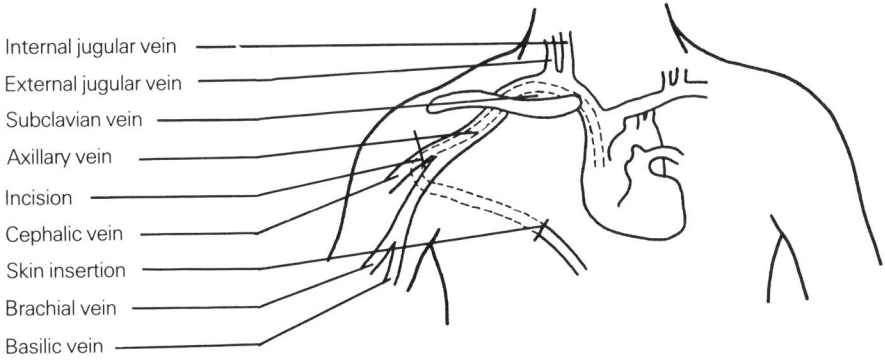

Figure 10.1   The ideal position and site for inserting the catheter

The catheter may be inserted directly into the vein or it may be tunnelled beneath the skin for a short distance before entering the vein. Skin tunnelling is usually performed if the catheter is intended to provide long term access to the vein as it reduces the risk of infection entering the vein from the skin insertion site. Any infection that develops around the catheter at the skin surface can be observed and treated before it reaches the vein. The fibrous tissue which develops around the subcutaneous catheter acts as a barrier to invading organisms. The Hickman wide bore catheter has a Dacron cuff which lies in the skin tunnel and, with the fibrous tissue that surrounds it, this acts as a very effective barrier against infection. The Hickman catheter or an equivalent silicone catheter suitable for skin tunnelling, e.g. the Nutricath, is used if there is a likelihood of the patient being discharged with his central line in place.

The Insertion Procedure

Ideally this is performed under full aseptic conditions, preferably in theatre, under general anaesthetic, local anaesthetic or heavy sedation.

The doctor inserts the catheter. The nurse's responsibilities are as follows:

1   To provide the patient with explanations and reassurance, e.g. teaching of the Valsalva manoeuvre (see below)
2   To ensure correct positoning of the patient, i.e. in the supine position or Trendelenburg position with the head down and roll of towel along the spinal column
3   To prepare fluids, to test the patency of the catheter and to prime the administration and extension sets
4   To prepare the local anaesthetic and dressing preparation, if required
5   To prepare any other equipment.

Checking the Position of the Catheter

The position of the catheter must be checked by X-ray before any drugs or fluids are infused. Normal saline, however, may be infused at a rate of 10-20 ml per hour to keep the catheter patent.

Hazards of Catheter Insertion

There are several potential hazards associated with the insertion of a central venous catheter:

1 Sepsis
2 Air embolism
3 Pneumothorax
4 Hydrothorax
5 Haemorrhage
6 Haemothorax
7 Brachial plexus injury
8 Thoracic duct trauma
9 Misdirection or kinking
10 Catheter embolism
11 Thrombosis.

Prevention of these complications depends largely on a careful insertion technique and strict asepsis. The risk of air embolism is reduced if the patient lies in the Trendelenburg position. This increases the venous filling and aids in performing the Valsalva manoeuvre during the procedure.

The Valsalva Manoeuvre

This may be performed by conscious patients to aid the insertion of the catheter. The patient is placed in a supine or Trendelenburg position. He/she is asked to breathe in and then to try to force the air out with mouth and nose closed. This increases the intrathoracic pressure so that the return of blood to the heart is momentarily reduced and the veins in the neck region become engorged. A distention of the vein up to 2.5 cm can be achieved in this way.

Principles of Catheter Care

Asepsis

Strict asepsis must be maintained to prevent the entry of bacteria into the system, especially at the site of insertion of the catheter. Sterile gloves should be worn whenever the insertion site is exposed and the giving set should be changed every 24 hours. Extension sets are only changed when the dressing is changed. The sterile dressing over the insertion site may be left in place for up to a week. However, the dressing may be changed more frequently should it become soiled or wet or if the patient complains of soreness or develops a pyrexia. An aseptic technique must be employed when the dressing is changed and the site should be checked for inflammation and oedema. Attention must also be given to the condition of the skin. When the dressing is changed, changing of the daily giving set and any extension set should be carried out at the same time.

Maintaining the Closed System

If equipment becomes disconnected, air embolism or profuse blood loss may occur. Luer locks provide a more secure connection and ideally all equipment should have these, e.g. giving sets and extension sets. Care should be taken to clamp the line firmly when changing equipment and connections should always be double checked. Precautions should also be taken to prevent the introduction of air into the system when making additions to, or when taking blood from, the central line.

Parenteral Nutrition

If a central venous catheter has been inserted for the purpose of total parental nutrition, then no other use should be made of it. In other words it should not be used for administration of drugs, blood and blood products or for blood sampling (Flannigan 1982).

Removal of Catheter

Skin-tunnelled Catheters

Removal of the skin-tunnelled catheter is performed by a member of the medical staff using strict aseptic technique. The patient is placed in the same position as for insertion of the catheter. Removal entails removing the anchoring suture and applying firm, steady pressure to the line. The entry and exit point should be covered immediately with an airtight dressing, pressure applied for approximately 5 minutes and the site left covered for at least 24 hours. The catheter tip is sent for bacteriological investigations. If a Hickman catheter with a Dacron cuff is in position, it may be necessary for this to be excised before applying traction on the catheter.

Catheters not Skin Tunnelled

If a catheter is not tunnelled through the skin, a member of the nursing staff may remove it, but only if he/she feels confident about this and adheres to a strict aseptic procedure.

Reading Central Venous Pressure

Central venous pressure (CVP) is the pressure within the superior vena cava or within the right atrium. CVP measurements reflect the relationship between the blood volume and cardiac competence (Figure 10.2).

Purpose of CVP Readings

1 To serve as a guide to fluid balance in seriously ill patients
2 To estimate blood volume deficits
3 To assist in monitoring circulatory failure.

Measuring CVP

The CVP measurement should be taken from a site in line with the right atrium (see Figure 10.3). Either of the sites indicated in the figure may be used, but it

Cardiac competence
(reduced ventricular
function raises CVP)

Blood volume (increased
venous return raises CVP)

Central
venous
pressure
(CVP)

Intrathoracic and
intraperitoneal
pressure (increase
in pressure raises
CVP)

Venous tone (increased
tone raises CVP)

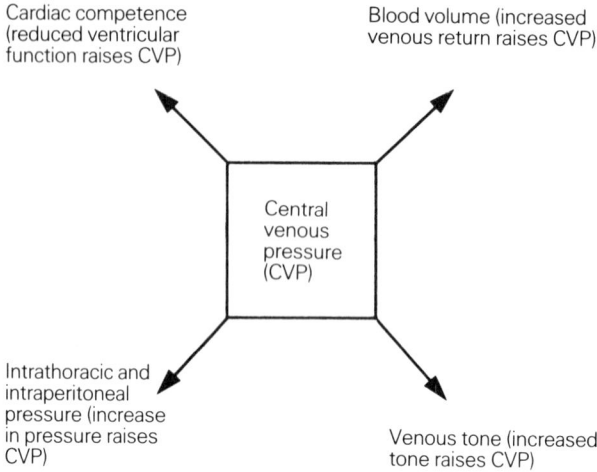

Figure 10.2   Determinants of central venous pressures

should be established at the outset of the readings which point is to be used as there is a pressure difference of about 5 cm water between them. It is useful to mark the chosen site for future readings and to note this site both on the CVP recording chart and in the care plan for the patient.

The normal values for CVP readings are: 0-5 cm water at the sternal angle and 5-10 cm water at the mid-axilla.

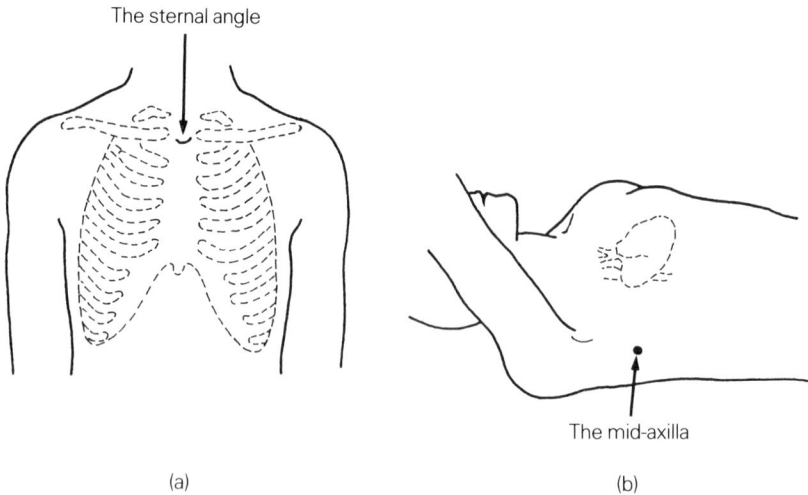

The sternal angle

The mid-axilla

(a)

(b)

Figure 10.3   Measuring central venous pressure. **a** The sternal angle. **b** The midaxilla

Discharging Patients with a Central Catheter in Position

Patients discharged with catheters in position should have skin-tunnelled lines. The patient and relatives or friends must be instructed and supervised in the technique of heparinizing the catheter before discharge. Sufficient equipment must be supplied to the patient to last from the time of discharge until the next outpatient appointment or admission.

The following equipment will be required:

1   A luer lock spigot with which to seal the end of the line and spares. These usually contain an intermittent latex injection port, or, more rarely, a noninjectable cap.
2   A clamp should be placed on the catheter.
3   A supply of Hepsal 50 IU per 5 ml. Alternatively a supply of ampoules of sterile normal saline 10 ml and a bottle of heparin 5000 IU per 5 ml may be provided.
4   Swabs saturated with isopropyl alcohol 70%, to clean the top of the heparin bottle
5   A pot of chlorhexidine in alcohol 70% to sterilize the catheter caps for reuse if they are of the noninjectable type
6   Sterile disposable forceps to remove the spigot from the chlorhexidine solution
7   A supply of sterile 10 ml syringes
8   21g needles (green) to draw up heparin and saline
9   25g needles (orange) to inject heparinized saline through the intermittent saline injection port, if present
10 Sterile gloves for use while handling the open end of the line.

On discharge, the catheter should be well established and the Dacron cuff covered with fibrous tissue, thus sealing off the catheter insertion site to the skin. The exit site may not require a dressing unless the patient requests it. In this case sterile topical swabs and hypoallergenic tape may be added to the above list.

The patient's technique and confidence while caring for the catheter should be assessed before discharge and the importance of correct calculation and asepsis stressed.

References and Further Reading

Brunner L S Suddarth D S (1982) Lippincott Manual of Nursing Practice, 3rd edition, J B Lippincott, pp. 271-274
Flannigan M (1982) Intravenous feeding, 2, Nursing Mirror 154 (17): 48-52
Janes E Marks M (1982) A Nurse's Guide to Parental Nutrition, S G Mason
Wood S (1982) Parenteral nutrition, Nursing 2 (4): 105-107

GUIDELINES: READING CENTRAL VENOUS PRESSURE

Equipment

1 Spirit level
2 Manometer
3 Three-way tap

Procedure

Action	Rationale
1 Explain the procedure to the patient.	1 To obtain the patient's consent and cooperation.
2 Ascertain the point of CVP reading, i.e. sternal angle or mid-axilla. If the patient agrees, this point should be marked on the patient and noted in the care plan chart for future reference.	2 CVP must always be read from the same point because the sternal angle reading is about 5 cm water higher than the mid-axilla reading.
3 Assist the patient to get into a recumbent or semirecumbent position to a maximum angle of 45°.	3 The position of the patient must allow the baseline of the manometer to be level with the patient's right atrium. If the patient is upright or is lying on his/her side, the right atrium will not be in line with the sternal angle or the mid-axilla.
4 Position the manometer so that the base-line is level with the right atrium.	4 To obtain an accurate CVP reading the base-line and the right atrium must be level.
5 Loosen the securing screw and slide the scale up or down until the base-line figure lies next to the arm of the spirit level (Figure	

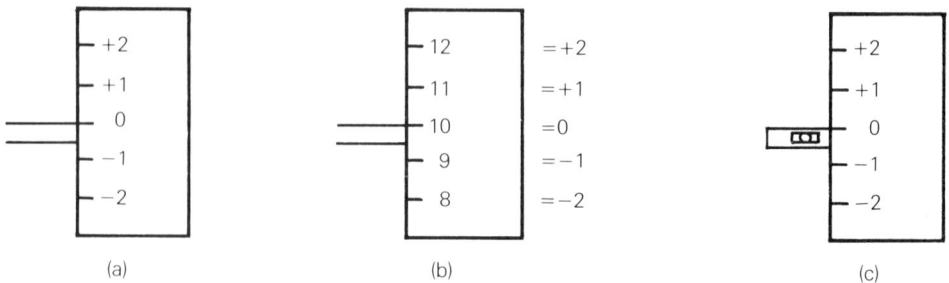

(a)   (b)   (c)

Figure 10.4a and **b** Setting the baseline. **c** Checking the baseline

Action	**Rationale**
10.4a). This figure may be 0 but is usually taken as +10 if the CVP reading is more than 2 cm below zero (Figure 10.4b).	Most scales do not extend below 2 cm, therefore the height of the scale must be altered to obtain a reading.
6 Check at base-line and right atrium are level by extending the arm of the spirit level to the sternal angle or to the mid-axilla. Move the manometer until the bubble is between the parallel lines of the spirit level (Figure 10.4c).	
7 Flush the line well by allowing the intravenous fluid to run through into the patient.	7 To ensure the patency of the line and to check for leaks, kinks, blockages, etc.
8 Turn off the three-way tap to the patient. Allow the manometer to fill slowly (Figure 10.5).	8 To allow the intravenous fluid to run into the manometer. To avoid **a** Bubbles, which cause inaccurate readings. **b** Overfilling of, and spillage from, the manometer that would put the patient at risk from infection.

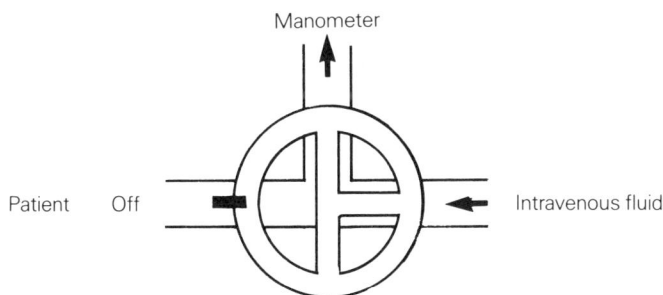

Manometer

Patient   Off   Intravenous fluid

Figure 10.5 Turn off the 3-way tap to the patient

9 Turn off the three-way tap to the intravenous fluid (Figure 10.6)	9 To allow fluid from the manometer to enter the patient's right atrium.
10 When the level of fluid in the manometer ceases to drop, and rises and falls with the patient's respirations, this is the CVP reading.	10 The pressure of the column of water in the manometer now equals the pressure in the right atrium.

Action	**Rationale**

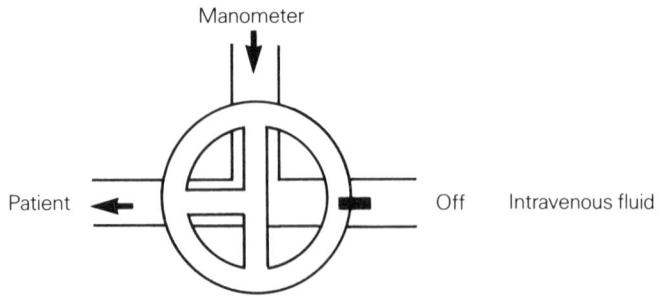

Figure 10.6   Turn off the 3-way tap to intravenous fluid

11 Turn off the three-way tap to the manometer (Figure 10.7).	11 To restore the intravenous line.

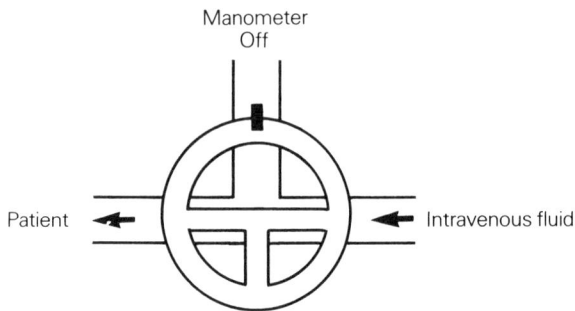

Figure 10.7   Turn off the 3-tap to manometer

12 Readjust the infusion rate.	
13 Record the CVP measurement on the appropriate chart. Compare this measurement with the patient's acceptable CVP limits as stated by the doctor or anaesthetist.	13 Acceptable CVP values vary with the patient and his/her overall condition. Deviations from these limits may require urgent medical intervention.

GUIDELINES: CHANGING THE DRESSING OVER A CENTRAL VENOUS CATHETER

Equipment

1   Sterile dressing pack
2   Hickman clamp soaking in a solution such as Hibitane *or* sterile artery

forceps and sterile topical swabs
3   Fluids for cleaning the wound
4   Appropriate hand hygiene preparation
5   Appropriate skin disinfectant solution, such as povidone iodine (Betadine)
6   Thin adhesive polyurethane film, such as OpSite spray or wound dressing
7   Intravenous giving set and extension set
8   Appropriate intravenous infusion solution
9   Sterile padded dressing
10 Hypoallergenic tape
11 Wound swab or sterile syringe
12 Sterile gloves
13 Surgical mask, if necessary
14 Disposable plastic apron

Note: Acetone is not used to defat the skin around the catheter because of the danger of acetone corroding the silicone material.

Procedure

Action	Rationale
1 Explain the procedure to the patient.	1 To obtain the patient's consent and cooperation.
2 Perform the dressing using an aseptic technique.	2 To prevent further infection. (For further information on asepsis, see the procedure on aseptic technique, pages 10-11.)
3 Screen the bed. Assist the patient into supine or Trendelenburg position.	3 To allow dust and airborne organisms to settle before the wound and the sterile field are exposed. To help prevent air embolus.
4 Wash your hands with an appropriate solution, such as soap and water or Hibiscrub. Put on the disposable plastic apron. Put on the surgical mask, if necessary. Place all equipment required for the dressing on the bottom shelf of a clean dressing trolley.	
5 Prime the giving set, keeping the luer lock sterile.	5 So that the infusion is ready for use when the current giving set is discontinued.
6 Take the trolley to the patient's bedside, disturbing the screens as little as possible.	6 To minimize airborne contamination.
7 Open the outer cover of the sterile dressing pack and slide the contents onto the top shelf of the trolley.	

Action	**Rationale**
8 Open the sterile field using the corners of the paper only. Using the forceps in the pack, arrange the sterile field with the handles of the instruments in one corner.	8 So that areas of potential contamination are kept to a minimum.
9 Attach a plastic disposable bag to the side of the trolley, below the level of the top shelf.	9 So that contaminated material is below the level of the sterile field.
10 Open the other sterile packs, tipping their contents gently on to the centre of the sterile field. Pour lotions into gallipots or an indented plastic tray.	
11 Loosen the old dressing gently, touching only the tape, etc., securing it.	11 So that the dressing can be lifted off easily with the forceps.
12 Clean your hands with an alcohol-based hand wash solution, such as Hibisol.	12 Hands may have become contaminated by handling the outer packs, etc.
13 Using forceps, or sterile disposable gloves if the dressing is large or bulky, remove the old dressing and discard it together with the forceps or gloves into the plastic bag.	
14 If the site is red or discharging, take a swab or syringe sample for bacteriological investigation. Routine samples should be taken weekly for patients having total parenteral nutrition and twice weekly for susceptible patients.	14 For identification of pathogens.
15 Clean the wound as necessary, working from the inside to the outside of the area and dealing with the cleanest parts of the wound first.	15 To minimize the risk of infection spread from a 'dirty' to a 'clean' area.
16 Spray the site with a skin disinfectant solution, such as Betadine.	
17 Apply a thin adhesive poly-urethane film, such as OpSite spray, or a wound dressing.	17 To provide an airtight seal over the insertion site and to prevent the entry of bacteria.
18 Discontinue the infusion in progress. Clamp the catheter using a Hickman clamp if the catheter is of silicone or artery forceps over	18 To prevent entry of air or leakage of blood when the catheter is disconnected. Swabs prevent cracking of a plastic catheter by

Action	**Rationale**
sterile topical swabs if it is of plastic.	artery forceps.
19 Clean your hands with an alcohol-based hand wash solution, such as Hibisol. Put on sterile gloves.	19 To minimize the risk of introducing infection into the catheter.
20 Ask the patient to perform the Valsalva manoeuvre. Disconnect the catheter from the old giving set and extension set and connect the prepared new set. Check that no air bubbles are present in the system. Unclamp the catheter and continue infusion.	20 To reduce the risk of air embolism.
21 Apply a sterile padded dressing, moulding it into place so that there are no folds or creases.	
22 Tape the extension set into a position comfortable for the patient.	22 To ensure the patient's comfort and to minimize the risk of accidental dislodging of the catheter.
23 Ensure that the drip rate is satisfactory.	
24 Fold up the sterile field, place it in the plastic disposal bag and seal the bag before moving the trolley.	24 To prevent environmental contamination.
25 Draw back the curtains.	
26 Dispose of waste in appropriate bags.	

GUIDELINES: TAKING BLOOD SAMPLES FROM A CENTRAL VENOUS CATHETER

Only nurses holding a certificate of competence, or nurses supervised by a suitably qualified nurse, should perform this procedure.

Equipment

1 Hickman clamp or artery forceps and sterile topical swabs
2 Small gallipot containing a solution such as Hibitane
3 Sterile 10 ml syringe
4 Sterile syringe of appropriate size for sample required and sterile needles
5 Blood sample bottles
6 Sterile gloves
7 Appropriate hand hygiene preparation

Procedure

<table>
<tr><th>Action</th><th>Rationale</th></tr>
<tr>
<td>1 Explain the procedure to the patient.</td>
<td>1 To obtain the patient's consent and cooperation.</td>
</tr>
<tr>
<td>2 Perform the dressing using an aseptic technique.</td>
<td>2 To prevent infection. (For further information on asepsis see the procedure on aseptic technique, pages 10–11.)</td>
</tr>
<tr>
<td>3 Assist the patient into a supine or Trendelenburg position.</td>
<td>3 To help prevent air embolus.</td>
</tr>
<tr>
<td>4 Wash your hands with an appropriate solution, such as soap and water or Hibiscrub.</td>
<td></td>
</tr>
<tr>
<td>5 Prepare a tray or trolley and take it to the bedside.</td>
<td></td>
</tr>
<tr>
<td>6 If intravenous fluid infusion is in progress, discontinue the infusion.</td>
<td></td>
</tr>
<tr>
<td>7 Clamp the catheter with a Hickman clamp if the catheter is of silicone or with artery forceps over sterile topical swabs if it is of plastic.</td>
<td>7 To prevent entry of air or leakage of blood via the catheter. Swabs prevent the artery forceps cracking a plastic catheter.</td>
</tr>
<tr>
<td>8 Open the syringe packets.</td>
<td>8 So that the syringes are readily accessible.</td>
</tr>
<tr>
<td>9 Clean your hands with an alcohol-based hand wash solution, such as Hibisol. Put on sterile gloves.</td>
<td>9 To minimize the risk of introducing infection into the catheter.</td>
</tr>
<tr>
<td>10 Disconnect the giving set from the catheter and cover the end of the set with the syringe cover or remove the catheter cap and place it in a gallipot containing a solution such as Hibitane.</td>
<td>10 To reduce the risk of contaminating the end of the giving set or the catheter cap while they are not attached to the catheter.</td>
</tr>
<tr>
<td>11 Attach a 10 ml syringe to the catheter. Release the clamp and withdraw 5–10 ml of blood.</td>
<td>11 To remove blood, heparin and intravenous fluids from the 'dead space' of the catheter. Samples from this 'dead space' are likely to cause inaccuracies in blood tests.</td>
</tr>
<tr>
<td>12 Reclamp the catheter and discard the sample and syringe.</td>
<td></td>
</tr>
<tr>
<td>13 Attach a new syringe of appropriate size. Release the clamp and withdraw the required amount of blood.</td>
<td>13 The original 10 ml syringe is not reused in order to reduce the risk of infection and the possibility of inaccuracies in the blood sample.</td>
</tr>
<tr>
<td>14 Reclamp the catheter and detach the syringe. Reconnect the giving set, unclamp the catheter and recommence infusion or</td>
<td>14 Unused catheters are heparinized to prevent blood clotting within them. The 'dead space' of the average Hickman catheter is 2.5</td>
</tr>
</table>

Action	Rationale
Heparinize line, replace the catheter cap from the gallipot and release the clamp.	ml and a minimum concentration of 50 IU heparin is needed to prevent clotting within this space. This may be given using either 0.5 ml heparin 1000 IU/ml in 9.5 ml saline, or 5.0 ml Hepsal (heparinized saline) 50 IU per 5 ml. Use sterile gloves to inject the heparin or saline solution in order to reduce the risk of introducing infection. Clamp the catheter before all of solution has been inserted and force the remaining saline in. This creates a positive pressure in the catheter, so preventing backflow of blood and any coagulation.

15 Put the blood sample into the appropriate bottle(s) and send to the laboratory with the necessary forms.

GUIDELINES: REMOVAL OF CATHETERS NOT SKIN TUNNELLED

Only nurses holding a certificate of competence, or nurses supervised by a suitably qualified nurse, should perform this procedure.

Equipment

1 Sterile dressing pack
2 Hickman clamp soaking in a solution such as Hibitane or sterile artery forceps and sterile topical swabs
3 Fluids for cleaning wound
4 Appropriate hand hygiene preparation
5 Appropriate skin disinfectant solution, such as povidone iodine (Betadine)
6 Sterile gloves
7 Surgical mask, if necessary
8 Wound swab or sterile syringe
9 Sterile scissors or stitch cutter
10 Small sterile specimen container
11 Collodion
12 Sterile padded dressing
13 Additional sterile topical swabs
14 Disposable plastic apron

Procedure

Action	Rationale
1 Explain the procedure to the patient.	1 To obtain the patient's consent and cooperation.
2 Perform the dressing using an aseptic technique.	2 To prevent infection. (For further information on asepsis see the procedure on aseptic technique, pages 10-11.)
3 Screen the bed. Assist the patient into a supine or Trendelenburg position	3 To allow dust and airborne organisms to settle before the wound and the sterile field are exposed. To help prevent air embolus.
4 Wash your hands with an appropriate solution, such as soap and water or Hibiscrub. Put on a disposable plastic apron. Put on a surgical mask, if necessary. Place all the equipment required for the dressing on the bottom shelf of a clean dressing trolley.	
5 Take the trolley to the patient's bedside, disturbing the screens as little as possible.	5 To minimize airborne contamination.
6 Open the outer cover of the sterile dressing pack and slide the contents on to the top shelf of the trolley.	
7 Open the sterile field using the corners of the paper only. Using the forceps in the pack, arrange the sterile field with the handles of the instruments in one corner.	7 So that areas of potential contamination are kept to a minimum.
8 Attach a disposable bag to the side of the trolley, below the level of the top shelf.	8 So that contaminated material is below the level of the sterile field.
9 Open the other sterile packs, tipping their contents gently on to the centre of the sterile field. Pour lotions into gallipots or an indented plastic tray.	
10 Loosen the old dressing gently, only touching the tape, etc., securing it.	10 So that the dressing can be lifted off easily with forceps.
11 Using forceps, or sterile disposable gloves if the dressing is large or bulky, remove the old dressing and discard it together with forceps or gloves into the plastic bag.	

Action	**Rationale**
12 If the site is red or discharging, take a swab or syringe sample for bacterological investigation.	12 For identification of pathogens.
13 Clean the wound as necessary, working from the inside to the outside of the area and dealing with the cleanest parts of the wound first.	13 To minimize the risk of infection spread from a 'dirty' to a 'clean' area.
14 Spray the site with a skin disinfectant solution, such as Betadine.	
15 Remove the top of the collodion bottle.	15 So that the collodion is easily accessible.
16 Discontinue the infusion in progress. Clamp a silicone catheter by using a Hickman clamp and a plastic catheter with artery forceps over sterile topical swabs.	16 To prevent entry of air or leakage of blood when the catheter is disconnected. Swabs prevent cracking of a plastic catheter by artery forceps.
17 Clean your hands with an alcohol-based hand wash solution, such as Hibisol. Put on sterile gloves.	17 To minimize the risk of introducing infection into the catheter.
18 Cut and remove the skin suture securing the catheter, if applicable.	
19 Disconnect the catheter from the giving set and the extension set.	
20 Ask the patient to perform the Valsalva manoeuvre.	20 To reduce the risk of air embolus.
21 Cover the insertion site with a thick pad of several sterile topical swabs.	21 Swabs are used to discourage the entry of organisms into the insertion site and to absorb any leakage of blood.
22 Hold the catheter with one hand near the point of insertion and pull firmly and gently. As the catheter begins to move, press firmly down on the site with the swabs. Maintain pressure on the swabs for about 5 minutes after the catheter has been removed.	22 Pressure is applied to prevent haemorrhage and to encourage resealing of the vein wall. It also prevents entry of air into the vein. Continued pressure is necessary to allow time for the puncture in the vein to close.
23 When the site has stopped bleeding, after about 5 minutes of pressure on the swabs, pour some collodion on to a sterile padded dressing.	
24 Discard the swabs and apply the	

Action	Rationale
sterile padded dressing and collodion to the site. Fix them in place with hypoallergenic tape.	
25 Ensure that the dressing is secure.	
26 Make the patient comfortable.	
27 Cut off the tip of the catheter and place it in a sterile pot for bacteriological investigation.	27 To detect any infection related to the catheter and thus provide necessary treatment.
28 Fold up the sterile field, place it in the plastic disposal bag and seal the bag before moving the trolley.	28 To prevent environmental contamination.
29 Draw back the curtains.	
30 Dispose of waste in appropriate bags.	

NURSING CARE PLAN

Problem	Cause	Suggested Action
1 Dyspnoea, chest pain or cyanosis	1 Hydrothorax, pnuemothorax or haemothorax due to insertion technique	1 Inform a doctor. Arrange for a chest X-ray. Assist with chest drainage, if necessary.
2 Change in pulse rate and rhythm after insertion of catheter	2 Cardiac irritability or cardiac rupture due to insertion technique	2 Inform a doctor.
3 Dyspnoea, chest pain, tachypnoea, disorientation, cyanosis, raised CVP, coma, cardiac arrest	3 Air embolism due to air entering circulation during the insertion procedure or via the catheter	3 Observe the patient closely, put him/her in a left side Trendelenburg position. Give oxygen or external cardiac compression.
4 Catheter-related septicaemia	4 **a** Poor asepsis **b** Over-flooding of the manometer, causing contamination	4 Culture of the patient's blood is required. Take a swab of the infusion site, employing strict asepsis and minimum handling of equipment. Administer antimicrobials as prescribed. Observe the patient closely.
5 Unable to draw back blood	5 **a** Catheter tip occluded by vein wall	5 Position patient on side where catheter is inserted, and ask him her to perform the

Problem	Cause	Suggested Action
		Valsalva manoeuvre.
	b Catheter blocked by blood clots due to (1) Infusion being too slow or switched off (2) Heparinization not having been carried out previously	**b** Inject 1000 IU/ml heparin (1 ml) and 1 ml normal saline into the catheter. Clamp and leave for 15 minutes. Attempt to aspirate with a 5 ml or 10 ml syringe to remove the clots. Irrigate with 5 ml heparinized saline. Repeat if necessary.
6 Leakage of fluid on to dressing	6 **a** Loose connection in system **b** Cracking of catheter or hub	6 **a** Check and tighten connections. **b** Report to intravenous nursing staff and/or medical staff.
7 Catheter required for many functions, e.g. blood sampling and extra drug administration	7 Limited routes of access available to satisfy the patient's requirements	7 Simplify regimes and methods of administration. Use of adaptors and administration. Use adaptors and administration sets available for this purpose.
8 Fluid overload resulting in dyspnoea, oedema, raised pulse rate and blood pressure	8 **a** Infusion too fast. **b** Inaccurate fluid monitoring **c** Metabolic disorders	8 Use flow control devices. Keep accurate records of the patient's fluid balance and weight. Revise the patient's fluid intake regime. Inform a doctor.
9 Inaccurate CVP readings	9 **a** Patient in a position different from that in which the initial reading was taken **b** Reference point on the patient not observed **c** Faulty pressure reading technique	9 **a** Position should be documented in the patient's records. **b** Zero of the manometer must be level with the patient's right atrium at the point marked on the patient, i.e. mid-axilla or sternal angle. **c** If the CVP reading is outside the limits deemed acceptable for

Problem	Cause	Suggested Action
		that patient and it is considered to be an accurate reading, re-check it after 15 or 30 minutes and inform a doctor if unchanged.
10 Elevated CVP	10 **a** Increased intrathoracic pressure caused by coughing, increased movement or pain **b** Lower extremities elevated	10 **a** Encourage coughing before taking the reading. Ensure that the patient is comfort-able and pain free. **b** Position the patient so that he/she is lying in a supine position. Give reassurance and/or sedation as necessary.
	c Patient having intermittent positive pressure ventilation	**c** Read the CVP at the end expiratory level (lowest point of fluctuation). This will always be higher than the 'normal' reading.
	d Anxiety and/or restlessness	**d** Verify the cause of the anxiety/restlessness.
	e Blood in progress via the CVP line	**e** Flush the line well with normal saline and reread.
	f Shivering and/or muscular spasm, e.g. postanaesthetic reaction	**f** Assess the patient's general condition, e.g. pulse, blood pressure, temperature. Check that the patient is warm enough. Inform a doctor.
11 Low CVP reading	11 **a** Leak in the system or equipment adjusted inaccurately **b** Changing of the patient's position from recumbent to semi-recumbent	11 **a** Check and readjust the system. **b** Reread with the patient in the original position.
12 Potential pulmonary embolus due to catheter tip embolus. Symptoms include chest pain, cool clammy skin, haemo-ptysis, tachycardia, hypotension.	12 Occasionally occurs after the removal of the catheter, especially the skin-tunnelled type	12 All skin-tunnelled catheters must be removed by medical staff. Notify a doctor immediately if the patient develops any of the related symptoms.

Problem	Cause	Suggested Action
13 Bleeding at the insertion site following removal of the catheter	13 Opening in the vein wall	13 Apply pressure over the site with sterile topical swabs. Cover the site with collodion and an occlusive dressing when the bleeding has stopped. Patients prescribed warfarin or heparin will require a longer period of pressure to compensate for the prolonged clotting time.

11

CYTOTOXIC DRUGS: HANDLING AND ADMINISTRATION

GENERAL INTRODUCTION

REFERENCE MATERIAL

In recent years there has been increasing concern about the occupational hazards associated with the handling of cancer chemotherapeutic agents. Certain cytotoxic drugs have been shown to have mutagenic, carcinogenic and teratogenic effects in both animals and man when given at therapeutic levels. On the basis of the evidence available at the present time, risks to personnel involved in reconstituting and administering cytotoxic drugs fall into two categories:

1 The proven local effects caused by direct contact with the skin, eyes and mucous membranes. These include

   a Dermatitis
   b Inflammation of mucous membranes
   c Pigmentation
   d Blistering associated with Mustine
   e Other apparently allergic reactions.

These hazards have been recognized for a number of years and protection using goggles and PVC gloves has been advised.

2 The potentially harmful short or long term systemic effects due to inhalation or ingestion of cytotoxic drugs during preparation. With the majority of compounds there is little or no absorption through intact skin. Systemic complaints from handlers include

   a Lightheadness   e Alopeica
   b Dizziness   f Coughing
   c Nausea   g Pruritis
   d Headache   h General malaise.

The working conditions where these were experienced were not desirable, i.e. a small, unventilated medicine closet. No formal collection of data was performed and the author readily admits to gathering information on an anecdotal basis.

There have been a number of studies in which the urine of cytotoxic drug handlers, including nurses, has been collected and screened for mutagenic activity using an accepted test (Ames et al. 1975). Although alterations in cell structure have been detected in many of the published works, this appears to be transient and of a low level. It has yet to be demonstatedd whether it is harmful and if this level of mutagenesis can be equated with carcinogenesis. Few conclusions can be drawn from results and more recent work has brought the validity of the test into doubt.

In summary, the local hazards of contact with cytotoxic drugs are well documented and it is only sensible to take precautions to prevent them. While the long term risks remain undefined, it is prudent to avoid any unnecessary exposure. This can be done by formulating locally agreed, practical policies in line with national guidelines, where available. Any guidelines should cover the following areas:

1   *Preparation of compounds* — environment, staff training, staff protection, technique, equipment
2   *Administration of drugs* — staff training, staff protection, technique, equipment
3   *Disposal* — of drugs, equipment and waste
4   *Accidents* — spillage and contamination of nurse, doctor or patient
5   A system for *monitoring and recording* any effects on hospital staff.

Note: The administration of intravenous medications is an area where the role of the nurse is being extended. For further information see the procedure on intravenous drug administration (pp. 205-222).

References and Further Reading

Ames B N et al. (1975) Methods for detecting carcinogens and mutagens with the *Salmonella*/mammalian microsome mutagenicity test, Mutation Research 31: 347-364

Anderson R et al. (1981) Assesment of exposure of hospital pharmacy personnel handling cancer chemotherapy agents, Paper presented at the 16th Annual American Society of Hospital Pharmacists Midyear Clinical Meeting, New Orleans, 7 December 1981.

Anderson R et al. (1982) Risk of handling infectable antineoplastic agents, American Journal of Hospital Pharmacy 39: 1881-1887

Bauman B Duvall E (1980) An unusual accident during the administration of chemotherapy, Cancer Nursing 3 (4): 305

Calvert A H (1981) The long term sequelae of cytotoxic therapy, Cancer Topics July/August

Crudi C B (1980) A Compounding Dilemma: I've Kept the Drug Sterile but Have I Contaminated Myself? National Intravenous Therapy Association

Falck K et al. (1979) Mutagenicity in urine of nurses handling cytotoxic agents, Lancet i: 1250

Galleli J F (1982) Evaluating the potential hazard of handling antineoplastic drugs, American Journal of Hospital Pharmacy 39: 1887

Hoffman D M (1980) The handling of antineoplastic drugs in a major cancer center, Hospital Pharmacy 15: 302

Knowles R S Virden J E (1980) Handling of injectable antineoplastic agents, British Medical Journal 2: 589-591

Ladik C F et al. (1980) Precautionary measures in the preparation of antineoplastics, American Journal of Hospital Pharmacy 37: 1184

Nguyen T V et al. (1982) Exposure of pharmacy personnel to mutagenic antineoplastic drugs, Cancer Research 42: 4792-4796

Nurses Action Group (1981) Beware of the drug, Nursing Mirror 152 (6): 22-25

Royal College of Nursing Oncology Nursing Society (1982) Report of the Working Party Established to Investigate the Involvement of Nurses in the Handling and Administration of Cytotoxic Drugs, Royal College of Nursing

Salvatore J (1981) Cancer chemotherapy agents: handling and disposal, American Journal of Intravenous Therapy and Clinical Nutrition 8 (2): 6

Speechley V (1982) Better safe than sorry, Nursing Mirror 154 (15): 11

Stuart M (1981) Sequence of administering vesicant cytotoxic drugs Part A, Oncology Nursing Forum 9 (1) Winter

Thomsen K Mikkelsen H (1975) Protective gloves used for handling nitrogen mustard contact, Dermatitis 1: 268-269

Tortorici M P (1980) Precautions followed by personnel involved with the preparation of parental antineoplastic medication, Hospital Pharmacy 15: 293

Vennitt S et al. (1983) Monitoring exposure of nursing and pharmacy personnel to cytotoxic drugs: urinary mutation assays and urinary platinum as markers of absorption, Lancet 1: 74-76

Waksvik H et al. (1981) Chromosome analyses of nurses handling cytostatic agents, Cancer Treatment Reports 65 (7/8): 607

Wilson J P Solimando D A (1981) Antineoplastics: a safety hazard, American Journal of Hospital Pharmacy 38: 624

Working Party of the Pharmaceutical Society of Great Britain on the Handling of Cytotoxic Drugs (1983) Guidelines for the handling of cytotoxic drugs, Pharmaceutical Journal 230 (6215): 230-231

INTRAPLEURAL INSTILLATION OF CYTOTOXIC DRUGS

Definition

Pleural effusion is a common complication of malignant disease and poses a considerable management problem. Such effusions are usually very distressing to the patient, causing progressive discomfort, inanition, dyspnoea and death from respiratory insufficiency. Effective palliation is, therefore, an important aspect in maintaining or improving the quality of life of the patient.

REFERENCE MATERIAL

Normal lung anatomy is altered dramatically by the presence of pleural effusion (Figure 11.1). In health there is less than 5 ml of transudate fluid present which acts as a lubricant and hydraulic seal between the visceral and parietal pleurae. Various conditions, e.g. infection and various neoplasms, upset this mechanism.

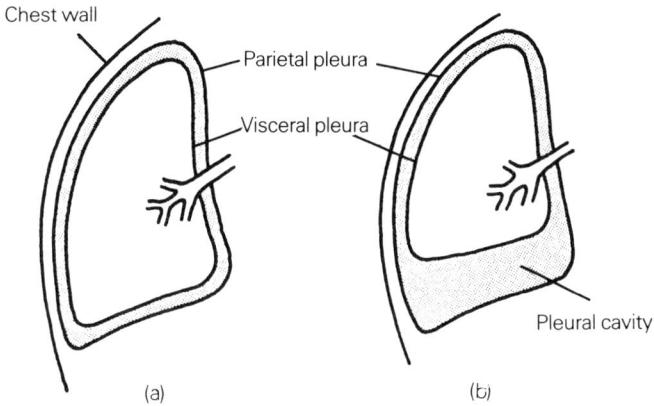

Figure 11.1 Lung anatomy. **a** Normal lung anatomy showing pleura. **b** Lung demonstrating presence of plerual effusion

The most common neoplasms causing malignant pleural effusions are those of

1   The breast
2   The lung
3   The gastrointestinal tract
4   Lymphoma
5   The prostate
6   The ovary
7   Sarcoma.

Wood (1981) states that 50% of patients with primary lung or breast carcinoma will develop effusions at some stage. Such patients may survive for months and even years.

A number of methods have been used to treat malignant pleural effusions. They include the following:

1   Surgical ablation of the pleural space
2   Tube thoracostomy
3   Repeated thoracentesis
4   Systemic chemotherapy
5   Radiotherapy
6   Instillation of sclerosing agents into the pleural space. Such agents include

a Talc powdrage
b Radioactive phosphorus
c Tetracycline (Wallach 1975)
d Cytotoxic drugs (thiotepa, bleomycin, nitrogen mustard, cyclo-phosphamide)

Trials carried out over the past 30 years have used a variety of techniques. The most significant changes during this period have been the use of a catheter or tube instead of a needle for both the drainage and instillation and the extension of the time allowed for drainage both before and after instillation of the drug.

All the studies state that the patient should be turned following instillation of the drug to ensure its complete distribution over the pleural surfaces. The timing used varies. Only one paper (Wood 1981) gives a detailed procedure. The necessity for such turning is based on clinical observation. No studies have been done comparing the results from patients who were turned with patients who were not.

Reports of studies using this technique emphasize that the procedure itself is painful and may cause pyrexia. There are also the problems and inherent dangers related to the insertion and management of the drainage tube, e.g. infection, pneumothorax, etc.

Furthermore, many of these patients will have other signs and symptoms of metastatic disease and the nursing problems arising from these will need to be identified and the appropriate care planned.

References and Further Reading

Anderson C et al. (1972) The treatment of malignant pleural effusions, Cancer 33:916-922

Groesteck H et al. (1962) Intracavitary Thio-tepa for malignant effusions, Surgery 28:90-95

Taylor L (1962) A catheter technique for intrapleural administration of alkylating agents: a report of ten cases, American Journal of the Medical Sciences 244(6):706-716

Wallach H (1975) Intrapleural tetracycline for malignant pleural effusions, Chest 68:510-512

Wood H (1981) Developments in the support of patients with malignant pleural effusions, in Cancer Nursing Update, edited by R Tiffany, Ballière Tindall, pp. 69-76

GUIDELINES: PROTECTION OF NURSING STAFF WHEN HANDLING CYTOTOXIC DRUGS

Action	Rationale
1 Reconstitution of cytotoxic drugs should take place in a well ventilated room. Doors and	1 To prevent any unnecessary airborne exposure from possible powder or droplet aerosols

Action	Rationale
windows should be closed to prevent draughts.	released
2 Where possible, the area should not be used for other purposes during the time that preparation is taking place. Ideally, these drugs should be prepared within a vertical laminar air flow cabinet.	2 As above.
3 The area should contain a sink and running water.	3 To clean surfaces and/or skin if spillage and/or contamination occurs.
4 The surface should be smooth and impermeable.	4 To enable cleaning of surfaces to be undertaken easily and quickly.
5 Reconstitution should take place in a plastic tray or equivalent vehicle.	5 To enable containment of spillage and ease of cleaning.
6 Nursing staff should receive instruction in the techniques of reconstitution and the reasons for their recommendation.	6 To ensure that staff are safe to practise and are aware of the risks involved.
7 Contact with the injection solution can largely be avoided by the use of PVC gloves such as Triflex or Travenol gloves.	7 Only poly(vinyl chloride), i.e. PVC, has been demonstrated to be impermeable to all cytotoxic agents.
8 All cuts and scratches should be covered	8 To prevent infiltration of the skin if damage to gloves occurs.
9 Antibiotic compounds can cause irritation in some individuals. Gloves should be worn as a precautionary measure if signs of sensitization have developed previously.	
10 Use goggles or protective glasses.	10 To prevent contact between drugs and the eyes. If the nurse wears glasses these should provide approximately 90% protection.
11 Wash after use.	11 To prevent cross-infection and/or cross-contamination.
12 Use a good quality face mask when reconstituting dry powder, especially when in ampoule form, e.g. bleomycin.	12 To prevent inhalation of any powder released during reconstitution.
13 Put on a disposable plastic apron.	13 To provide a barrier between the drug and the handler.
14 Ampoules should be held away from the face and covered with a piece of sterile topical swab when breaking them.	14 To prevent contamination of the gloves or skin. To prevent formation of aerosols or liberation of powder.

Action	**Rationale**
15 Airways, i.e. an extra needle, should always be used to vent vials.	15 To prevent pressure differentials which can cause separation of the needle and syringe used for preparation. In more extreme circumstances vial cap and the vial have separated, and explosion of a vial has been reported.
16 The diluent should be slowly introduced down the wall of the vial or ampoule.	16 To ensure that the powder is thoroughly wet before agitation and is not released into the atmosphere.
17 Needles should be capped before the expulsion of air or the tip should be covered with a sterile topical swab or the air should be expelled into the vial or ampoule.	17 To prevent aerosol formation.
18 Gloves and goggles should continue to be worn during administration as the nurse is handling the drugs and may still be contaminated. Gloves should be washed if contaminated and changed if damaged. Goggles should be washed if contaminated.	18 To prevent contamination at a later stage of the procedure.
19 Contamination of the skin, mucous membranes and eyes should be treated promptly. All areas should be washed with copious amounts of tap water or normal saline. Eye wash may be available.	19 To prevent any local damage to tissue.
20 Infiltration of skin with a vesicant agent should be treated as an extravasation and ice applied immediately.	20 To prevent any local damage to tissue.
21 If erythema and/or other local reaction occurs in any circumstances, contact the occupational health unit or a member of the medical staff so that appropriate treatment may be advised.	21 To prevent further damage and/or complications.
22 Contact the occupational health unit if any unusual local or systemic symptoms occur after contact with cytotoxic drugs.	22 To aid with recording and monitoring of staff.

Action	**Rationale**
23 Contact the occupational health unit if pregnancy is suspected or confirmed.	23 To discuss future work patterns and any anxiety that may be felt.

GUIDELINES: PROTECTION OF THE ENVIRONMENT

Action	**Rationale**

Spillage

1 Act immediately.	1 Any spillage may become a health hazard.
2 Put on PVC gloves.	2 To protect your hands.
3 If there is a visible powder spill, wear a face mask of good quality.	3 To prevent inhalation of powder.
4 Wipe up the remains with a damp cloth or paper towel and place them in a high risk waste disposal bag.	4 To absorb all spillage and prevent dispersal. To ensure careful handling and disposal by incineration.
5 Wash contaminated surfaces with copious amounts of water and any exposed skin areas with soap and cold water.	5 To ensure that all spillage is cleaned up.
6 Dispose of any washing materials.	6 To ensure that all contaminated material is sent for incineration.

Disposal

1 'Sharps' should be placed in the special container provided.	1 To ensure incineration and to prevent laceration and/or innoculation during transit or disposal.
2 Dry waste, intravenous administration sets and other contaminated material should be placed in high risk waste disposal bags.	2 To ensure careful handling and disposal by incineration.
3 Excess drug solutions should be flushed into the drainage system using copious amounts of cold water.	3 To ensure adequate dilution of any cytotoxic drugs.
4 Reusable trays and other equipment should be washed with copious amounts of water followed by disinfectant.	4 To prevent cross-infection and cross-contamination.

GUIDELINES: INTRAVENOUS ADMINISTRATION OF CYTOTOXIC DRUGS

Action

Rationale

	Action		Rationale
1	Continue to wear any protective clothing used during the preparation of the drug. Contaminated and/or damaged clothing should be replaced before continuing.	1	To protect nursing staff from harm.
2	Use an aseptic technique throughout.	2	To prevent local and/or systemic infection. Patients are frequently immunosuppressed and at greater risk.
3	Check the following with another nurse: **a** Correct dilution of drug **b** Correct dose of drug **c** Correct route and method of administration.	3	To ensure that the patient is given the correct drug in the prescribed dose, using the appropriate diluent, and by the correct route.
4	Explain the procedure to the patient.	4	To obtain the patient's consent and cooperation.
5	Inspect the infusion or injection site.	5	To detect any phenomena, e.g. phlebitis, that would render the vein unusable.
6	Establish the patency of the line using normal saline.	6	To determine whether the vein will accommodate the extra fluid flow and remain patent.
7	Ensure the correct administration speed.	7	To prevent speed shock.
8	Be aware of the immediate effects of the drug.	8	To know what to observe for during adminstration. To be prepared to manage any side effects.
9	Administer drugs in the correct order, i.e. vesicant agents first.	9	To ensure that those agents likely to cause tissue damage are given when the venous integrity is greatest, i.e. at the beginning.
10	Observe the vein.	10	To detect any problems at the earliest moment.
11	Observe for signs of extravasation, e.g. pain and swelling at the site of injection.	11	To prevent any unnecessary damage to soft tissue, and to enable the remainder of the drug(s) to be given correctly at some other site. To enable prompt treatment to be given, therefore minimizing local damage, and possibly preserving venous access for future treatment.

Action	Rationale
12 Flush the line between drugs and after administration.	12 To prevent drug interaction. To prevent leakage along the path of the cannula or from the puncture site.
13 Be aware of the patient's comfort throughout the procedure.	13 To minimize trauma to the patient. To involve the patient in treatment and detect any side affects and/or problems that may then be avoided at the next treatment.
14 Record details of the administration in the appropriate documents.	14 To prevent any duplication of treatment. To provide a point of reference in the event of any queries.
15 Protect the patient from contact with the drugs by	
a Placing a plastic sheet or small incontinence pad or equivalent under the sterile towel	**a** To provide a waterproof barrier and protect the skin.
b Inserting the needle carefully into the injection site of the giving set or into the bung	**b** To prevent exiting on the other side and contaminating or innoculating the patient.
c Careful changing of syringes	**c** To avoid leakage and contamination of the nurse or the patient.
d Securing a good bond between needle and syringe	**d** To prevent separation, which may occur due to pressure required for administration, resulting in contamination.
e Checking the injection site or bung at the end of the procedure	**e** To ensure that there is no leakage.
f Acting promptly if any contamination is noted and washing the area with cold water or saline.	**f** To prevent any local reaction on skin or mucous membranes, etc.

ADMINISTRATION OF CYTOTOXIC DRUGS BY OTHER ROUTES

ORAL ADMINISTRATION OF CYTOTOXIC DRUGS

Nurses dispensing tablets or capsules should do this using a non-touch technique. If tablets have to be counted, this should be done using a triangle, which should be washed after use.

Many tablets are coated and this protects the drug in its inner core. There is no handling risk if these coatings are not broken.

A small number of tablets are compressed powders, but where there is no free powder visible there is no risk.

It is important that these tablets are not crushed.

Capsules are free from risk if they have not been opened or have not either been broken or leaked. They should not be crushed or opened.

Any visible spillage should be dealt with as previously directed (see page 119).

INTRAMUSCULAR AND SUBCUTANEOUS INJECTION OF CYTOTOXIC DRUGS

Preparation and reconstitution of drugs should be in line with the preceding guidelines (see pages 116-119). Although handling of the drugs is less in this situation, the nurse should continue to wear his/her gloves to administer the injection. Spillage and disposal of equipment should be dealt with as previously directed (see page 119).

Recommendations about administration should be carefully followed, e.g. deep instramuscular injection and care taken not to leak drugs on to the the skin.

GUIDELINES: ADMINISTRATION OF INTRAPLEURAL DRUGS

Action	Rationale
Instillation of Drug	
1 Explain the procedure to the patient.	1 To obtain the patient's consent and cooperation.
2 Administer premedication to the patient if ordered.	2 To relieve anxiety and pain.
3 Prepare equipment.	
4 Assist the doctor with instillation.	
5 Leave the tube clamped.	5 To prevent back flow of the drug instilled.
Rotation of Patient	
1 Turn the patient in the following rotation: a Left side b Flat c Right side d Prone.	1 To ensure that the drug instilled coats and washes the pleural cavity completely.
2 Carry out the rotations as follows: a 5 minutes in each position, repeated once, equals 40 minutes	

Action	Rationale
b 30 minutes in each position, repeated once, equals 4 hours **c** 1 hour in each position equals 4 hours.	
3 Assess for pain every 2-4 hours and administer analgesics as necessary.	3 To keep the patient free from pain
4 Record the vital signs every 15 minutes for 1 hour, then every hour until stable, then 4 hourly.	4 To observe for pyrexia, a common side effect that may be indicative of the onset of infection or pneumathorax.

Drainage of Thoracotomy Tube

Action	Rationale
1 Make the patient comfortable in whichever position suits him/her.	
2 Unclamp the chest tube.	2 To allow drainage of the drug instilled.
3 Maintain underwater seal drainage until a volume of less than 50 ml drainage in 24 hours for two consecutive days or for a maximum of 7 days is achieved. (For further information see the procedure on intrapleural drainage, pages 196-202	3 To allow drainage of the drug instilled.
4 Record the colour and amount of drainage in the appropriate documents.	4 To monitor the effectiveness of therapy.

GUIDELINES: INTRAVESICAL INSTALLATION OF CYTOTOXIC DRUGS

Equipment

1 60 ml bladder syringe and needle adapter
2 18 or 20 ml sterile syringe
3 Drug and diluent, e.g. sterile water
4 PVC gloves, such as Triflex gloves
5 Large gauge needles
6 Clinically clean tray
7 Protective eye glasses or goggles
8 Swabs saturated with isopropyl alcohol 70%
9 Gate clip

10   Catheter bag, if catheter is to remain in position
11   Sterile towel

If the patient is not already catheterized, include catheterization equipment. (For further information see the procedure on urinary catheterization, pages 449—453.)

Procedure

Action	Rationale
1 Explain the procedure to the patient.	1 To obtain the patient's consent and cooperation.
2 Check the patient's blood count for that day before the first administration of the drug. The blood count will not need checking for subsequent administrations given within that week. Do not introduce the drug and inform the medical staff if the white blood cell count is below 3000 and/or the platelet count is below 100 000.	2 Absorption of the drug through the bladder wall may cause some myelosuppression.
3 Prepare the drug:	
a Check the prescription on the patient's drug chart with another nurse.	**a** To comply with hospital policy and legal requirements. To minimize the risk of error.
b Wash your hands. Put on safety goggles and PVC gloves, such as Triflex gloves.	**b** To protect the eyes and hands of the nurse from accidental spillage of the drug.
c Dilute the drug as prescribed and draw up into the bladder syringe using a needle adapter.	**c** So that the drug is ready for instillation.
d Put a cover over the syringe tip and place the syringe in a clean receiver.	**d** Keep the end of the syringe closed to prevent leakage of the drug and to discourage the entry of organisms.
4 If the patient has not got a catheter in position, catheterize him/her and empty the bladder of urine.	4 See the procedure on urinary catheterization (pages 449-453). To prevent dilution of the drug.
5 Place the necessary equipment on a clean trolley or tray.	
6 Take the trolley to the patient's bedside and screen the bed.	
7 Put on PVC gloves.	7 To protect the nurse's hands from drug spillage.

Action	Rationale
8 Place a sterile towel under the end of the catheter. Clamp the catheter and disconnect the urine drainage bag.	8 To gain access to the catheter. To prevent urine from soiling the bed.
9 Remove the cover from the syringe and insert the nozzle into the end of the catheter. Release the clamp and inject the drug slowly.	9 Rapid injection of drug and diluent would be uncomfortable for the patient.
10 When the correct volume of drug has been instilled, clamp the catheter and disconnect the syringe.	10 To prevent drainage of the drug from the bladder.
11 If the catheter is to stay in position, connect the catheter to a new drainge bag. Otherwise withdraw water from the catheter balloon using a 10 or 20 ml syringe and remove the catheter using gentle traction.	11 To maintain closed systems and to reduce the risk of entry of bacteria. If the patient does not require the catheter, it may be removed. Infection is more likely if the catheter is left in position.
12 Make the patient comfortable and ensure that he/she knows about changing his/her position during the next hour while the drug is in the bladder.	12 To ensure that all of the bladder mucosa contacts the drug.
13 If the patient is unable to turn himself/herself, the nurses should position him/her as necessary.	13 To prevent the development of pressure sores. For intravesical drug installation to people in outpatient departments the journey home is usually sufficient to coat the bladder mucosa.
14 When the drug has been in the bladder for exactly 1 hour request the patient to micturate. If a catheter is in position, release the clamp so that the drug and urine drain into the catheter bag.	14 One hour is the time specified for intravesical drugs to induce the maximum therapeutic effect with minimum side effects.

NURSING CARE PLAN: INTRAVESICAL DRUG ADMINISTRATION

Problem	Cause	Suggested Action
1 No drainage of urine when the catheter is inserted	1 Bladder is empty or the catheter is in the wrong place, e.g. in the urethra or in a false track. False tracks may develop after repeated cytoscopy or bladder surgery.	1 Do not inflate the balloon but tape the catheter to the skin to keep it in position. Check when the patient last micturated. Encourage the patient to drink a few glasses of fluid. Do not give the drug until urine flow is seen or correct positioning of the catheter is established. Inform a doctor if no urine has drained during the next 30 minutes.
2 Haematuria	2 Trauma of catheterization or loosening of blood clots following cytoscopy by fluid injected into the bladder	2 Inform a doctor. Observe the patient for signs of clot rentention, shock, haemorrhage or fluid retention. Encourage the patient to drink fluids.
3 Leakage from around the catheter following administration of the drug	3 Catheter slipping out of the bladder or bladder spasm caused by the drug	3 Check the position of the catheter. Inform a doctor if leakage persists. Protect the patient's skin by wrapping sterile topical swabs around the catheter. Estimate the volume lost by leakage.
4 Patient unable to retain the requisite drug volume in the bladder for the time required	4 Low bladder capacity; weak sphincter muscles; unstable detrusor muscle causing uncontrolled bladder contractions	4 Note actual duration of the drug in the bladder and inform a doctor.
5 Patient has pain during installation of the drug or while the drug is in the bladder.	5 Drug injected too quickly; volume of drug and diluent too great for comfort;	5 Allow the drug to drain out and/or stop installation if the pain is severe. Inform a

Problem	Cause	Suggested Action
	drug painful to raw areas in the bladder; drug causes painful spasm of the bladder	doctor. Administer Entonox if apppropriate (see pages 156-160) and have analgesics prescribed for subsequent administration.
6 Patient unable to pass urine after the drug has been in situ for the required length of time	6 Anxiety; poor bladder tone; prostatism	6 Reassure the patient. Encourage the patient to drink fluids.
7 Urine does not drain from the catheter when the clamp is released	7 **a** Catheter wrongly placed **b** Catheter blocked with clots and/or debris	7 **a** Check the position of the catheter. **b** Perform bladder lavage.

12

DRUG ADMINISTRATION

Legislation

The range of substances which are controlled in some way or an another by law is extensive. Three broad categories may be identified:

1 Narcotic drugs
2 Poisons
3 Medicines

In the United Kingdom preparations must conform to certain standards as specified in the *British Pharmacopoeia* and the *British Pharmacopoeia Codex.*

The law relating to the above-mentioned categories is contained in three statutes. Anyone working in the National Health Service will require a working knowledge of these three statutes, and of the body of regulations made under them, if they are to meet their legal obligations in their particular fields.

The Misuse of Drugs Act, 1971

This Act lists the drugs to be controlled and classifies them for the purpose of the Act. It prohibits virtually all activities with controlled drugs and thereby creates a series of criminal offences for which it specifies penalties and law enforcement procedures. It authorizes certain activities with controlled drugs for professional medical (including dental and veterinary) use which would otherwise be unlawful. These authorized activities are themselves subject to control.

In addition, the Act confers on the Secretary of State at the Home Office a variety of powers made under the Act to prevent the misuse of drugs, and it creates the Advisory Council on the Misuse of Drugs.

A classification of the therapeutic value of the controlled drugs is required for setting limits on what medical use they may be put to. This is achieved by dividing them into four schedules:

1 Controlled drugs combined with other substances in such small amounts that they are not liable to produce dependence or cause harm if misused, except any preparation for injection
2 The opiates and the major stimulants (amphetamines)
3 Minor stimulants, not considered to be as harmful as the opiates and hallucinogens
4 Hallucinogenic drugs (e.g. lysergic acid diethylamine, LSD) and cannabis.

Authorization of Activities Otherwise Unlawful   Such authorization may be considered in three cases:

1 *Administration of controlled drugs (Regulation 7)* Any person, irrespective of qualification, may administer a Schedule 1 drug to any other person provided that no offence is committed. A doctor or dentist or someone acting under their direction may administer any drug in Schedule 2 or 3 to any patient. Schedule 4 substances may not be administered by anyone who does not possess a special licence to do so issued by the Secretary of State. Such licences are issued only for research and scientific purposes.
2 *Production and supply of Schedule 1, 2 and 3 drugs (Regulations 8 and 9)* Provided that he/she is acting in his/her capacity as such, among those who may supply or offer to supply a Schedule 1, 2, or 3 drug to any person who may lawfully possess it are a sister or acting sister in charge of a ward, theatre or other department in a hospital or nursing home where the drug is supplied to him/her by a person responsible for dispensing and supply of medicines in that hospital. A sister or acting sister in charge of a ward, etc., may supply a drug only for administration to a patient in that ward, etc., and under the direction of a doctor or dentist.
3 *Possession of controlled drugs (Regulation 10)* There is no restriction on a Schedule 1 drug. Any person may have in his/her possession a Schedule 2 or 3 drug for administration for medical, dental or veterinary use under the directions of a practitioner, provided that it was not obtained under false pretences.

Requirements Concerning Documentation   These requirements may be considered under five headings:

1 *Supplies of Schedule 2 and 3 drugs from a hospital pharmacy to a ward (Regulation 14)* A requisition is required where the person in a hospital or nursing home who is responsible for the dispensing and supply of medicines supplies a controlled drug to a sister or acting sister in charge of the ward, theatre or other department. The requisition must be in writing, must be signed by the recipient and must specify the total quantity of drug to be supplied. The requisition must be marked by the supplier as having been complied with (to prevent it being used twice) and retained in the pharmacy. The recipient must also keep a copy.

2 *Correct form of prescription (Regulation 15)* For the treatment of a patient in a hospital or a nursing home, it is not necessary to include the name and address of the person treated if the prescription is written on the patient's card or case notes. The prescription must be written in indelible ink and signed and dated by the person issuing it. When drugs are issued on a patient's discharge or in an outpatient department the issuer must also specify, in his/her own handwriting, the dose to be taken, the strength of the preparation and the total quantity to be supplied. This information must be given in figures and in words to prevent alteration. If the prescription implies that the material is to be dispensed in instalments, it must state the amount of each instalment and their intervals.

3 *The markings of bottles, etc. (Regulation 18)* Where a controlled drug in Schedule 2 or 3 is supplied, it must be in a bottle, etc., that is clearly marked either with the amount of drug therein, or the number of dose units and the quantity of drug in each unit.

4 *Drug registers (Regulations 19 and 20)* Anyone authorized to supply Schedule 2 or Schedule 4 drugs must in respect of those drugs keep a register in which are entered in chronological order details of the quantities of drugs both obtained and supplied. Separate registers or a separate part of the register must be kept for each class of drug. (There is no legal requirement that such a register be kept by a sister or acting sister of a ward or other department. However, the Aitken Report recommended that the sister or acting sister should keep such a register and, in practice, this is the case.) The following rules must be observed in maintaining the register:

a Each page should indicate at its head which class of drugs it refers to.
b Entries must be made on the day of the transaction or, where that is impossible, at the very latest on the next day.
c There must be no cancellations, alterations or obliterations. Correction must be made by way of a dated footnote or marginal note.
d All entries must be indelible.
e The register should not be used for any other purpose.
All registers and order forms must be kept for a period of two years from the last date of entry.

5 *Safe custody of controlled drugs (Regulation 3)* All controlled drugs must be kept in a locked safe, cabinet or room constructed and maintained so as to prevent unauthorized entry and the regulations define in detail the required construction of such safes, etc.

Summary Hospital wards and departments are authorized to keep a stock of controlled drugs. These can be obtained by the use of a written order on a special duplicate form, signed by the sister or acting sister in charge of a ward, etc., for safe keeping and use. They can only be given to a patient on a doctor's written prescription, which should, in indelible ink, give the date, the patient's full name, ward and hospital, the preparation's name, strength and dose, and the time at which it is to be given. If the dose is to be repeated, the minimum interval that must elapse between doses must be recorded. All doses are recorded on the prescription sheet and in the stock record book.

Controlled drugs, when supplied to a ward, etc., are signed for by the sister or acting sister in charge of that ward, etc., and are then kept in a locked cupboard reserved for their exclusive use, the key to which is kept by the sister or acting sister in charge of the ward, etc. A record is kept of the stocks and of their individual use. All prescriptions, order forms and record books must be kept for a period of two years from the last date of entry. Surplus stock is returned to the pharmacy for destruction by the appropriate personnel, but expired mixtures may be destroyed in the ward by the sister or acting sister in charge of the ward, if witnessed by a pharmacist. If a fractional dose is given, the surplus is discarded and the fact witnessed and recorded together with the actual amount given to the patient.

The Poisons Act, 1972

This Act deals only with nonmedicinal poisons. However toxic a substance may be, it is not poison for the purpose of this Act if it is not on the Poisons List. The Act deals with four related aspect of poisons control:

1   The establishment of a Poisons Board
2   The listing of controlled poisons
3   The controls of the sale of listed poisons
4   The system of inspection to enforce the provisions of the Act.

Some substances on the Poisons List also have medicinal uses. When sold as medicinal products they are controlled under the Medicines Act, 1968.

The Medicines Act, 1968

This Act covers both human and animal medicines. The Act is comprehensive, covering virtually every possible activity concerned with a medicinal product and also some related areas such as retail pharmacies and the British Pharmacopoeia. In National health Service hospitals, adherence to the Act means that purchase of medicines is normally by a pharmacist or, failing this, by a nurse or doctor. Medicines must be stored in a suitable environment so that they reach the patient in a stable condition. Containers must be labelled according to the law and issued and administered in accordance with a written prescription signed by a doctor or dentist. The adverse use or misuse of medicines is thus prevented by having trained health care professionals involved in their control and administration. The Act may be divided into seven broad categories:

1   The administrative system
2   The licensing system

3   The sale and supply of medicines to the public
4   The retail pharmacies
5   Packing and labelling
6   The promotion of medicines
7   The *British Pharmacopoeia.*

Section II of the licensing system of this Act permits a registered nurse or a certified midwife to assemble a medicinal product without the need for a manufacturer's licence. 'Assembly' is defined as either enclosing a medicinal product with or without other medicinal products of the same description in a container to be labelled before sale or supply or, if already enclosed, labelled before sale or supply.

Types of Medicinal Preparations

The types of drug preparation used in therapeutics can be divided into five main groups, each group having subdivisions within it.

Oral Preparations

Oral liquid preparations must be shaken well to ensure thorough mixing and uniform concentration. If a sediment forms after pouring, it should be stirred immediately before swallowing. Oral preparations should be poured into the appropriate container, on a flat, solid surface, at eye level.

Mixtures   Aqueous solutions or suspensions of drugs in water, together flavouring or suspending agents.

Elixers and Syrups   Clear, flavoured and sometimes sweetened solutions of drugs, often suitable for administration of small doses to children.

Tinctures   Alcoholic solutions of the active principles of crude drugs.

Emulsions   Mixtures of oil in water, rendered homogenous by the addition of other substances known as emulsifying agents.

Linctuses   Sweet, syrup-like preparations of drugs used in the treatment of coughs. They should be sipped and swallowed slowly without dilution.

Tablets   Tablets have the advantage over mixtures of affording an accurate dose. Many tablets are coated to improve stability and appearance and contain additives to ensure disintegration and absorption. In cases where the drug is a gastric irritant or is broken down by gastric acid, an enteric coating may be used. This coating is designed to permit the tablet to pass unchanged into the intestines where absorption takes place. Some long acting tablets contain the drug in the interstices of a porous plastic core from which the active compound is slowly released as the tablet passes along the alimentary tract. Any tablet that is not scored should not be crushed or broken. This is particularly important in the case of cytotoxic drugs as it can lead to contamination. Sublingual, chewable and effervescent tablets are also available.

Capsules   Small containers made of hard gelatin. They are useful as a means of administering drugs with an unpleasant taste and are also popular as containers for orally active antibiotics. Capsules should not be broken or opened.

Lozenges   Lozenges consist of drugs incorporated into a flavoured base and are designed to dissolve slowly in the mouth.

Pastilles   Pastilles are solid products intended to dissolve slowly in the mouth for local treatment of the mouth and throat.

Rectal and Vaginal Preparations

Enemas   Solutions administered into the rectum as laxatives or retention enemas.

Suppositories   Solid pellets for rectal administration. They may contain an active drug and may have a long action, because of slow absorption; alternatively they may permit the use of a drug that has gastric irritant properties, although some may still have a local or systemic effect.

Pessaries   Solid products for vaginal administration and designed to have a local action.

Injections

A preparation intended for injection is a sterile solution, suspension or emulsion of a drug designed for parenteral administration. Injections are used to administer drugs which may be inactive or not tolerated orally or to produce rapid, localized or prolonged action depending on the method of administration. Injections may be prepared for administration by intradermal, subcutaneous, intramuscular, intravenous, intra-arterial, intrathecal or intra-articular routes. The intramuscular route is employed for most injections as absorption is fairly rapid.

Subcutaneous Injections   These are given into the highly vascular layer beneath the epidermis and drugs are fairly rapidly absorbed by this route.

Intradermal Injections   These are mainly for diagnostic tests.

Intravenous Injections   These range from small volume direct drug administration to large volume infusions.

Intrathecal Injections   These may be used when the drug concerned does not penetrate the blood/brain barrier.

Intra-articular Injection   This term refers to the injection of a solution into a joint.

Intra-arterial Injections   These are given directly into an artery for peripheral conditions.

Subconjunctival Injection   Some drugs may be given by this procedure in ophthalmology.

Topical Applications

Topical applications comprise a wide range of products intended for local application to the body and include the following:

Creams   Semisolid emulsions containing a high proportion of water. Creams are used where a highly occlusive effect is not required and bland creams are applied for their emollient, cooling or moistening effects.

Liniments   Thin creams or oily preparations of drugs applied to the skin by rubbing. They should not be applied to broken skin.

Lotions   Solutions or suspensions of drugs for application to the skin, wounds or mucous membranes.

Ointments   Semisolid preparations intended for application to the skin.

Pastes   Stiff ointments often containing large amounts of powdered ingredients, e.g. zinc oxide.

Collodions   Collodions are painted on to the skin and allowed to dry to leave a flexible film over the site of application. They may be used to seal cuts or to hold a dissolved drug in contact with the skin for a prolonged period of time.

Gels   Semisolid or solid preparations made using a suitable gelling agent. This term may also be applied to viscous suspensions for oral use, e.g. aluminium hydroxide gel.

Paints   Liquid preparations for application with a brush to the skin or mucous surfaces. The vehicle may evaporate, leaving a film of drug on the skin.

Inhalations

Inhalation once referred solely to the inhalation of volatile constituents of such products as tincture of benzoin. Modern inhalation products are chiefly bronchodilators presented for oral inhalation as aerosols. These aerosols contain a metered dose of the drug in solution in a pressurized container with an inert gas as the propellant. When the pressure is released, the dose is discharged as a fine spray which, if inhaled orally, is carried deep into the lungs. The lung surface area available for absorption is so large that the response to a dose is almost as rapid as that following an injection.

Solutions

Solutions are liquid preparations containing one or more ingredients, usually dissolved in water. They may be sterile or nonsterile. For example, aqueous solutions or antiseptics and solutions for internal administration are usually nonsterile. Injections are an example of sterile solutions.

Lipsomes

A recent development in the administration of drugs is by the use of lipsomes. These are small vesicles, bounded by layers of phospholipids, glycolipids or other substances, depending on the method of manufacture. Small quantities of drug can be encapsulated in these lipsomes. This permits the use of smaller doses, a decrease in toxicity and rapidity of degradation and the possibility of achieving a localizing effect on a target organ or tissue. Lipsome-encapsulated drugs are not commercially available at the time of writing.

Adamson (1978) gives a useful outline of the ways in which medical preparations are formulated in the United Kingdom.

Storage

Certain principles may be discerned when discussing the storage of medicinal preparations. Those relating to controlled drugs and scheduled poisons have been mentioned above.

All medicinal preparations should be stored in locked cupbards and kept under conditions which conform with any applicable requirements and any manufacturers' recommendations. Labels should be legible and firmly attached. Contents should never be transferred from one container to another. Stocks should be checked regularly. Ideally, pharmacists should check ward stocks routinely. Excessive stocks are wasteful and dangerous in that most drugs deteriorate with storage. Expiry dates must be noted and the preparation returned to the pharmacy. Controlled drugs and scheduled poisons must be checked in the presence of a witness at frequent intervals according to hospital policy (daily, weekly) and any discrepency reported to the appropriate senior nurse.

General recommendations for storage of preparations appear in the *British Pharmacopoeia Codex:*

1 *Aerosol preparations* require storage away from heat and sunlight.
2 *Creams* may deteriorate under the influence of temperature change and to avoid bacterial contamination should not be kept longer than 14 days after dilution.
3 *Eye drops* should not be used for more than 1 month after opening at home or for much shorter periods when used in hospital.
4 *Mixtures* may be less stable after dilution than the undiluted preparations.
5 *Tablets* need physical protection to prevent breakage, although sugar coating may prevent many of the effects of light and moisture. Effervescent tablets should be stored dry and dispensed in their original container.
6 *Capsules* need cool storage to avoid untoward changes in the gelatin component.

The *British National Formulary* gives guidance on the storage of individual preparations. The term 'a cool place' means one with a temperature of not more than 15°C (but above freezing point) and 'room temperature' a range from 15 to 25°C.

1   *Antibiotic injections or mixtures*   have a limited shelf life after reconstitution and most are best kept between 2 and 10°C, e.g. in a domestic refrigerator but not a deep freeze. Some injections must be used immediately after reconstitution, while for others the *British National Formulary* recommends precise limitations on storage.

2   *Corticosteroid preparations* may be particularly sensitive to light. Ultraviolet light and fluorescent lighting degrade prednisolone in solution and serious deficiencies in commercial hydrocortisone creams and lotions have also been noted.

3   *Bacterial vaccines, toxoids and toxins*   deteriorate at temperatures approaching 20°C, and should be portected from light at a temperature of 2-10°C (but not frozen).

4   *Viral and rickettsial vaccines*   require similar storage conditions to those for bacterial vaccines; their shelf life varies from, for example, 18 months for influenza vaccine to 14 days for smallpox vaccine. Improper handling of measles vaccine is probably an important cause of vaccine failure, as it also used to be with smallpox vaccine.

Manufacturers' data sheets for many products give specific recommendations on storage.

Table 12.1 lists those drugs which may be particularly susceptible to deterioration under adverse storage conditions (e.g. strong light or heat) and includes those which meet most emergency needs in general practice.

Table 12.1   Drugs particularly susceptible to deterioration

Adrenaline solution	Idoxuridine solution
Aminophylline suppositories	Insulin solution
Asprin tablets	Isoprenaline tablets and solution
Choline theophyllinate tablets	Nystatin, all formulations
Diamorphine solution	Oxytocin, all formulations
Ergometrine solution	Paraldehyde (store in complete darkness)
Ergotamine solution	Phenylephrine solution
Glyceryl trinitrate tablets	Sulphacetamide solution
Heparin solution	Suxamethonium solution

For scheduled poisons, a standard locked drug cupboard is recommended which contains a small inner cupboard with a separate lock and key for controlled drugs. Some cupboards have a red warning light which is turned on whenever the main door is open. A standard locked medicine trolley that can be taken to the patient's bedside is recommended for storage of preparations in current use. It is common practice for individual prescriptions to be dispensed in containers marked with the patient's name, the drug and the quantity. The trolley should be secured with a lock and chain when not in use, preferably in the ward nursing office.

Administration

The effective and safe administration of drugs to patients demands a partnership between the various health professionals concerned, i.e. doctors, pharmacists and nurses. The nurse is responsible for the correct administration of prescribed drugs to patients in his/her care. To achieve this the nurse must have a sound knowledge of the use, action, usual dose and side effects of the drugs being administered. Various studies have shown that this is not always the case. Markowitz et al. (1981) came to the conclusion that not only nurses but doctors and pharmacists in the survey hospital needed to upgrade their knowledge of the drugs they prescribed or administered. They then went on to suggest that inadequate practitioner knowledge may contribute to the incidence of preventable adverse drug reactions in hospitals. Francis (1980) examined the number of 'hidden', i.e. undeclared, medication errors committed by nurses. In the survey hospital it was found that nurses made ten times more of such errors than they reported.

Observation of the patient receiving medication is important. No drug produces a single effect. The combined effect of two or more drugs taken together may be different from the effects when taken separately. The effectiveness of any drug should be noted and any signs of resistance or dependence reported. Side effects may vary from slight symptoms to severe reaction and any signs must be brought to the attention of the appropriate personnel.

The nurse must also be aware of the hazards involved in handling drugs, detergents and alcohols. Nurses Action Group (1981) attempts to highlight some hazards and offers advice on how nurses should protect themselves from some of the more common preparations found in hospitals.

Wherever possible, patients should be encouraged to be responsible for storing and administering their own medication. Falconer (1971), in her study, found that patients were able to cope proficiently with the administration of their medication. Even mildly confused patients, who were, initially, judged to be unsuitable for self-medication, were able to become independent after a period of instruction and supervision. Roberts (1978), in her study of self-medication in the elderly, reported that no patient took another's medication. Most patients kept their medicines in handbags or other places of safety. The common factor among those who failed to comply was that of ingnoring the tablets altogether. There was no evidence of overdosage.

Injections

Injection is defined as the act of giving medication by use of a syringe and needle.

Newton and Newton (1979) identify eight routes for the use of parenteral injection:

1	Intra-arterial	5	Intralesional
2	Intra-articular	6	Intramuscular
3	Intracardiac	7	Intravenous
4	Intradermal	8	Subcutaneous

Intrathecal routes are employed when the prescribed drug is unable to cross the blood/brain barrier. These authors also include a useful table of the tissues, sites and types of needle used, the amount of medication usually injected and the medications commonly administered via these routes.

Sites of Injection

Site selection is predetermined for intra-arterial, intra-articular, intracardiac, intralesional and intrathecal injections. The choice of the remaining sites will normally depend on the desired therapeutic effect and the patient's safety and comfort.

Intradermal   Chosen sites are the ventral forearms and the scapulae. Observation of an inflammatory reaction is a priority, so the best sites are those that are highly pigmented, thinly keratinized and hairless.

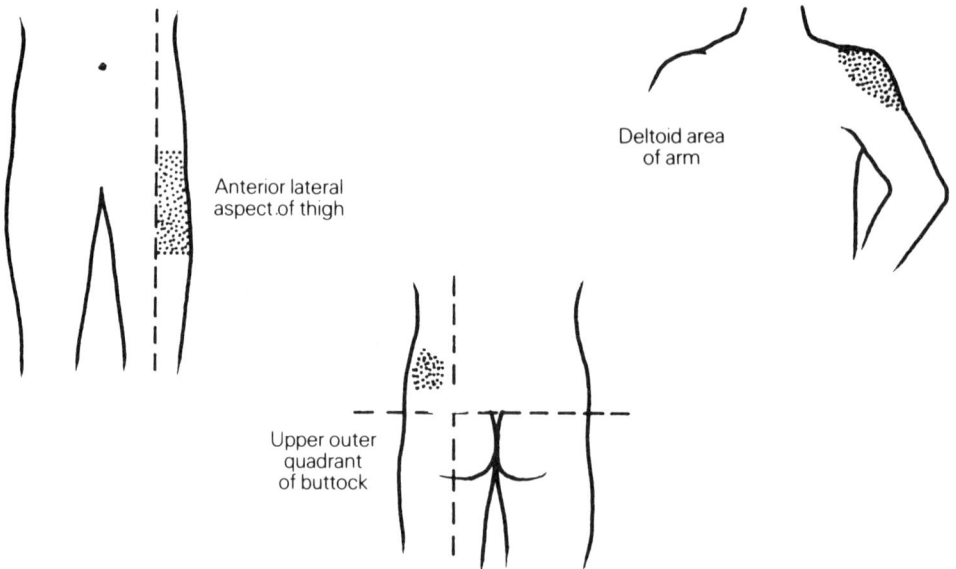

Figure 12.1   Sites for intramuscular injections

Subcutaneous Chosen sites are the lateral aspects of the upper arms, and thighs, the abdomen in the umbilical region, the back and the lower loins. Slow absorption is a priority so ideal sites are those poorly supplied with sensory nerves. Rotation of these sites decreases the likelihood of irritation and ensures improved absorption.

Intramuscular Intramuscular injections are given at five sites (see Figure 12.1):

1 *Mid-deltoid* Used for the injection of such drugs as narcotics, sedatives, absorbed tetanus toxoid, vaccines, epinephrine in oil and vitamin B_{12}. It has the advantage of being easily accessible whether the patient is standing, sitting or lying down. It is also a better site than the gluteal muscles for small volume (less than 2 ml) rapid onset injections. Because the area is small, it limits the number and size of the injections that can be given at this point.

2 *Gluteus medius* Used for deep intramuscular and Z-track injections. The gluteus muscle has the lowest drug absorption rate. The muscle mass is also likely to have atrophied in elderly, nonambulent and emaciated patients. This site carries with it the danger of the needle hitting the sciatic nerve and the superior gluteal arteries.

3 *Gluteus minimus* Used for antibiotics, antiemetics, deep intramuscular and Z-track injections in oil, narcotics and sedatives. It is best used when large volume intramuscular injections are required and for injections in the elderly, nonambulant and emaciated patient as the site is away from major nerves and vascular structures.

4 *Rectus femoris* Used for antiemetics, narcotics, sedatives, injections in oil, deep intramuscular and Z-track injections. It is the preferred site for infants and for self-administration of injections.

5 *Vastus lateralis* Used for deep intramuscular and Z-track injections. This site is free from major nerves and blood vessels. It is a large muscle and can accommodate repeated injections.

Skin preparation

McConnell (1982) quotes the two most common solutions for preparing the skin for injection as ethyl alcohol and the iodophors, such as povidone iodine (Betadine). If using the iodophors, the nurse must check beforehand that the patient is not allergic to iodine. An iodophor must not be used to prepare the skin for an intradermal injection as the solution discolours the skin and this makes it difficult to assess any expected reaction.

When cleaning the skin, the use of friction together with a circular motion is recommended. The nurse should begin at the centre of the chosen site and progress outwards. The antiseptic must be allowed to dry thoroughly before injection, otherwise the antiseptic may be forced into the tissue with the injection.

Recent research, however, has questioned the value of skin preparation prior to injection. Dann (1969) has shown that there is no experimental evidence that skin bacteria are introduced into the deeper tissues by injection, thereby causing infection. Antiseptics in current use cannot act in the time allowed in practice (5 seconds on average) and cannot possibly cause complete sterility. Over a period of 6 years, during which time more than 5000 injections were given to unselected patients via all the injection routes, without using any form of skin preparation, no single case of local and/or systemic infection was reported. Only before injections where strict asepsis is needed, as in intrathecal or intra-articular injections, is skin preparation required. Koivistov and Felig (1978) carried out a survey into the need for skin preparation before giving an insulin injection and found that skin preparation did reduce skin bacterial count but was not necessary to prevent infection at the injection site.

Needle Bevel

Three categories of needle bevel are available:

1 *Regular* For all intramuscular and subcutaneous injections.
2 *Intradermal* For diagnostic injections and other injections into the epidermis.
3 *Short* Tends to be used rarely. It is recommended only for transferring medication from container to syringe.

Needle Size

Lenz (1983) states that when choosing the correct needle length for intramuscular injections it is important to assess the muscle mass of the injection site, the amount of subcutaneous fat and the weight of the patient. Without such an assessment, most injections intended for gluteal muscle are deposited in gluteal fat. The following are suggested by the author as ways of determining the most suitable size of needle to use:

Deltoid and vastus lateralis muscles The muscle to be used should be grasped between thumb and forefinger to determine the depth of the muscle mass or the amount of subcutaneous fat at the injection site. One half of the distance between thumb and forefinger will be the appropriate length of the needle required to penetrate into that muscle.

Gluteal muscles The layer of fat and skin above the muscle should be gently lifted with the thumb and forefinger for the same reasons as before. Use the patient's weight to calculate the needle length required. Lenz recommends the following guide:

31.5 - 40 kg	2.5 cm needle
40.5 - 90 kg	5 - 7.5 cm needle
90+ kg	10 - 15 cm needle

Injections and Pain

McConnell (1982) and Newton and Newton (1979) set out, in point form, techniques which may reduce the discomfort experienced by the patient. Kruszewski et al. (1979) focus on ways in which positioning can help to minimize pain. Field (1981), in an interesting article, attempts to answer the question what it is like to give an injection and goes on to explore the meaning and use of language relating to injections, the feelings involved in preparing and administering injections, and the meaning of the patient's response to the nurse.

Intravenous Drug Administration

The administration of intravenous medications is an area where the role of the nurse is being increasingly extended. For further information, see the procedure on intravenous drug administration (pages 213-222).

Intra-arterial Drug Administration

Injection of drugs into an artery is a rare and hazardous procedure. The introduction of the cannula or catheter must be performed with care as the vessel may go into spasm, causing pain and occlusion. This could result in necrosis of an organ or part of a limb. Injection of irritant chemicals increases the risk of spasm and its sequentiae. In patients with some forms of cancer, however, arterial catheterization is occasionally performed when it is desirable to deliver a high concentration of a drug to a tumour mass. The most common procedures are catheterization of the hepatic artery and isolated limb perfusion.

References and Further Reading

Adamson L (1978) Control of medicines in the UK, Nursing Times 74: 973-975

Bayliss P F C (1980) Law on Poisons, Medicines and Related Substances, 3rd edition, Ravenswood Publications

Central Health Services Council (1958) Report of Joint Sub-Committee on the Control of Dangerous Drugs and Poisons in Hospitals. Chairman J K Aitken, HMSO

Dale J R Appelbe G E (1979) Pharmacy, Law and Ethics, 2nd edition, The Pharmaceutical Press

Dann T C (1969) Routine skin preparation before injection: an unnecessary procedure, Lancet ii: 96-97

Dorr R Fritz W (1980) Cancer Chemotherapy Handbook, Kimpton

Drugs and Therapeutics Bulletin (1977) Storage and shelf life of drugs: when is it important? Drugs and Therapeutics Bulletin 15 (21): 81-83

Falconer M (1971) Self administered medication, Hospital Administration in Canada 13 (5): 28-30

Field P A (1981) A phenomenological look at giving an injection, Journal of Advanced Nursing 6 (4): 291-296

Fink J L (1983) Preventing lawsuits, Nursing Life 3 (2): 27-29

Francis G (1980) Nurses' medication 'errors': a new perspective, Supervisor Nurse 11 (8): 11-13

Hopkins S J (1983) Drugs and Pharmacology for Nurses, 8th edition, Churchill Livingstone, pp. 13-17

King E M et al. (1981) Illustrated Manual of Nursing Techniques, 2nd edition, J B Lippincott, pp. 331-337

Koivistov V A Felig P (1978) Is skin preparation necessary before insulin injection? Lancet i: 1072-1073

Kruszewski A Z et al. (1979) Effect of positioning on discomfort from intramuscular injections in the dorsogluteal site, Nursing Research 28 (2): 103-105

Lenz C L (1983) Make your needle selection right to the point, Nursing (US) 13 (2): 50-51

Loebl S et al. (1980) The Nurse's Drug Handbook, 2nd edition, John Wiley, pp. 10-22

Lydiate P W H (1977) The Law Relating to the Misuse of Drugs, Butterworth

McConnell E A (1982) The subtle art of really good injections, Research Nurse 45 (2): 25-34

Markowitz J S et al. (1981) Nurses, physicians, and pharmacists: their knowledge of hazards of medication, Nursing Research 30 (6): 366-370

Marks M (no date) Neoplatin Cisplatin: A Nurse's Guide, Mead Johnson, p. 7

Newton D W Newton M (1979) Route, site and technique: three key decisions in giving parenteral injections, Nursing (US) 9 (7): 18-25

Nurses Action Group (1981) Health and safety 3. Beware the drug, Nursing Mirror 152: 22-25

Pearson R M Nestor P (1977) Drug interactions, Nursing Mirror 145: Supplement XI

Roberts R (1978) Self medication trial for the elderly, Nursing Times 74 (23): 976-977

Thomas S (1979) Practical nursing — medicines: care and adminstration, Nursing Mirror 148: 28-30

Wade A (1980) Pharmaceuticals Handbook, 19th edition, Pharmaceuticals Press

Whincup M H (1982) Legal Rights and Duties in Medical and Nursing Service, 3rd edition, Ravenswood Publications

GUIDELINES: ORAL DRUG ADMINISTRATION

Equipment

1 Medicine trolley
2 Jug of water
3 Tumblers
4 Graduated medicine containers
5 Bowl with warm soapy water
6 Roll of paper towel
7 Disposable waste bag
8 Two spoons

Procedure

Action	Rationale
1 Wash your hands.	1 To prevent cross-infection.
2 Ensure that the medicine trolley is prepared before beginning the procedure.	2 To prevent interruption of the procedure once it has begun.
3 Carry out the procedure in the company of another nurse. One nurse should be a qualified nurse. The other nurse, preferably, should be a student.	3 To minimize error. To create a learning situation.
4 Before administering any presribed drug, check that it is due and has not been given already. Check that the information contained in the prescription chart is complete, correct and legible.	4 To protect the patient from harm.
5 Select the required medication and check the expiry date.	5 Treatment with medication that is outside the expiry date is dangerous. Drugs deteriorate with storage. The expiry date indicates when a particular drug is no longer pharmacologically efficacious.
6 Empty the required dose into a medicine container. Avoid touching the preparation.	6 To prevent cross-infection. To prevent harm to the nurse.
7 Take the medication and the prescription chart to the patient. Check the patient's identity and the dose to be given.	7 To prevent error.
8 Evaluate the patient's knowledge of the medication being offered. If this knowledge appears to be faulty or incorrect, offer an explanation of the use, action, dose and potential side effects of the drug or drugs involved.	8 A patient has a right to information about treatment.
9 Administer the drug as prescribed.	
10 Offer a glass of water, if allowed, to facilitate swallowing the medication.	
11 Record the dose given in the prescription chart and in any other place made necessary by legal requirement or hospital policy.	11 To meet legal requirements and hospital policy.

Action	Rationale
12 Place the used medicine container and tumbler in the bowl of warm, soapy water.	
13 Administer irritating drugs with meals or snacks.	13 To minimize their effect on the gastric mucosa.
14 Administer drugs that interfere with foods, or drugs destroyed in significant proportions by digestive enzymes, between meals or on an empty stomach.	14 To prevent interference with the absorption of the drug.
15 Do not break a tablet unless it is scored. Break scored tablets with a file.	15 Breaking may cause incorrect dosage, gastrointestinal irritation or destruction of a drug in an incompatible pH.
16 Do not interfere with time release capsules and enteric coated tablets. Instruct patients to swallow these whole and not to chew them.	16 The absorption rate of the drug will be altered.
17 Sublingual tablets must be placed under the tongue and buccal tablets between gum and cheek.	17 To allow for correct absorption.

Controlled Drugs

1 Two nurses must be involved in the administration of a controlled drug, one of whom must be a registered general nurse.	1 To comply with the legal obligations and hospital policy.
2 Select the correct drug from the controlled drug cupboard.	
3 Check the stock against the last entry in the ward record book.	
4 Check the appropriate dose against the prescription sheet.	
5 Return the remaining stock to the cupboard and lock the cupboard.	
6 Enter the date and the patient's name in the ward record book.	
7 Take the prepared dose to the patient, whose identity is checked.	
8 Administer the drug after checking the prescription chart again. Once the drug has been administered, the prescription chart is signed by the nurse responsible for administering the medication.	

Action	Rationale

9 The dose, time of administration and the signatures of the two nurses are entered against the patient's name in the ward record book.

GUIDELINES: ADMINISTRATION OF INJECTIONS

Equipment

1   Sterile tray or receiver in which to place drug and equipment
2   19g needle(s) to ease reconstitution and drawing up
3   21, 23 or 25g needle, size dependent on route of administration
4   Syringe(s) of appropriate size for amount of drug to be given
5   Swabs saturated with isopropyl alcohol 70%
6   Sterile topical swab, if drug is presented in ampoule form
7   Sterile wool balls, if drug is presented in vial or dry powder form
8   Drug(s) to be administered
9   Patient's prescription chart, to check dose, route, etc.
10 Recording sheet or book as required by law or hospital policy
11 Any protective clothing required by hospital policy for specific drugs, such as antibiotics or cytotoxic drugs.

Procedure

Action	Rationale
1 Collect and check all equipment.	1 To prevent delays and enable full concentration on the procedure.
2 Check that the packaging of all equipment is intact.	2 To ensure sterility. If seal is damaged discard.
3 Wash your hands.	3 To prevent contamination of medication and equipment.
4 Prepare needle(s), syringe(s), etc., on a tray or receiver.	
5 Inspect all equipment.	5 To check that none is damaged; if so discard.
6 Consult the patient's prescription sheet, and ascertain the following: **a** Drug **b** Dose **c** Date and time of administration **d** Route and method of administration **e** Diluent as appropriate **f** Validity of prescription **g** Signature of doctor.	6 To ensure that the patient is given the correct drug in the prescribed dose using the appropriate diluent and by the correct route.

Action	**Rationale**
7 Check all details with another nurse.	7 To minimize any risk of error.
8 Select the drug in the appropriate size of container, and check the expiry date.	8 To reduce wastage. To prevent an ineffective or toxic compound being administered to the patient.
9 Proceed with the preparation of the drug, using protective clothing if advisable.	

Single Dose Ampoule: Solution

1 Inspect the solution for cloudiness or particulate matter. If this is present, discard and follow hospital guidelines on what action to take, e.g. return drug to pharmacy.	1 To prevent the patient from receiving an unstable or contaminated drug.
2 Tap the neck of the ampoule gently.	2 To ensure that all the solution is in the bottom of the ampoule.
3 Cover the neck of the ampoule with a sterile topical swab and snap it open. If there is any difficulty a file may be required.	3 To aid asepsis. To prevent aerosol formation or contact with the drug which could lead to a sensitivity reaction. To prevent injury to the nurse.
4 Inspect the solution for glass fragments; if present, discard.	4 To prevent injection of foreign matter into the patient.
5 Withdraw the required amount of solution, tilting the ampoule if necessary.	5 To avoid drawing in any air.
6 Replace the guard on the needle and tap the syringe to dislodge any air bubbles. Expel air.	6 To prevent aerosol formation, etc. To ensure that the correct amount of drug is in the syringe.
7 Alternatives to expelling the air with the needle guard in place include the following: **a** Covering the needle tip with sterile cotton wool or topical swab **b** Using the ampoule or vial to receive any air and/or drug.	
8 Change the needle.	8 To reduce the risk of infection. To avoid tracking medications through superficial tissues. To ensure that the correct size of needle is used for the injection.

Action	Rationale

Single Dose Ampoule: Powder

1 Tap the neck of the ampoule gently.

2 Cover the neck of the ampoule with a sterile topical swab and snap it open. If there is any difficulty a file may be required.

3 Add the correct diluent carefully down the wall of the ampoule.

4 Agitate the ampoule and inspect the contents.

5 When the solution is clear withdraw the prescribed amount, tilting the ampoule if necessary.

6 Replace the guard on the needle and tap the syringe to dislodge any air bubbles. Expel air.

7 Change the needle.

Rationale

1 To ensure that any powder lodged here falls to the bottom of the ampoule.

2 To aid asepsis. To prevent contact with the drug which could cause a sensitivity reaction. To prevent injury to the nurse.

3 To ensure that the powder is throughly wet before agitation and is not released into the atmosphere.

4 To dissolve the drug.
To detect any glass fragments or particulate matter. If present, continue agitation or discard as appropriate.

5 To avoid drawing in air.

6 To prevent aerosol formation, etc. To ensure that the correct amount of drug is in the syringe.

7 To reduce the risk of infection. To avoid tracking medications though superficial tissues. To ensure that the correct size of needle is used for the injection.

Multidose Vial: Solution

1 Inspect the solution for cloudiness or particulate matter. If this is present, discard. Follow hospital guidelines on what action to take, e.g. return drug to pharmacy.

2 Clean the rubber cap with the chosen antiseptic and let it dry.

3 Insert a 19g needle into the cap to vent the bottle (Figure 12.2a).

4 Withdraw the prescribed amount of solution, and inspect for pieces of rubber which may have 'cored out' of the cap (Figure 12.2b)

Rationale

1 To prevent patient from receiving an unstable or contaminated drug.

2 To prevent bacterial contamination of the drug.

3 To prevent pressure differentials which can cause separation of needle and syringe.

4 To prevent the injection of foreign matter into the patient.

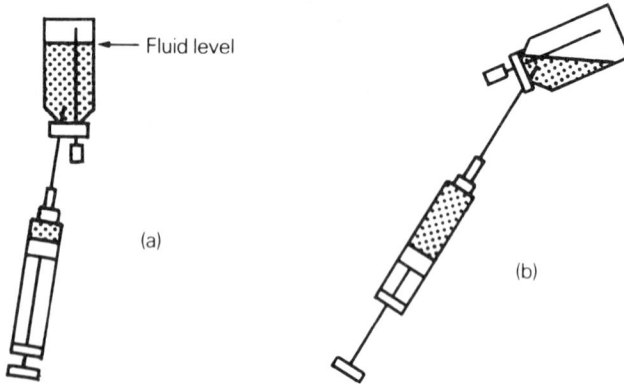

Fluid level

(a)

(b)

Figure 12.2 a To remove reconstituted solution, insert syringe needle then invert vial. Ensuring that tip of second needle is above fluid, withdraw the solution. **b** Remove air from syringe without spraying into the atmosphere by injecting air back into vial

Action

Rationale

Note: Coring can be minimized by inserting the needle into the cap, bevel up, at an angle of 45-60°. Before complete insertion of the needle tip, lift the needle to 90° and proceed (Figure 12.3).

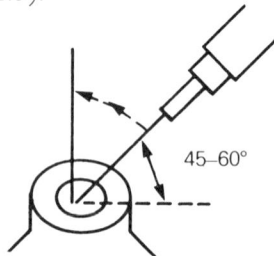

45–60°

Figure 12.3 Method to minimize coring

5 Replace the guard on the needle and tap the syringe to dislodge any air bubbles. Expel air.

6 Change the needle.

5 To prevent aerosol formation. To ensure that the correct amount of drug is in the syringe.

6 To reduce the risk of infection. To avoid possible trauma to the patient if the needle has barbed. To avoid tracking medications through superficial tissues. To ensure that the correct size of needle is used for the injection.

Action	**Rationale**

Multidose Vial: Powder

1 Clean the rubber cap with the chosen antiseptic and let it dry.

2 Insert a 19g needle into the cap to vent the bottle (Figure 12.4a).

3 Add the correct diluent carefully down the wall of the vial.

4 Remove the needle and the syringe.

5 Place a sterile wool ball over the venting needle (Figure 12.4b).

1 To prevent bacterial contamination of the drug.

2 To prevent pressure differentials, which can cause separation of needle and syringe.

3 To ensure that the powder is thoroughly wet before it is shaken and is not released into the atmosphere.

5 To prevent contamination of the drug or the atmosphere.

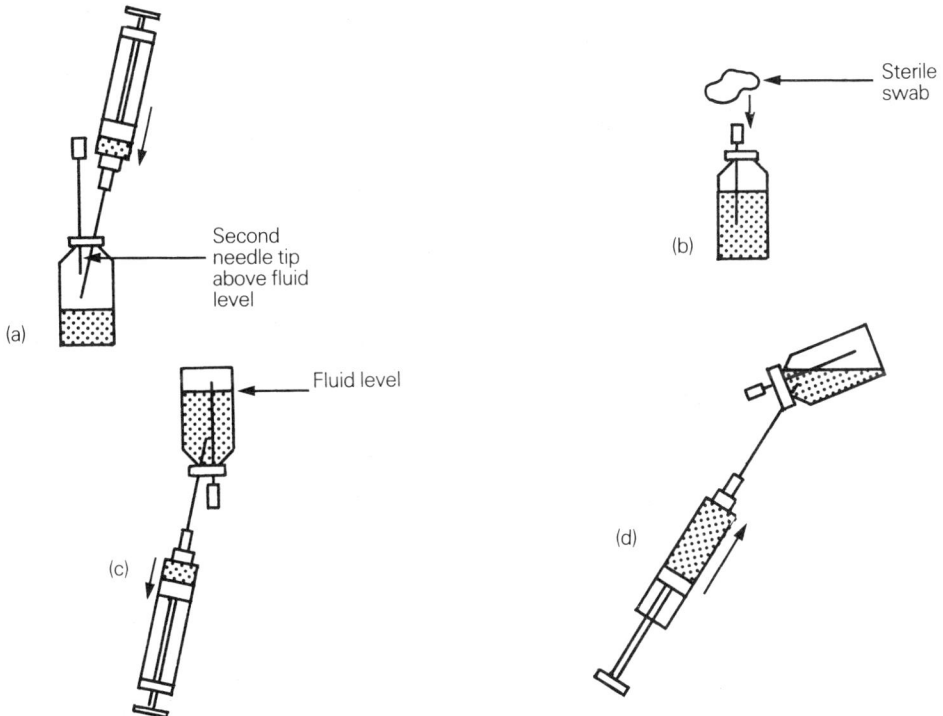

Figure 12.4 Suggested method of vial reconstitution to avoid environmental exposure. **a** When reconstituting vial, insert a second needle to allow air to escape when adding diluent for injection. **b** When shaking the vial to dissolve the powder, push in second needle up to luer connection and cover with a sterile swab. **c** To remove reconstituted solution, insert syringe needle then invert vial. Ensuring that tip of second needle is above the fluid, withdraw the solution. **d** Remove air from syringe without spraying into the atmosphere by injecting air back into vial

Action	**Rationale**
6 Shake well and inspect the contents.	6 To dissolve the drug. To detect any particulate matter or rubber pieces.
7 When the solution is clear, clean the rubber cap and withdraw the prescribed amount (Figure 12.4c, d).	
8 Inspect again for pieces of rubber which may have been 'cored out' of the cap.	8 To prevent injection of foreign matter into the patient.
Note: Coring can be minimized by inserting the needle into the cap bevel up at an angle of 45-60°. Before complete insertion of the needle tip, lift the needle to 90° and proceed. (See Figure 12.3.)	
9 Replace the guard on the needle and tap the syringe to dislodge any air bubbles. Expel air.	9 To prevent aerosol formation. To ensure that the correct amount of drug is in the syringe.
10 Change the needle.	10 To reduce the risk of infection. To avoid possible trauma to the patient if the needle has barbed. To avoid tracking medications through superficial tissues. To ensure that the correct size of needle is used for the injection.
11 Label any amount remaining in a multidose vial, and add the date of reconstitution if appropriate.	11 To encourage economy. To ensure that the drug is discarded when the expiry date is passed.
12 Discard any waste, making sure that it is placed in the correct containers, e.g. 'sharps' into a designated receptacle.	12 To ensure safe disposal and to avoid laceration or other injury to staff. After the injection, needle and syringe must also be safely disposed of for the above reasons and to prevent reuse of equipment.
13 Check again that the amount of drug in the syringe corresponds with the patient's prescription chart.	
14 Check that all the necessary equipment is in the tray or receiver with the correct gauge of needle, etc.	

Action	**Rationale**

15 Proceed to the patient.

Note: The nurse may encounter other presentations of drugs for injection, e.g. vials with a transfer needle, and should follow the manufacturer's instructions in these instances.

Subcutaneous Injections

Action	Rationale
1 Explain the procedure to the patient.	1 To obtain the patient's consent and cooperation.
2 Assist the patient into the required position.	
3 Expose the chosen site.	
4 Choose the correct needle size.	4 To minimize the risk of missing the subcutaneous tissue and any ensuing pain.
5 Clean the chosen site with a swab saturated with isopropyl alcohol 70%.	5 To reduce the number of pathogens introduced into the skin by the needle at the time of insertion. (For further information on this action see the relevant material in the Reference Materials section, pages 128-141.)
6 Grasp the skin firmly.	6 To elevate the subcutaneous tissue.
7 Insert the needle into the skin at an angle of 45° and release the grasped skin.	7 Injecting medication into compressed tissue irritates nerve fibres and causes the patient discomfort.
8 Pull back the plunger. If no blood is aspirated, depress the plunger and inject the drug slowly. If blood appears, withdraw the needle, replace it and begin again. Explain to the patient what has occurred.	8 To confirm that the needle is in the correct position. To prevent pain and ensure even distribution of the drug.
9 Withdraw the needle rapidly. Apply pressure to any bleeding point.	9 To prevent haematoma formation.
10 Record in the appropriate documents that the injection has been given.	
11 Dispose of the equipment in the required fashion.	11 To ensure safe disposal and to avoid laceration or other injury to staff.

Action	**Rationale**

Intramuscular Injections

1 Explain the procedure to the patient.	1 To obtain the patient's consent and cooperation.
2 Assist the patient into the required position.	
3 Expose the chosen site.	
4 Clean the chosen site with a swab saturated with ispopropyl alcohol 70%.	4 To reduce the number of pathogens introduced into the skin by the needle at the time of insertion. (For further information on this action see the relevant material the Reference Materials section, pages 128-141.)
5 Stretch the skin around the chosen site.	5 To facilitate the insertion of the needle and to displace the subcutaneous tissue.
6 Holding the needle at an angle of 90°, quickly plunge it into the skin. Leave a third of the shaft of the needle exposed.	6 To ensure that the needle penetrates the muscle. To facilitate removal of the needle should it break.
7 Pull back the plunger. If no blood is aspirated, depress the plunger and inject the drug slowly. If blood appears, withdraw the needle, replace it and begin again. Explain to the patient what has occurred.	7 To confirm that the needle is in the correct position. To prevent pain and ensure even distribution of the drug.
8 Withdraw the needle rapidly. Apply pressure to any bleeding point.	8 To prevent haematoma formation.
9 Record in the appropriate documents that the injection has been given.	
10 Dispose of the equipment in the required fashion.	10 To ensure safe disposal and to avoid laceration or other injury to staff.

GUIDELINES: ADMINISTRATION OF RECTAL AND VAGINAL PREPARATIONS

Equipment

1 Disposable glove
2 Topical swabs
3 Lubricating jelly
4 Prescription chart

Procedure

Action **Rationale**

Rectal Preparations

For further information about the administration of rectal medication see the relevant sections of procedure on bowel care (pages 62-67).

Vaginal Pessaries

Action	Rationale
1 Explain the procedure to the patient.	1 To obtain the patient's consent and cooperation.
2 Select the appropriate pessary and check it with the prescription chart and another nurse.	2 To ensure that the correct medication is given to the correct patient at the appropriate time.
3 Assist the patient into the appropriate position, either left lateral with buttocks to the edge of the bed or supine with knees drawn up and legs parted.	3 To facilitate the correct insertion of the pessary.
4 Wash your hands and put on gloves.	4 To prevent cross-infection.
5 Apply lubricating jelly to a topical swab and from the swab on to the pessary.	5 To facilitate insertion of the pessary and ensure the patient's comfort.
6 Insert the pessary along the posterior vaginal wall and into the top of the vagina. *Note:* This procedure is best performed late in the evening when the patient is unlikely to get out of bed.	6 To ensure that the pessary is retained and that the medication can reach its maximum efficiency.
7 Wipe away any excess lubricating jelly from the patient's vulval and/or perineal area with a topical swab.	7 To promote patient comfort.
8 Make the patient comfortable and apply a fresh sanitary pad.	8 To absorb any excess discharge.
9 Record in the appropriate documents that the pessary has been given.	

GUIDELINES: TOPICAL APPLICATIONS OF DRUGS

Equipment

1 Flat wooden spatulae
2 Sterile topical swabs
3 Applicators

Procedure

Action	Rationale
1 Explain the procedure to the patient.	1 To obtain the patient's consent and cooperation.
2 Use aseptic technique if the skin is broken.	2 To prevent local or systemic infection.
3 Remove semisolid or stiff preparations from their containers with a flat wooden spatula. Use a different spatula each time if more of the preparation is required.	3 To prevent cross-infection.
4 If the medication is to be rubbed into the skin, the preparation should be placed on a sterile topical swab. The wearing of gloves may be necessary.	4 To prevent cross-infection. To protect the nurse.
5 If the preparation causes staining, advise the patient of this.	5 To ensure that adequate pre-cautions are taken beforehand and to prevent unwanted stains.

GUIDELINES: ADMINISTRATION OF DRUGS IN OTHER FORMS

Procedure

Action	Rationale

Inhalations

1 Seat the patient in an upright position if possible.	1 To permit full expansion of the diaphragm.
2 Administer only one drug at a time unless specifically instructed to the contrary.	2 Several drugs used together may cause undesirable reactions or they may inactivate each other.
3 Measure any liquid medication with a syringe.	3 To ensure the correct dose.
4 Clean any equipment used after use.	4 To prevent infection.

Gargles

1 Throat irrigations should not be warmer than 49 °C.	1 Any liquid warmer than 49 °C will destroy or damage tissue.

Nasal Drops

1 Have paper tissues available.	1 To wipe away secretions and/or medication.

Action	**Rationale**
2 Clean the patient's nasal passages.	2 To ensure maximum penetration for the medication.
3 Hyperextend the patient's neck.	3 To obtain the best position for insertion of the medication.
4 Avoid touching the external nares with the dropper.	4 To prevent the patient from sneezing.
5 Request the patient to maintain his/her position for 1-2 minutes.	5 To ensure full absorption of the medication.
6 Each patient should have his/her own medication and dropper.	6 To prevent cross-infection.

Eye Medications

For further information see the procedure on eye care (pages 170-175).

Ear Drops

1 Ask the patient to lie on his/her side with the ear to be treated uppermost.	1 To ensure the best position for insertion of the drops.
2 Warm the drops to body temperature if allowed.	2 To prevent trauma to the patient.
3 Pull the cartilagenous part of the pinna backwards and upwards.	3 To prepare the auditory meatus for instillation of the drops.
4 Allow the drops to fall in the direction of the external canal.	4 To ensure that the medication reaches the target.
5 Request the patient to remain in this position for 1-2 minutes.	5 To allow the medication to reach the eardrum and be absorbed.

13

ENTONOX ADMINISTRATION

Definition

Entonox is a gaseous mixture of 50% oxygen and 50% nitrous oxide which acts as an analgesic agent when inhaled. The mixture remains stable at temperatures of above —6°C.

The Entonox cylinder is coloured blue and has white segments on the shoulder. The apparatus consists of the cylinder, the Bodok seal, inhalation tubing and the handpiece. Either a mask or a mouthpiece may be used (Figure 13.1).

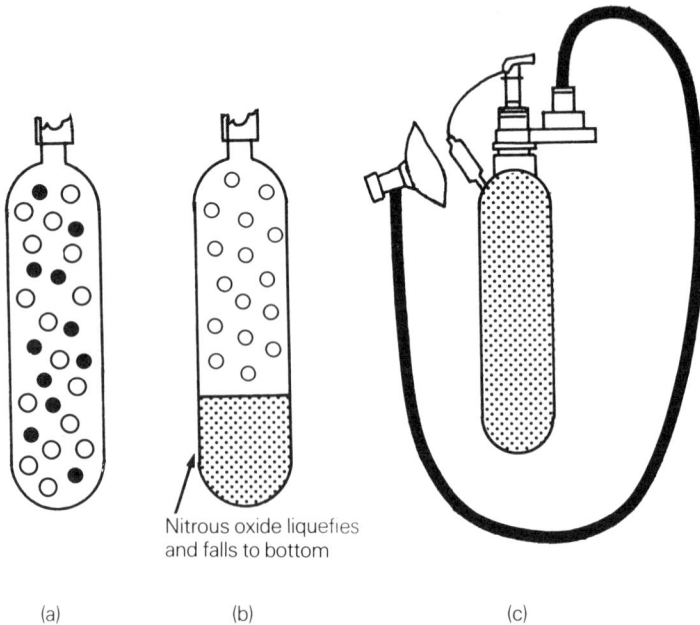

Nitrous oxide liquefies and falls to bottom

(a)   (b)   (c)

Figure 13.1 Entonox cylinder. The apparatus consists of the cylinder, the Bodok seal, inhalation tubing and the handpiece. Either a mask or a mouthpiece may be used

Indications

The use of Entonox is indicated prior to or during a number of painful procedures:

1 Changing packs, drains and dressings
2 Removal of sutures from sensitive areas, e.g. the vulva
3 Re-dressing burns, where an occlusive or open technique is not used
4 Invasive procedures such as catheterization and sigmoidoscopy
5 Childbirth
6 Removal of radioactive intracavity gynaecological applicators
7 Following myocardial infarction (Entonox provides safe analgesia as well as supplementary oxygen)
8 Altering the position of a patient who is in pain
9 Manual evacuation of the bowel to relieve constipation
10 Traumatic injuries
11 Applying orthopaedic traction
12 Physiotherapy procedures, particularly postoperatively.

Contraindications

Its use is contraindicated in the following cases and situations:

1 Maxillofacial injuries, as the patient may not be able to hold the mask tightly to the face or to use the mouthpiece adequately
2 Head injuries with impairment of consciousness
3 Heavily sedated patients
4 Intoxicated patients
5 Pneumothorax, as it will increase the problem
6 The 'bends', as nitrous oxide escapes into the bloodstream and increases the size of the nitrogen bubbles in the tissues
7 Laryngectomy patients, as they will be unable to use the apparatus
8 Administration over continous periods of longer than 48-72 hours as leucopoenia may occur
9 Temperatures below −6 °C as separation of the gases occurs.

REFERENCE MATERIAL

The relief of pain for patients undergoing painful procedures is often not adequately met. The reasons for this are varied and range from the inability of professional personnel adequately to measure how much pain a patient is suffering to the difficulty of judging at the outset how painful a procedure will prove to be to a patient. Nurses are able to administer analgesics only if the doctor has specifically prescribed their use. Many procedures can only be assessed as painful once their performance has begun. At this stage it is difficult either to wait for a doctor to prescribe analgesics or to wait for a prescribed analgesic to take effect. In these situations an analgesic that could be prescribed. and administered by nurses, would take rapid effect, would be equally rapidly excreted from the body and would have few side effects is the ideal. Entonox meets all these criteria.

Comparison of Opiates and Entonox

Opiates	Entonox
1 Usually have to be given by injection — an added discomfort for the patient. There is also the risk of local or systemic infection.	1 Inhaled, i.e. a painless procedure.
2 May take up to 1 hour to become effective.	2 Rapid onset, i.e. $1\frac{1}{2}$-2 minutes.
3 Effects then last for approximately 1 hour more.	3 Effects wear off rapidly, i.e. in approximately 2-5 minutes.
4 Need to be prescribed by a doctor.	4 Can be prescribed by an appropriately qualified trained nurse or physiotherapist.
5 Side effects include respiratory and cardiovascular depression, emesis, drowsiness and thus an inability to cooperate.	5 Side effects are few and self-limiting as the gas is self-administered. Recovery from side effects such as drowsiness and amnesia is rapid.
6 Tend to decrease peripheral circulation in patients suffering from shock due to their effect on the cardiovascular system.	6 The extra oxygen in Entonox increases peripheral circulation oxygenation in patients suffering from shock.

Principle of Administration

Entonox is designed for self-administration by the patient. The apparatus works as a demand unit; i.e. gas can only be obtained by the patient inhaling and producing a negative pressure. When the patient exhales, the gas flow stops. The patient must hold the mask firmly over his/her face to produce an airtight fit before the gas will flow. Expired gases escape by the expiratory valve on the hand piece. Alternatively a mouthpiece can be used. It is essential to adhere to this method of self-administration as it is impossible for the patient to overdose him/herself because if he/she becomes drowsy he/she will relax his/her grip on the hand set and the gas flow will cease when no negative pressure is applied.

A smaller dose than normal of an opiate may be given to augment the effects of Entonox. This should be given in sufficient time to take effect before the procedure begins.

Entonox has an oxygen content two and a half times that of air and is, therefore, a good way of giving extra oxygen as well as providing analgesia.

Personnel Qualified to Teach and Supervise the Use of Entonox

Only those staff who have been trained and supervised in the use of Entonox should be allowed to train and supervise patients. Usually these will be

1   Registered general nurses or certified midwives
2   Physiotherapists.

References and Further Reading

Diggory G (1979) Entonox and its role in nursing care, Nursing (April): 28-31
Entonox (1975) Abstracted proceedings of the symposium on Entonox organized by the Department of Anaesthesia, St Bartholomew's Hospital
Msi J (1981) The use of Entonox for the relief of pain experienced by cancer patients, in Cancer Nursing Update, edited by R Tiffany, Ballière Tindall, pp. 185-187

Audiovisual Aids

Entonox in Hospitals, BOC's Audio Visual Services, 42 Upper Richmond Road, West London SW14 8DD

GUIDELINES: ENTONOX ADMINISTRATION

Equipment

1   Entonox cylinder and head
2   Face mask or mouthpiece

Procedure

Action	Rationale
1 Check to see if there is gas in the Entonox cylinder by turning the tap in an anticlockwise (⌒) direction.	
2 Examine the gauge to determine how much gas is in the cylinder.	2 To ensure an adequate supply of gas throughout the procedure.
3 Ensure that the patient is in as comfortable a position as possible.	
4 Demonstrate how to use the apparatus by holding the mask tightly to your face and breathing in and out regularly and deeply. A hissing sound will indicate that the patient is inhaling the gas.	4 To ensure that the patient understands what to do before any painful procedure commences. To reassure the patient of the nontoxic effects of the gas. To provide a correct role model.

Action	Rationale
5 Allow the patient to practise using the apparatus.	5 To enable the patient to adopt the correct technique and observe the analgesic effect of the gas before the procedure commences.
6 Encourage the patient to breathe gas in and out for at least 2 minutes prior to commencing any painful procedure.	6 To allow sufficient time for an adequate circulatory level of nitrous oxide to provide analgesia. (When the patient inhales, gas enters first the lungs then the pulmonary and systemic circulations. It takes 1-2 minutes to build up reasonable concentrations of nitrous oxide in the brain.)
7 During the procedure keep encouraging the patient to breathe in and out regularly and deeply.	7 To maintain adequate circulatory levels, thus providing adequate analgesia.
8 At the end of the procedure observe the patient until the effects of the gas have worn off.	8 Some patients may feel a transient drowsiness or giddiness and should be discouraged from getting out of bed until these effects have worn off. It is rare for the patient to experience transient amnesia.
9 Turn off the Entonox supply from the cylinder by turning the tap in a clockwise ( ) direction. The gauge should then read 'Empty'.	9 To avoid potential seepage of gas from the apparatus.
10 Depress the diaphragm under the valve to express residual gas.	
11 Wash the face mask, expiratory valve and hand piece in a neutral detergent.	11 To minimize the risk of cross-infection.

NURSING CARE PLAN

Problem	Cause	Suggested Action
1 Patient not experiencing adequate analgesic effect	1 a Entonox cylinder empty b Apparatus not properly connected c Patient not inhaling deeply enough	1 a Check before procedure commences. c Encourage patient to breathe in until a hissing noise can be heard from the cylinder.

Problem	Cause	Suggested Action
	d Patient inhaling pure oxygen, i.e. cylinder has been stored below −6 °C and nitrous oxide has liquified and settled at the bottom of the cylinder. (All cylinders should be stored horizontally at a temperature of 10 °C or above for 24 hours before use.)	**d** Initially safe, but later patient may inhale pure nitrous oxide and be asphyxiated. Discontinue the procedure. Ensure adequate warming of the cylinder and inversion of the cylinder to remix the gases adequately.
	e Not enough time has been allowed for nitrous oxide to exert its analgesic effect.	**e** Allow at least 2 minutes of Entonox use before commencing the procedure.
2 Patient experiences generalized muscle rigidity	2 Hyperventilation during inhalation	2 Discontinue Entonox and allow the patient to recover. Explain the procedure again, stressing deep and regular inspiration. Try a mouthpiece instead of a mask.
3 Patient unable to tolerate a mask	3 Smell of rubber, feeling of claustrophobia	3 Try a mouthpiece.
4 Patient feels nauseated, drowsy or giddy	4 Effect of nitrous oxide accumulation	4 Discontinue Entonox administration — the effect will then rapidly disappear.
5 Patient afraid to use Entonox	5 Associates gases with previous hospital procedures, e.g. anaesthesia before surgery	5 Demonstrate use and thus its nontoxic effects.

14

EYE CARE

Indications
Eye care may be necessary under the following circumstances:
1 To relieve pain and discomfort
2 To prevent infection.

REFERENCE MATERIAL
The patient can be instructed to carry out many of the procedures involved in eye care him/herself. However, the nurse is often involved in caring for the

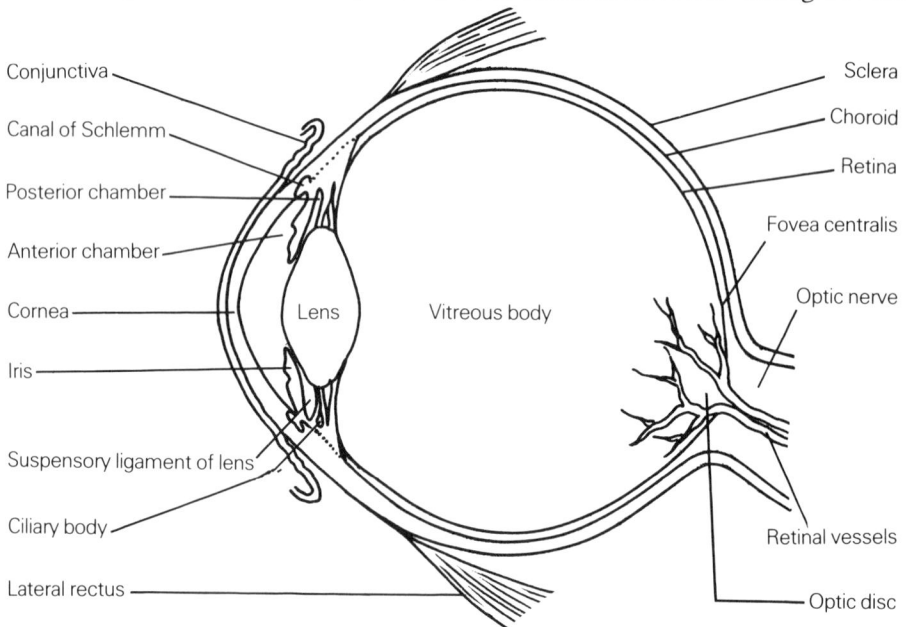

Figure 14.1 Anatomy and physiology of the eye

postoperative, very ill or unconscious patient. Infection can easily be transmitted, by careless technique, from one eye to the other. In some cases this can lead to loss of sight.

Anatomy and Physiology

The eyeball is protected from injury by the bony cavity of the orbit, the conjuctiva, the lacrimal apparatus, the eyebrows, the eyelids and eyelashes.
  The eyeball itself has three layers (see Figure 14.1):

1 The outermost, composed of the cornea and sclera
2 The middle, composed of the choroid, ciliary body and iris (uveal tract)
3 The innermost, composed of the retina, macula lutea (yellow spot) and fovea centralis.

The function of the outer coat is protective. The middle layer is vascular and pigmented, while the innermost contains the light-sensitive nerve endings which are concerned with vision, i.e. the rods and cones.

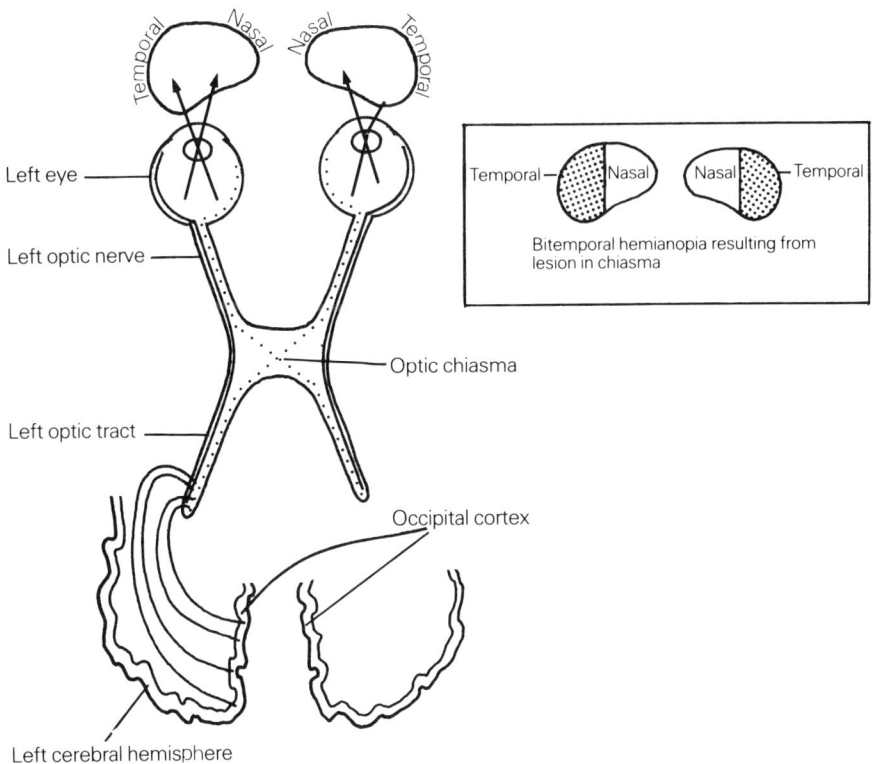

Figure 14.2 Visual pathways and visual fields

The blood vessels of the retina are readily seen with an ophthalmoscope. Abnormal changes in these vessels can be indicative of both generalized diseases, such as diabetes and hypertension, and diseases of the eye itself.

The optic nerve (cranial nerve II) has two tracts which cross over at the optic chiasma. Each tract supplies the opposite side of the body. These tracts enter the eyeball to the side of the macula lutea. This area is known as the optic disc and is an area of no vision (blindspot) (see Figure 14.2).

The inside of the eyeball is divided by the lens into an anterior and posterior chamber. The anterior chamber is filled with a clear, watery fluid called the aqueous humour and the posterior chamber by a jelly-like substance called the vitreous humour which gives the eyeball its shape.

The tears are produced in the lacrimal gland (Figure 14.3). Their function is to wash over the eyeball, removing any foreign substances and providing antisepsis by the action of the enzyme lysozyme. Lysozyme ruptures the cell walls of bacteria and causes their lysis or death. The tears drain through the lacrimal puncti into the nasolacrimal duct. In health, the surface of the eye should always be slightly moist.

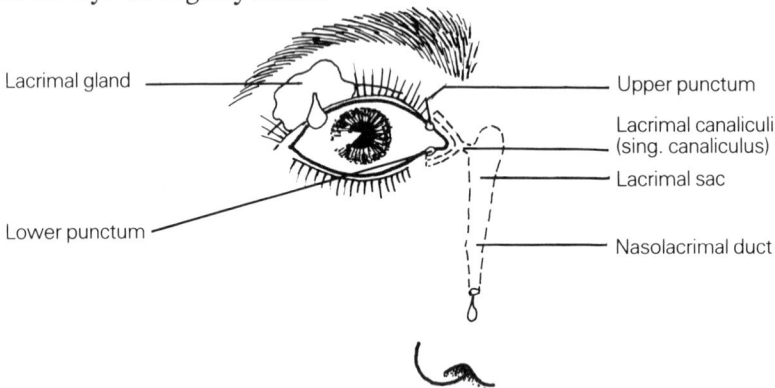

Figure 14.3   Lacrimal apparatus

The cornea has no blood vessels and is dependent on the tears and aqueous humour for its nourishment.

General Principles of Eye Care

Aseptic technique is not always essential when performing eye care, but the positions of the patient and the nurse in relation to the light source are vital in order for the procedure to be carried out safely and efficiently.

Position of the Patient

Where possible the patient should be lying down with his/her head tilted backwards and his/her chin pointing upwards. This enables ease of access to the eyes. It is also easier for the patient to maintain the head in this position when lying down.

Position of the Nurse

If possible the nurse should work from behind the patient's head. This gives him/her ease of access to both eyes and any equipment used can be kept out of the patient's line of vision. With the nurse behind him/her the patient is also more able to cooperate and less likely to try to follow the nurse's movements with his/her eyes.

Position of the Light Source

A good light source before commencing eye procedures is necessary in order to be able to assess carefully the state of the eyes and to avoid damaging their delicate structures during the procedure. The light should be above and behind the nurse or to his/her side. Light should never be allowed to shine directly into the patient's eyes as this will be painful and harmful to the patient.

Instillation of Drops

Most types of drops are instilled into the outer side of the lower fornix as the conjuctiva is less sensitive than the cornea and the outer side avoids loss of the drops into the nasolacrimal passage. Exceptions to this are as follows:

1 *Drops used to lubricate the cornea*   These should be directed on to the cornea. Oil-based drops produce less corneal reaction than aqueous ones as they do not feel as cold to the cornea when administered.
2 *Anaesthetic drops*   The first drops should be instilled into the conjunctiva and then directly on to the cornea until the patient is no longer able to feel the drops.
3 *Drops used to treat the nasal passages*   These should be instilled at the punctal end of the eye.

The number of drops to be instilled depends on the type of solution used and its purpose. Usually one drop only is ordered and will be sufficient if it is instilled in the correct manner. The exceptions to the 'one drop' rule are

1 *Oil-based solutions, e.g. paroleine*   This is used for lubricating the eyeball and several drops are usually ordered.
2 *Anaesthetic drops*   It is usual to instill two or three drops at a time at intervals, until the drop cannot be felt on the eye.

The dropper should be held as close to the eye as possible without touching either the lids or the cornea, i.e. approximately 2.5 cm. This will avoid corneal damage and the risk of infection. If the drop falls from too great a distance it is difficult to control and will also be uncomfortable for the patient.

There are a variety of droppers and bottles, including pipettes, pipettes incorporated into the eye drop bottle, plastic bottles and single dose packs. Pipettes are easy to use but need drying and sterilizing between doses. The disposable varieties are also expensive. The bottles that incorporate a pipette have an advantage in that the flow of drops is easily controlled. Plastic bottles can be squeezed and so avoid the need for a pipette but again, they are expensive. Ideally, single dose containers should be used if they do not prove too expensive for routine use.

Eye Irrigation

The most common use of eye irrigation is for the removal of a caustic substance from the eye. This should be done as soon as possible to minimize damage. The procedure is also used as a preoperative preparation or to remove infected material. The lotion most commonly ordered is normal saline. Boracic lotion in a solution of 4% may also be used. In an emergency, water may be used.

Care of an Insensitive Eye

Any interference with the sensory nerve supply to the eye, such as unconsciousness, will cause the eye surface to become insensitive. The blink reflex is often lost, the eye surface becomes dry and the cornea may be damaged. Corneal ulcers, scarring and loss of vision may be the end result.

When a patient has lost these protective reflexes it is the duty of the nurse to institute measures to replace them. The treatment aims at keeping the eye surface clean by swabbing, lubricating the surface, the instillation of oil-based drops, such as paroleine, and protecting the cornea by closing the eyelids. In certain cases the lids may be kept closed by the use of a nonallergenic tape. Eye pads should be avoided as the eye may open beneath them, rubbing or scratching the cornea. Frequency of care is determined by the needs of the individual patient.

Eye Medications

Drugs may be given either systemically or topically to exert an effect on the eye. However, if given systemically the prescribing doctor needs to take account of the physiological barrier and the blood/aqueous barrier which exists within the eye and which is selective in allowing drugs to pass into the intraocular fluids. Permeability of this barrier may be altered in inflammatory conditions and following paracentesis.

Drugs applied locally meet some resistance at the tear film. The cornea allows the passage of water but not of drugs. This resistance may alter where there are corneal epithelial changes. Wetting agents may be employed to alter corneal permeability.

Many drugs will produce similar effects on a diseased or a healthy eye. Drugs for use in the eye are usually classified according to their action:

1 *Mydriatics and cycloplegics* These drugs produce their effects by paralysing the sphincter, by stimulating the dilator muscle of the pupil or

by a combination of both (see Figure 14.4). Atropine 1% is the most commonly used mydriatic. It is usually administered as drops but can be used as an ointment. It takes half an hour to dilate the pupil after instillation and about 2 hours to paralyse the sphincter. Its mydriatic effect may last for over a week and cycloplegia for 2-4 days.

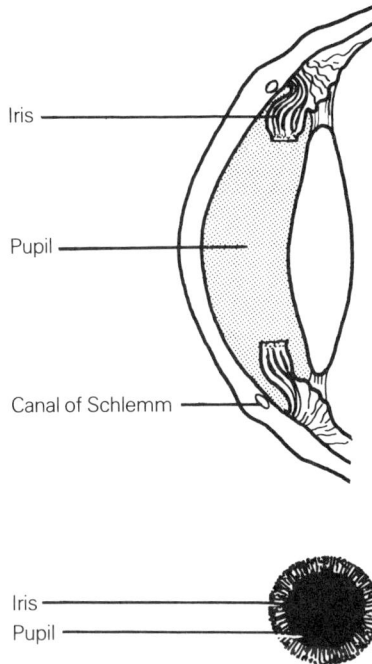

Figure 14.4 Effect of mydriatics

2 *Miotics* These drugs produce their effects by constricting the pupil and contracting the ciliary muscle (Figure 14.5). Miotics are used primarily in the treatment of glaucoma.

3 *Local anaesthetics* These render the eye and the inner surfaces of the lids insensitive. They are used prior to minor surgery, removal of foreign bodies and tonometry. Cocaine is less used now as some patients develop an idiosyncracy to it and may suddenly collapse after its use. Its effects do not wear off for at least half an hour after administration.

4 *Anti-inflammatories* These may be steroids, antihistamines or pyrazole derivatives, such as oxyphenabutazone 10%.

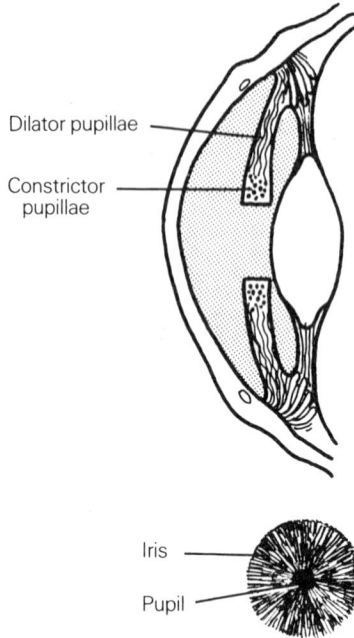

Figure 14.5   Effect of miotics

5   *Antibiotics*   Antibiotics can be used in the active treatment of infection and as prophylactics both pre- and postoperatively, following removal of a foreign body or following an injury. Antibiotic preparations in common use are framycetin 0.5%, sulphacetamide 10, 20 and 30%, neomycin 0.5% and chloramphenicol 0.5%.

6   *Artificial tears*   Where tear deficiency exists due to disease processes, treatment with radiation or reduction of the blink reflex, artificial lubricants such as methyl cellulose or hypromellose may be used.

Toxic Effects of Common Systemic Drugs on the Eye

As the eye may be the first place to show signs of systemic disease, so some systemic drugs may now show their toxic effects in the eye. These effects range from pruritis, irritation, redness, excess tear formation with overflow (epiphora), photophobia and blapharoconjunctivitis to disturbance of vision.

1   *Methotrexate and related antimetabolites*   These drugs affect the Meibornian glands, aggrevate seborrhoeic blepharitis, and produce photophobia, epiphora, periorbital oedema and conjunctival hyperaemia.

2   *5-Fluorouracil (5-FU)*   5-FU causes canalicular fibrosis and oculomotor disturbances (probably secondary to a local neurotoxicity affecting the brainstem).
3   *Antihistamines*   Antihistamines decrease tear production and may lead to 'dry eye', especially in patients with Sjorgen's syndrome or ocular pemphigus, in patients who wear contact lenses and in the elderly.
4   *Tamoxifen*   This drug can cause subepithelial, whirl-like, corneal deposits and retinal lesions.
5   *Indomethacin*   Indomethacin can cause corneal deposits and retinal pigmentary toxicity.
6   *Oral contraceptives*   These can stimulate corneal steeping and intolerance to contact lenses.
7   *Atropine, scopalamine and belladonna-like substances*   Such drugs cause mydriasis and cycloplegia.
8   *Corticosteroids*   Prolonged use of corticosteroids produces posterior subcapsular cataracts.
9   *Chloramphenicol*   Chloramphenicol treatment can led to optic neuritis.
10 *Ethambutol*   This drug can cause damage to the optic nerve.

References and Further Reading

Bryant W M (1981) Common toxic effects of systemic drugs on the eye, Occupational Health Nursing: 15-17
Chilman A M Thomas M (1978) Understanding Nursing Care, Churchill Livingstone, pp. 410-411
Darling V H Thorpe M R (1981) Ophthalmic Nursing, 2nd edition, Ballière Tindall, pp. 12-20, 27-32
Garland P (1975) Ophthalmic Nursing, 6th edition, Faber and Faber pp. 37-38, 42, 45, 50-68, 81-82
Percy E Smith W A M (1973) Ophthalmology (Ophthalmic Techniques) William Heinemann Medical Books, pp. 214-223
Phillips M (1982) Ophthalmic preparations, Nursing Mirror 155: 69-71
Rooke F C E Rothwell P J Woodhouse D F (1980) Ophthalmic Nursing — Its Practice and Management, Churchill Livingston, pp. 190-207
Smith J Nachazel D P (1980) Opthalmologic Nursing, Little, Brown, pp. 269-282
Wilson P (1976) Modern Ophthalmic Nursing, Edward Arnold, pp. 39-43, 57-61

GUIDELINES: EYE SWABBING

Equipment

1   Sterile dressing pack
2   Normal saline solution
3   Sodium bicarbonate solution

Procedure

Action	Rationale
1 Explain the procedure to the patient.	1 To obtain the patient's consent and cooperation.
2 Assist the patient into the correct position: **a** Head well supported and tilted back **b** Preferably the patient should be in bed or lying on a couch.	2 The patient needs to be discouraged from flinching or making unexpected movements and so should be in the most comforable position possible at the start of the procedure.
3 Ensure an adequate light source, taking care not to dazzle the patient.	3 To enable maximum observation of the eyes without causing the patient harm or discomfort.
4 Wash and dry your hands thoroughly.	4 Asepsis is essential, particularly where the patient has a damaged eye or has just had an operation on the eye. Infection can lead to loss of an eye.
5 Always treat the uninfected or uninflammed eye first.	5 To avoid cross-infection.
6 Using a slightly moistened wool swab, ask the patient to look up and swab the lower lid from the nasal corner outwards.	6 If the swab is too wet the solution will run down the patient's cheek. This increases the risk of cross-infection and causes the patient discomfort. Swabbing from the nasal corner outwards avoids the risk of swabbing discharge into the lacrymal punctum, or even across the bridge of the nose into the other eye.
7 Ensure that the edge of the swab is not above the lid margin.	7 To avoid touching the sensitive cornea.
8 Using a new swab each time, repeat the procedure until all discharge has been removed.	8 To avoid infection.
9 Swab with a dry swab.	9 Moist areas encourage bacterial growth.
10 Swab the upper lid by slightly everting the lid margin and asking the patient to look down. Swab from the nasal corner outwards and use a new swab each time until all discharge has been removed.	
11 Swab with a dry swab.	

Action	Rationale
12 Once both eyelids have been cleansed and dried, make the patient comfortable.	
13 Remove and dispose of equipment.	13 To avoid cross-infection.
14 Wash your hands.	
15 Record the procedure in the appropriate documents.	15 To monitor trends and fluctuations.

Note: For information about obtaining an eye swab for pathological investigations, see the appropriate section on specimen collection (pages 374-380).

GUIDELINES: INSTILLATION OF EYE DROPS

Equipment

1 Sterile dressing pack
2 Normal saline solution
3 Sodium bicarbonate solution
4 Appropriate eye drops. (Any preparation must be checked against the doctor's prescription by two nurses.)

Procedure

Action	Rationale
1 Explain the procedure to the patient.	1 To obtain the patient's consent and cooperation.
2 If there is any discharge, proceed as for eye swabbing.	2 To remove any infected material and thus ensure adequate absorption of the drops.
3 Check the following:	
a Prescription against bottle label	a To ensure that appropriate drops are instilled.
b For which eye the drops are prescribed	b To avoid cross-infection and instillation of the drug into the wrong eye.
c Expiry date on bottle.	c To ensure that medication is patent.
4 Assist the patient into the correct position, i.e. head well supported and tilted back.	4 To ensure that drops are instilled beneath the lower lid into the fornix and to avoid excess solution running down the patient's cheek.

Action	Rationale
5 Wash and dry your hands thoroughly.	5 Asepsis is essential, particularly when the patient has a damaged eye or has just had an operation on the eye. Infection can lead to loss of an eye.
6 Place a cotton wool swab on the lower lid against the lid margin.	6 To absorb any excess solution which may be irritating to the surrounding skin.
7 Ask the patient to look up immediately prior to instilling the drop.	7 This opens the eye and allows the drop to be instilled into the outer side of the lower fornix. If done too soon the patient may blink as the drop is instilled.
8 Ask the patient to close his/her eye. Keep the wool swab on the lower lid.	8 To ensure absorption of the fluid and to avoid excess running down the cheek.
9 Make the patient comfortable.	
10 Remove and dispose of equipment.	10 To avoid cross-infection.
11 Wash your hands.	
12 Record the procedure in the appropriate documents.	12 To monitor trends and fluctuations.

GUIDELINES: INSTILLATION OF EYE OINTMENT

Equipment

1 Sterile dressing pack
2 Normal saline solution
3 Sodium bicarbonate solution may be used to soften a crusted discharge
4 Appropriate eye ointment. (Any preparation must be checked against the doctor's prescription by two nurses.)

Procedure

Action	Rationale
1 Explain the procedure to the patient.	1 To obtain the patient's consent and cooperation.
2 If there is any discharge, and to remove any previous application of ointment, proceed as for eye swabbing.	2 To remove any infected material and previous ointment to allow for absorption of ointment.

Action	**Rationale**
3 Check the following: **a** Prescription against tube of ointment **b** For which eye the ointment is prescribed **c** Expiry date on tube.	**a** To ensure that appropriate ointment is applied. **b** To avoid cross-infection and administration of an inappropriate treatment. **c** To ensure that medication is patent.
4 Wash and dry your hands thoroughly.	4 To avoid infection.
5 Place a wool swab on the lower lid against the lid margin.	5 To absorb excess ointment which may be irritating to the surrounding skin.
6 Slightly evert the lower lid by pulling on the wool swab. Ask the patient to look up immediately prior to applying the cream.	6 To allow the application to be made inside the lower lid into the lower fornix.
7 Apply the ointment by gently squeezing the tube and, with the nozzle 2.5 cm above the lower lid, drawing a line along the inner edge of the lower lid from the nasal corner outward.	
8 Ask the patient to close his/her eye and remove excess ointment with a new wool swab.	8 To avoid excess ointment irritating the surrounding skin.
9 Warn the patient that, when he/she opens his/her eye, vision will be a little blurred for a few minutes.	
10 Make the patient comfortable.	
11 Remove and dispose of equipment.	11 To avoid infection.
12 Wash your hands.	
13 Record the procedure in the appropriate documents.	13 To monitor trends and fluctuations.

GUIDELINES: EYE IRRIGATION

Equipment

1 Sterile dressing pack

2 Irrigation fluid (usually sterile normal saline but, in an emergency, tap water may be used)
3 Receiver
4 Towel
5 Plastic cape
6 Irrigating flask
7 Hot water in a bowl to warm irrigating fluid to tepid temperature

Procedure

Action	Rationale
1 Explain the procedure to the patient.	1 To gain the patient's consent and cooperation.
2 Prepare the irrigation fluid to the appropriate temperature.	2 Tepid fluid will be more comfortable for the patient. The solution should be poured across the inner aspect of the nurse's wrist to test the temperature.
3 Assist the patient into the appropriate position: **a** Head comfortably supported with chin almost horizontal **b** Head inclined to the side of the eye to be treated.	3 To avoid the solution running either over the cheek into the eye or out of the eye and down the side of the nose.
4 Wash and dry your hands.	4 To avoid infection.
5 Remove any discharge from the eye by swabbing.	5 To prevent washing the discharge down the lacrimal duct or across the cheek.
6 Ask the patient to hold the receiver against his/her cheek below the eye being teated.	6 To collect irrigation fluid as it runs away from the eye.
7 Position the towel and plastic cape.	7 To protect the patient's clothing.
8 Hold the patient's eyelids apart, using your first and second fingers, against the orbital ridge.	8 The patient will be unable to hold his/her eye open once irrigation commences.
9 Do not press on the eyeball.	9 To avoid causing the patient discomfort or pain.
10 Warn the patient that the flow of solution is going to start and pour a little on to his/her cheek first.	
11 Direct the flow of the fluid from the nasal corner outwards.	11 To wash away from the lacrimal punctum.
12 Ask the patient to look up, down and to either side while irrigating.	12 To ensure that the whole area is washed.
13 Keep the flow of irrigation fluid constant.	

Action	**Rationale**
14 When the eye has been thoroughly irrigated, ask the patient to close his/her eyes and use a new swab to dry the lids.	
15 Take the receiver from the patient and dry his/her cheek.	15 If the receiver is removed first, solution may run down the patient's neck.
16 Make the patient comfortable.	
17 Remove and dispose of equipment.	17 To avoid infection.
18 Wash your hands.	
19 Record the procedure in the appropriate documents.	19 To monitor trends and fluctuations.

15

GASTRIC LAVAGE

Definition

Gastric lavage is the irrigation or washing out of the stomach with repeated flushing of an appropriate fluid. It is used to obtain a specimen of gastric contents and to remove poisons or other harmful substances, that were swallowed deliberately or accidentally, thus preventing further absorption.

Indications

Gastric lavage may be used under the following circumstances:

1 If the patient is seen within 4 hours of ingesting poisons or harmful substances.
2 If the patient is unconscious and the time of ingestion is not known.
3 In all cases of salicylate poisoning within 12 hours of ingestion.
4 For gastrointestinal haemorrhage (Evans 1981).

REFERENCE MATERIAL

The reliability of gastric lavage is debatable, advice on its use conflicting, and its value questionable (Burstom 1970; Matthew 1971; Stoddart 1975; Goth 1976). Blake et al. (1978) attempted to identify those factors that influenced the decision to perform gastric lavage in 236 cases of deliberate self-poisoning seen over a period of 6 months in one hospital. Of patients seen within 4 hours of ingesting the poison, 87% had a lavage performed irrespective of the number of tablets and the nature of the drug taken. Overall, 77% had a gastric lavage. Most of the late lavages were carried out for salicylate ingestion. The authors concluded that given the changing pattern of drugs used for attempted self-poisoning, at least 50% of patients were subjected to gastric lavage unnecessarily.

Gastric lavage is generally carried out by medical staff assisted by nurses. Registered general nurses in specialized units, mainly accident and emergency departments, may carry out the procedure without medical involvement after initial assessment.

Gastric Lavage Versus Induced Emesis

Research has shown (Beckett and Rowland 1965; Bell 1969; Chazan and Cohen 1969) that of the two methods for removing gastric contents in drug overdose, induced emesis is more effective than gastric lavage.

The issue is more complicated than this, however, for one method cannot be applied to the exclusion of the other in all cases. For drug-induced emesis, two agents are commonly used — ipecacuanha and apomorphine. Ipecacuanha is a centrally acting drug, its site of action being in the chemoreceptor zone in the medulla oblongata. As a result it takes from 20 to 25 minutes to produce an effect. If this fact is not appreciated, repeated doses may be given before the first dose has had time to work and this may result in protracted vomiting. A sufficient quantity of water (up to 10 glasses is quoted in the literature) must be given to produce emesis. Apomorphine produces vomiting within about 5 minutes and again water must be given to produce the required effect. The drug is administered subcutaneously or intramuscularly. It possesses narcotic properties and is contraindicated in patients who have ingested sedatives or hypnotics or who have respiratory problems. Induced emesis should only be used when the patient is alert and the development of lethargy and coma is unlikely. Unless the patient is awake the cough reflex may be depressed and this may result in the patient inhaling the vomitus. When a drug with strong antimetic properties has been ingested, e.g. chlorpromazine, induced emesis will have little or no effect and gastric lavage may become the method of choice.

Gastric lavage is contraindicated when a caustic or corrosive has been ingested because of the possibility of perforating the oesophagus when passing the tube. It is also contraindicated when strychnine has been ingested since stimulation while passing the tube into the stomach may precipitate convulsions. In patients brought to a hospital's emergency department several hours (4 hours is quoted in the literature) after the ingestion of drugs, gastric lavage is held to be of little value in that after such a period of time very little if any of the drug will remain in the stomach. Any drug that does remain may then be washed into the small intestines by the procedure. Gastric lavage within 6 hours is quoted by Evans (1981) as valuable in methanol poisoning. Drugs such as aspirin and glutethimide remain in the small intestines for long periods and act as a reservoir for continued absorption. Gastric lavage is useful at any time within 12 hours of ingestion in these cases.

Gastric Lavage Tubes

Cosgriff (1978) gives a brief illlustrated summary of some of the tubes used for gastric lavage in the United States of America. The tube of choice in the United Kingdom appears to be 30 gauge Jacques stomach tube (Matthew 1971; Evans 1981). This wide bore tube enables tablets, food with tablet particles adherent, and virtually all the contents of the stomach to be evacuated through it.

References and Further Reading

Arena J (1974) Poisoning: Toxicology, Symptoms, Treatment, 3rd edition, Charles C Thomas

Beckett A Rowland M (1965) Urinary excretion kinetics of amphetamine in man, Journal of Pharmacy and Pharmacology 17: 628

Bell D S (1969) Dangers of treatment of status epilepticus with diazepam, British Medical Journal 1: 159

Blake D R et al. (1978) Is there excessive use of gastric lavage in the treatment of self-poisoning? Lancet ii: 1362-1364

Budassi S A Barber J M (1981) Emergency Nursing: Principles and Practice, C V Mosby, pp. 1619-1620

Burstom G R (1970) Self-poisoning, Lloyd-Luke, p. 39.

Chazan J Cohen J (1969) Clincial spectrum of glutethimide intoxication, Journal of the American Medical Asssociation 208: 837

Cosgriff J H (1978) An Atlas of Diagnostic and Therapeutic Procedures for Emergency Personnel, J B Lippincott, pp. 157, 163, 165, 172

Cosgriff J H Anderson D L (1975) The Practice of Emergency Nursing, J B Lippincott pp. 158-159

Evans R (1981) Emergency Medicine, Butterworth, pp. 17, 19-20, 25, 229

Goth A (1976) Medical Pharmacology: Principles and Concepts, C V Mosby, p. 624

Matthew H (1971) Acute poisoning: some myths and misconceptions, British Medical Journal 1: 521

Stoddart J C (1975) Intensive Therapy, Blackwell Scientific Publications, p. 110

GUIDELINES: GASTRIC LAVAGE

Equipment

1 Sterile gastric tube with connector
2 Connecting tubing
3 Lubricating jelly
4 Tape
5 Syringe (50 ml)
6 Receiver
7 Litmus paper
8 Mouth gag
9 Funnel
10 Jug
11 Tepid water or prescribed irrigation fluid
12 Plastic sheet
13 Disposable paper sheets
14 Disposable plastic aprons
15 Disposable plastic gloves
16 Bucket

17 Suction equipment
18 Emergency resuscitation equipment

Procedure

Action	**Rationale**
1 Explain the procedure to the patient when possible.	1 To obtain the patient's consent and cooperation. (The efficacy of explanations is questionable, however, on the basis that an adult who has ingested a toxic substance deliberately is unlikely to want to cooperate with agents whose aim is to prevent suicidal gestures.)
2 Unconscious patients must be intubated.	2 To maintain a clear airway.
3 Place the patient on a firm surface, lying in the left lateral position with his/her head down (Figure 15.1) (A standard emergency department trolley should be available ideally.)	3 To maintain a clear airway.

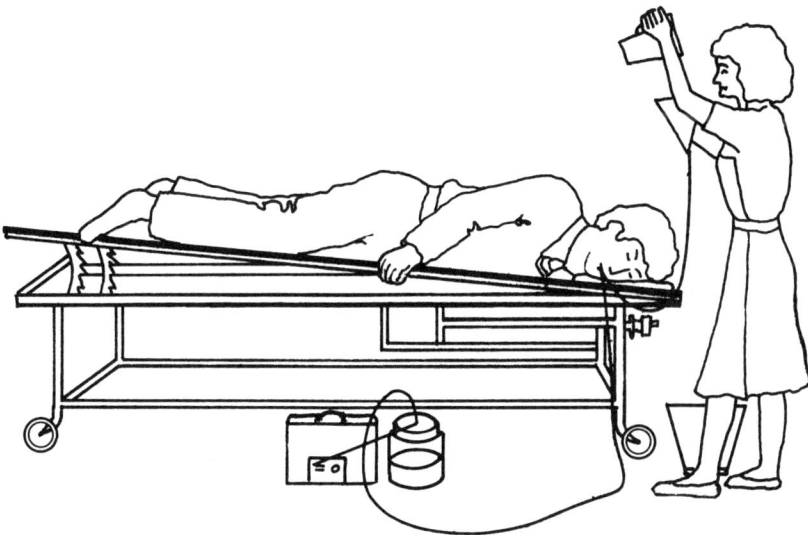

Figure 15.1 Gastric lavage

Action	Rationale
4 Remove any prostheses from the buccal cavity. Remove debris and/or vomitus from the buccal cavity with suction.	4 To maintain a clear airway.
5 Have emergency resuscitation equipment available.	5 Strong vagal stimulation can induce cardiac dysrhythmias and cardiopulmonary arrest.
6 Place a disposable sheet under the patient's head and a plastic sheet over the floor.	6 To protect nurse and patient should vomiting occur.
7 Lubricate the tube with jelly.	7 To facilitate passage of the tube.
8 If the patient is able to cooperate, ask him/her to sit up and swallow sips of water.	8 Swallowing will cause the epiglottis to close and prevent accidental passage of the tube into the trachea.
9 Secure the tube with tape once inserted.	9 To prevent dislodgement of the tube.
10 *Either* aspirate the tube before lavage begins and test the aspirate with litmus paper, *or* listen with a stethoscope over the stomach as air is introduced into the tube via a syringe.	10 To ensure that the tube is in the stomach.
11 Retain a specimen of aspirate in a labelled specimen bottle.	11 For analysis.
12 Instill, via a funnel, water, or the prescribed irrigation fluid, in volumes of 100-500 ml.	12 Approximately 500 ml of fluid is necessary to flatten out the rugae of the stomach so that the fluid may reach all parts of the mucous membrane.
13 Any fluid instilled must be tepid.	13 To prevent a sudden lowering of body temperature and possible shock.
14 Hold the funnel below the level of the patient. Once the required amount of fluid has been poured into the funnel, raise it gradually until the fluid empties into the stomach. Do not allow the contents of the funnel to empty.	14 To control the rate at which the fluid is instilled.
15 Lower the funnel and observe all the contents as they return from the stomach. Empty the contents into a bucket. If blood returns,	A siphoning action is needed to recall the contents of the stomach.

Action	Rationale

stop the procedure and inform the medical staff. Lavage until the returning fluid is clear.

16 Pinch the tube off and remove the tube quickly. Have suction at hand.

16 Gagging and possible vomiting may occur when the tube is removed. As the tube reaches the pharynx, any fluid left may escape and infiltrate into the lungs.

17 Provide oral hygiene facilities as required.

17 To maintain a clean, moist mouth. To prevent the accummulation of oral secretions. To prevent the development of mouth infection.

16

HEPATITIS B

Definition

Hepatitis B is a DNA virus that will replicate only in the livers of humans and chimpanzees.

REFERENCE MATERIAL

Epidemiology

Hepatitis B virus infection is caused by the transfer of the virus from an infected individual or article to a susceptible individual via the blood. The virus has also been detected in saliva and semen. This transfer normally occurs through one of the following means:

1   Accidental innoculation
2   An existing break in host skin
3   Spillage into the eyes or mouth.

Infectivity

An individual with acute hepatitis B is probably most infectious during the late incubation and prodromal periods. The incubation period of hepatitis B is about 2-5 months. There are three patterns of clinical response:

1   Some 30-40% of adults develop clinically apparent hepatitis.
2   Some 50-60% of adults remain asymptomatic but show serological evidence of infection.
3   Some 5-10% of adults develop chronic infection (HBs Ag carrier state).

Infections with hepatitis B virus are generally mild, presenting as a flu-like illness, approximately half of known cases being accompanied by jaundice. There is a fatality rate, however, of less than 1% and deaths are mainly due to fulminating liver failure. In the United Kingdom only 0.1% of the population are carriers. Less than 5% of infections in the United Kingdom progress to the carrier state. This state occurs most frequently after inapparent infections without a history of jaundice.

Diagnosis

Diagnosis is confirmed by blood test, i.e. a virological test requiring 10 ml of clotted blood. Three antigen-antibody systems are recognized as serological markers for diagnosis of present or past infection with hepatitis B virus:

1 Hepatitis B surface antigen (HBs Ag) denotes current hepatitis B infection. Antibody to hepatitis B surface antigen (anti HBs) denotes past infection and immunity to further infections.
2 Antibody to hepatitis B core antigen (anti HBc) denotes present or past hepatitis B virus infection and very high levels are found in hepatitis B surface antigen carriers.
3 Hepatitis Be antigen is detected both in the early period of acute hepatitis B infection and in some carriers. During recovery from an acute infection HBe Ag is usually replaced by anti HBe. (e antigen carriers are more infectious than surface antigen carriers.)

Screening Policy for Hepatitis B Surface Antigen

Screening of the entire hospital patient population would be an effective way to identify hepatitis B infection, but this would be costly and time-consuming in terms of the benefits derived. It is important, however, to screen patients before their admission to a transplant or renal unit.

In general, the best compromise is to test those patients belonging to groups in which there is a high prevalence of hepatitis B. This includes the following persons:

1 All new admissions who currently live or were born in countries where there is a high prevalance of hepatitis B, such as the developing countries
2 Drug addicts
3 Male homosexuals
4 Mentally subnormal patients in institutions
5 Multiple transfusion patients
6 All patients acutely or recently jaundiced
7 Tattooed individuals.

Vaccine

Prophylactic measures are the only means of combating the disease to date since no safe and effective antiviral agent for the treatment of hepatitis B has been discovered. Recently a vaccine has been prepared which confers active immunity for up to 2 years. The vaccine, however, is expensive (£63.50 for a course of three monthly injections, at 1984 prices) and it is in short supply. The vaccine does not offer protection against other forms of viral hepatitis. Guidelines for the use of the vaccine on the high risk groups have now been drawn up by the Department of Health and Social Security.

Education of the Patient and Hospital Staff

An explanation of the patient's diagnosis must be given to enable him/her to comply with any infection control measures. While ensuring maximum protection against infection spread, the patient must not be made to feel socially embarrassed or unduly alarmed by the precautions imposed.

All departments and staff who may be involved with the patient must be made aware of the diagnosis so that they can make their own precautionary arrangements, e.g. haematology and bacteriology. Hospital areas where personnel carry an increased risk of acquiring hepatitis B are

1   Transplant and haemodialysis units
2   Mental subnormality units
3   Intensive care and casualty units
4   Gastroenterology, haemophilia and infectious diseases units.

Dienstag and Ryan (1982) have shown that general ward nurses are at no greater risk of acquiring hepatitis B than the general population.

All specimens and specimen cards must be placed immediately in the plastic bags provided and labelled 'High Risk' so that the laboratory staff are made aware of the hazard.

References

Dienstag J L Ryan D M (1982) Occupational exposure to hepatitis B virus in hospital personnel: infection or immunization, American Journal of Epidemiology 115: 22-29

Grist N R (1981) Hepatitis and other infections in clinical laboratory staff, Journal of Clinical Pathology 34: 655-658

Hart C A (1983) Prevention of hepatitis B infections, Journal of Infection Control Nursing, Nursing Times 79 (4 May): 46, 48

Jeffries M (1982) Hepatitis B: vaccine fix, World Medicine 18 (1): 69-70, 72

Tedder R S (1980) Hepatitis B in hospitals, British Journal of Hospital Medicine 23 (3): 266, 275-276, 278-279

Working Party on the Clinical Use of Specific Immunoglobulin in Hepatitis B (1982) Use of immunoglobulin with high content of antibody to hepatitis B surface antigen (anti-HBs), British Medical Journal 285: 951-954

Yellowlees H Poole A A B (1982) Hepatitis B vaccine: guidance for use, DHSS Letter CM082 (13)

GUIDELINES: HEPATITIS B

Procedure

Action	Rationale
1 The patient may be nursed on an open ward unless there is a high risk of blood contamination of the ward environment.	1 If adequate precautions can be adhered to on an open ward, there is no need to isolate the patient.

Action	Rationale
2 The patient must be assessed daily to establish accurately any sites of bleeding. Changes in the patient's condition should be recorded in his/her care plan.	2 Sites of bleeding must be identified in order that the appropriate precautions can be taken.
3 An individual container for disposing of 'sharps' must be kept for the patient. The container must be labelled 'High Risk' and when half full it must be sealed and put into the appropriate bag. The bag is then securely stapled, marked 'High Risk' and sent for incineration.	3 Contaminated 'sharps' are a potential innoculation hazard to others, so particular caution must be taken in handling them. Overloaded 'sharps' containers may cause needles to pierce the walls of the container or even protrude through the top.
4 A personal disposable bag should be kept on a regular holder with a lid for the patient's disposable waste. When full this should be securely stapled shut, marked 'High Risk' and sent for incineration.	4 To confine potentially contaminated material, e.g. blood-stained tissues.
5 The patient's personal hygiene equipment must be clearly marked and kept at the bedside.	5 To prevent accidental usage of equipment by others.
6 Used linen that is not blood-stained is placed in the ward linen bags in the usual way.	6 Linen free from blood stains is not contaminated and may be dealt with in the normal manner.
7 The patient should use the ward bath or shower last and the area must be thoroughly cleaned afterwards.	7 To allow time for cleaning before the area is used by others.
8 During venepuncture or other procedures likely to cause bleeding, furniture, bedding and clothing in the adjacent area should be protected with polythene sheeting.	8 To prevent contamination of the environment with spilled blood.
9 All staff involved with the patient should cover any cuts or grazes on their hands with waterproof dressings.	9 Broken skin provides a portal of entry for the hepatitis virus in the event of contact with the patient's blood.
10 Routine daily cleaning procedures may be carried out as normal. Domestic staff are advised to wear gloves. It should be ascertained that domestic staff understand the potential hazard associated with blood contamination.	10 Explanation is necessary as the domestic staff may not understand the hazards involved or may over-react to the situation.

Action	Rationale

Accidental Innoculation or Spillage of Blood

1 Any accident involving skin penetration or heavy contamination of abraided skin or mucosal surfaces of staff should be recorded on an accident form and taken to bacteriology immediately. If the risk of infection from this incident is high, hepatitis B immunoglobulin must be given within 48 hours.

1 To protect personnel. To comply with legal and/or hospital requirements.

2 Blood spillage on to unbroken skin should be washed off with soap and running water. A scrubbing brush should not be used as this could break the skin. Complete an accident form as above.

2 To remove the source of potential contamination.

3 Accidential innoculation sites should be cleaned under running water, encouraged to bleed freely and then sealed. Complete an accident form, as above.

3 Bleeding helps 'wash' the innoculated virus out of the system.

4 Blood spilled on hard surfaces must be wiped up immediately with paper towels and the area washed well with a solution such as glutaraldehyde.

4 To prevent viral spread. Dried blood remains infectious for several days.

5 Linen stained with blood must be put in a suitable bag which is stapled shut and marked 'High Risk'. This must be incinerated and the linen room informed.

5 Blood-stained linen is highly infectious.

Precautions if Bleeding is Present

1 Disposable pillowcases and sheets must be used if there is a likelihood of blood spillage. A plastic pillowcase must be used to protect the pillow.

1 Blood-stained linen is highly infectious and cannot be reused. Disposable linen is therefore cheaper and more practical.

2 If bleeding is present in the mouth:
a Use disposable crockery and cutlery and discard, with any uneaten food, into the bedside disposal bag.

Action	Rationale
b Keep a personal food tray and water jug at the bedside.	
c Disposable mouth-care equipment, sputum pot and tissues should be kept at the bedside.	**c** The sputum may be contaminated with blood from the mouth, therefore precautions must include avoiding contact with the patient's sputum.
3 If haematuria or melaena is present: **a** Wear plastic gowns and gloves when handling excreta. **b** Keep a toilet and handbasin for the patient's sole use, if practicable. **c** If a toilet is not available for the patient's sole use, bedpans or urinals must be used. These should be washed in the usual manner in the bedpan washer and dried carefully. They should then be placed in the appropriate bag, marked 'High Risk', stapled securely shut and sent to the central sterile supplies department for autoclaving.	3 Blood present in the urine or faeces makes the patient's excreta a potential source of hepatitis B contamination.
4 If the patient has a wound or a break in the skin: **a** Cover the area adequately so that there is no seepage. **b** Used dressings should be securely sealed in a plastic bag before being disposed of in the appropriate bag. **c** All tapes, lotions and creams are kept solely for the patient's use. **d** The dressing trolley must be cleaned carefully before reuse. **e** Metal instruments should be cleaned scrupulously with soap and water and soaked in a solution such as glutaraldehyde for 3 hours. Instruments are then placed in the appropriate bag, marked 'High Risk', which is securely stapled shut and sent to central sterile supplies department.	4 To prevent the spread of the virus from dried or fresh blood.

Action	**Rationale**
5 If a patient who is bleeding has to be transported elsewhere, the porter involved should be provided with the following: **a** Disposable gloves and aprons **b** Disposable trolley sheets or chair covers **c** Cleaning equipment for the trolley or chair prior to use by the next patient.	5 To prevent the contamination of the porter or other patients.

Death of a Hepatitis B Patient

1 There should be minimal handling of the body.	1 To decrease the risk of infection of the nursing staff.
2 Nurses should wear disposable plastic aprons and gloves when handling the body.	
3 The body should be totally enclosed in a plastic bag specifically designed for highly contagious patients.	3 To reduce the risk to portering and mortuary staff.
4 The mortuary staff should be informed of the diagnosis.	
5 If the relatives wish to view the body, they must be advised not to touch it.	5 To prevent contamination.

17

HUMIDIFICATION

Definition
Humidification may be defined as increasing the moisture content of air. In health, inspired air is filtered, warmed and moistened by the ciliated lining and mucus produced in the upper respiratory pathways.

Indications
Humidification is indicated in the following cases:

1 Trauma
2 Pneumonia
3 Rhinitis
4 Surgery resulting in tracheostomy
5 Continuous oxygen therapy.

REFERENCE MATERIAL

Types of Humidifier
A wide variety of apparatus is now manufactured to provide the patient with humidified air. Such apparatus will warm, humidify and filter the air without recourse, necessarily, to an oxygen supply.

The following types of apparatus are among those widely used.

Blower Humidifier   An electrical machine which heats, filters and moistens the air without the need for an oxygen supply. The air reaches the patient by tubing attached to the tracheostomy tube.

Ohio Nebulizer   A large plastic reservoir for water which attaches to an oxygen flow meter. Humidified oxygen is supplied to the patient via a tracheostomy mask. These reservoirs can be resterilized.

Inspiron System Nebulizer   A small plastic reservoir which acts in a similar way to the Ohio nebulizer. This system is relatively inexpensive in comparison with the Ohio nebulizer and is disposable.

Room Humidifiers   Water reservoirs which, by means of electrical heating, produce a source of steam at the bedside. A room humidifier may be used in addition to any other means of humidification.

Additional Equipment

Tracheostomy

Roger's Spray   is used to assist humidification in patients with a tracheostomy. The spray is comprised of a small glass reservoir which projects a jet of sodium bicarbonate 1% or normal saline directly into the trachea. It is used prior to suctioning to loosen secretions and to stimulate the cough reflex. The patient should be taught to use this as soon as possible.

Laryngectomy

Three pieces of equipment are commonly met in association with patients with a laryngectomy.

Buchanan Bib   Mesh bib which ties around the neck and covers the tracheostomy. This protects the stoma from accidental entry of foreign bodies, dust, etc., and helps to warm the air entering the trachea. All patients with newly formed stomas should wear some type of protective bib.

Laryngo Foam   This is a disposable sponge which protects and moistens the tracheastome.

Swedish Nose   Swedish noses are small reservoirs that are attached directly to the tracheostomy tube. They are made by various firms. Expired air is collected from the patient while inspired air is warmed and filtered.

References and Further Reading

Ballantyne J C et al. (1978) Otolaryngology, 3rd edition, John Wright and Son

Cox S Jones G (1980) Head and neck nursing care, in Cancer Nursing: Surgical, edited by R Tiffany, Faber and Faber, pp. 163-191

Edels Y (1983) Laryngectomy — Diagnosis to Rehabilitation, Croom Helm

Freud R H (1979) Principles of Head and Neck Surgery, Appleton Century Crofts

Iveson Iveson J (1981) Students' forum. Tracheostomy, Nursing Mirror 153 (4): 30-31

McKelvie P L (1980) Surgical aspects of laryngectomy, in Laryngectomy Rehabilitation Seminars, Poole 1978, Abingdon 1980, National Society for Cancer Relief, pp. 80-81

Nursing (US) (1976) Up to date survey of tracheal tubes, Nursing (US) 5 (11): 66-72

Stell P M Moran A G (1978) Head and Neck Surgery, William Heinemann Medical Books

GUIDELINES: HUMIDIFICATION

Procedure

Action	Rationale
Immediate Postoperative Care, i.e. the First 24-48 Hours	
1 Fill a suitable nebulizer, such as an Ohio or Inspiron nebulizer, with sterile water and attach it to the oxygen supply. Set the oxygen rate at 4 litres per minute at 40%. Give a constant supply of humidified oxygen for 24-48 hours.	1 Constant humidification is required while new stoma adapts to the outside environment (especially for laryngectomy patients). Humidification also prevents the formation of crusts which are liable to obstruct the airway.
2 Spray sodium bicarbonate 1% into the trachea as necessary, using a spray such as Roger's spray or a syringe.	2 To loosen secretions prior to suction and to stimulate the cough reflex.
3 For patients in cubicles, a room humidifier may be placed at the bedside.	3 To provide a warm, humid environment.
Subsequent Care	
1 Give humidified oxygen as required. Usually patients need about 10-15 minutes of humidification every 4 hours. This may be adapted according to the patient's needs, e.g. throughout the night.	1 Patients begin to adapt to breathing through their tracheostomy after the first 24-48 hours. Some humidification is required according to individual needs and to prevent crust formation in the airway.
2 If the patient does not require oxygen, blow humidifiers may be used.	2 These provide humidified air without the need for an oxygen supply.
3 Teach the patient to keep his/her tracheostomy moist by using a spray such as Roger's spray or a syringe containing 1% sodium bicarbonate or normal saline, prior to suctioning.	3 To loosen secretions and to prevent crust formation. To prevent contamination. Sterile sodium bicarbonate and normal saline are supplied in small bottles which, if not fully used within 24 hours, should be changed. If a spray is used, such as Roger's spray, this should be washed and dried each day and resterilized once the patient is discharged.
4 Provide bibs, such as Buchanan bibs, for patients.	4 To protect stoma.

18

INTRAPLEURAL DRAINAGE

Definition
Intrapleural drainage is an underwater seal system of drainage that prevents the entry of air into the pleural space, thus avoiding pneumothorax.

Indications
Intrapleural drainage is indicated under two circumstances.

1 To remove matter from the pleural space or thoracic cavity:
   a Solids, e.g. fibrin or clotted blood.
   b Liquids, e.g. serous fluids, blood, pus, chyle or gastric juice
   c Gas, e.g. air from the lungs, trachea or oesophagus.
2 To allow the lung to re-expand following surgery.

REFERENCE MATERIAL

Anatomy and Physiology
The pleura is a thin sheet of tissue covering the undersurface of the ribs, diaphragm and the structures of the mediastinum. It continues over the surface of both lungs, thus forming a space known as the pleural space. The layer in contact with the surface of the lungs is known as the visceral pleura; that in contact with the thoracic wall, the parietal pleura. These two memberanes are continuous with each other but are separated by a thin serous fluid that allows the pleurae to slide smoothly over each other during respiration. In health the pleural space is a potential space only. This space has a negative pressure normally. The elastic tissues of the lungs and the chest wall continually pull in opposite directions, the lungs tending to recoil inwards and the chest wall outwards. As these opposing forces attempt to pull the visceral and parietal pleurae apart, they create a negative pressure in the pleural space. Pressures in the pleural space are approximately 8 mm H_2O during inspiration and 2 mm H_2O on expiration. A negative pressure of 54 mm H_2O can be measured during

forced inspiraiion; during forced expiration, e.g. coughing, a positive pressure of approximately 68 mm H_2O develops.

Any opening of the thoracic cavity results in a loss of negative pressure and the lungs collapse. Collections of fluids or materials can also cause the lung to collapse as these substances take up space, restricting expansion of the lungs and inhibiting cardiopulmonary function.

When a tube is inserted to remove air it is normally inserted fairly high in the intrapleural space as air is light and will usually rise. If a tube is inserted to remove liquids or debris, it is usually inserted fairly low in the intrapleural space on the premise that the substances are relatively heavy and will therefore fall due to gravity. If more than one tube is inserted, e.g. following intrathoracic surgery, to remove both air and fluid or debris, the higher, known as the apical drain, is used to remove air, and the lower, known as the basal drain, is used to remove liquid and debris.

Types of Chest Drain (see Figure 18.1)

Any system must be capable of removing whatever collects in the pleural space more rapidly than it accummulates.

Single Bottle Water-seal System

In this system the end of the drainage tube from the patient's chest is covered by a layer of water that permits drainage and prevents lung collapse by sealing out the atmosphere. Drainage depends on gravity, the mechanics of respiration and, if necessary, suction by the addition of a controlled vacuum. The tube from the patient should extend approximately 2.5 cm below the level of the water in the container.

Two-bottle Water-seal System

This system consists of the same water-seal chamber with the addition of a manometer bottle. Drainage is similar again to the single bottle system. Suction, however, is controlled by containing sufficient fluids to establish the degree of vacuum required. Effective drainage depends on gravity and the amount of suction added as controlled by the manometer bottle.

Three-bottle Water-seal System

The initial chamber in this system collects the drainage, so that the fluid in the water-seal chamber stays constant as drainage accumulates. This has an advantage over the above-mentioned systems in that as the chest drainage collects in the water-seal chamber the resistance of flow from the pleural space is increased. When the fluid in the water-seal chamber equals the amount of fluid in the manometer bottle, any effective suction is cancelled. In this system drainge depends on gravity and the amount of suction added as controlled by the manometer. The suction system maintains a negative pressure throughout the closed drainage system. The manometer bottle regulates the amount of vacuum in the system.

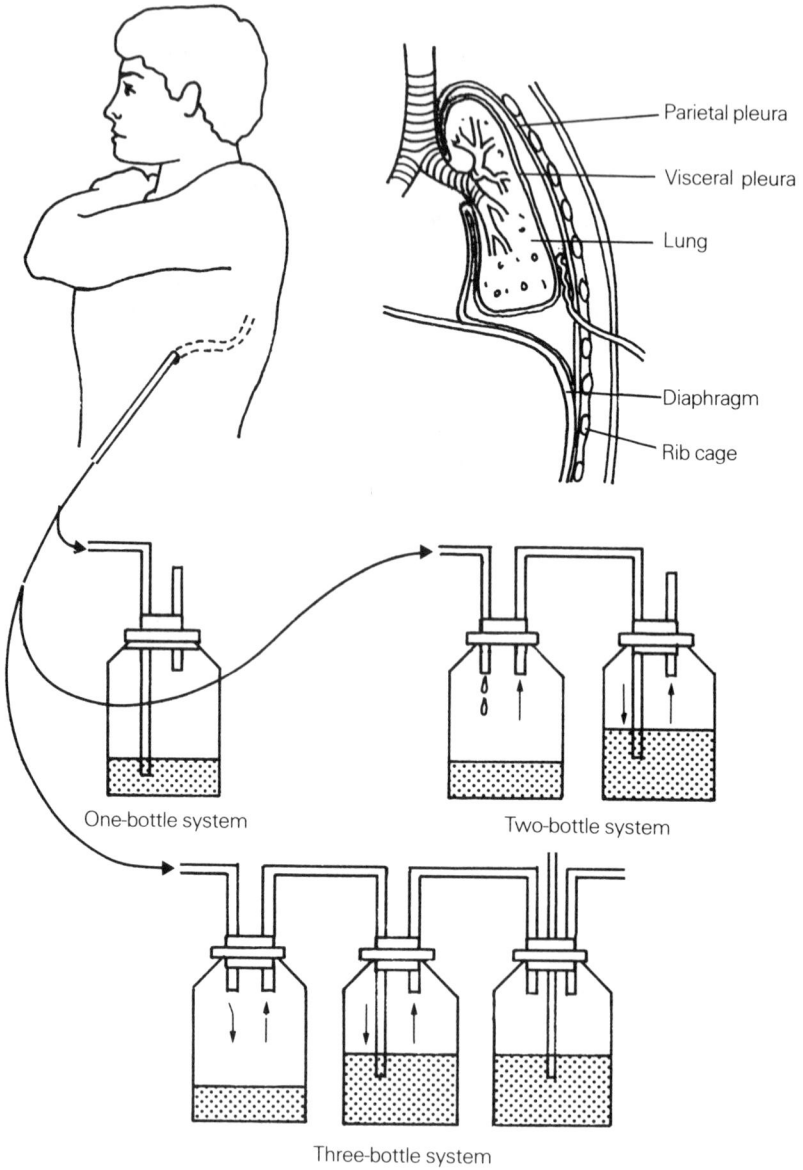

Parietal pleura

Visceral pleura

Lung

Diaphragm

Rib cage

One-bottle system

Two-bottle system

Three-bottle system

Figure 18.1 One-, two-, and three-bottle chest drainage systems

The Argyle 'Double Seal' System

This system consists of four chambers and is portable (see Figure 18.2). The second chamber is the collection chamber and is divided into three subchambers. The next chamber is the water-seal chamber. It is essentially U-shaped . The last chamber is the suction control chamber. Again this is U-shaped. The extra chamber in an Argyle unit is also a water-seal chamber. The patient's air passes through the third chamber into the suction source. If, however, the passage into the suction source is accidentally obstructed, the patient's air will pass instead through the first chamber into the atmosphere. The first chamber provides a safety vent of the patient's air.

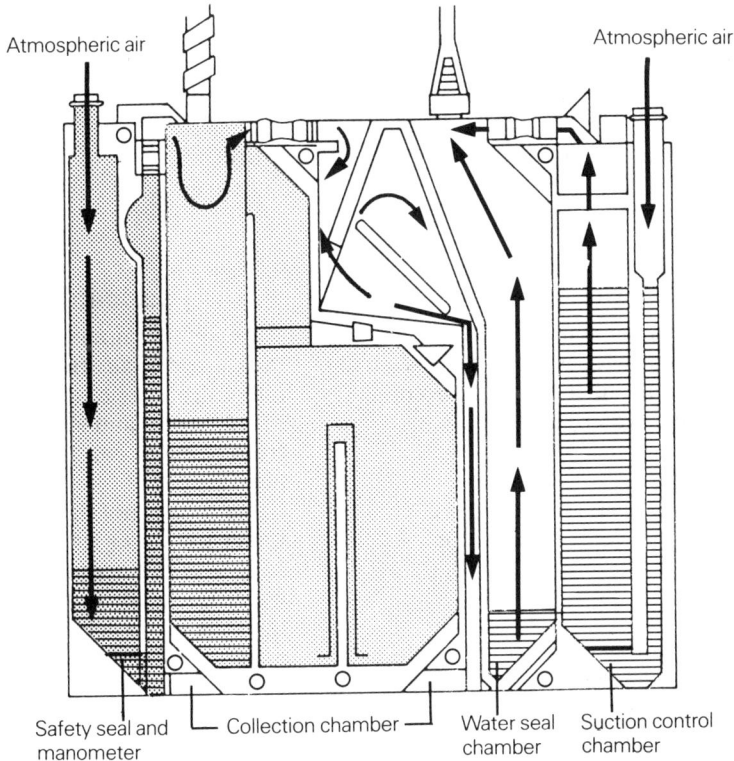

Atmospheric air

Atmospheric air

Safety seal and manometer

Collection chamber

Water seal chamber

Suction control chamber

Figure 18.2 Argyle double seal system

References

Brunner L S Suddarth D S (1982) The Lippincott Manual of Medical-Surgical Nursing, Harper and Row, pp. 354-366

Brunner L S Suddarth D S (1982) The Lippincott Manual of Nursing Practice, 3rd edition, J B Lippincott, pp. 224-277

Cohen S Stack M (1980) Programmed instruction: how to work with chest tubes, American Journal of Nursing 80: 685-712

Erickson R (1981) Chest tubes: they're really not that complicated, Nursing (US) 11 (5): 34-43

Erickson R (1981) Solving chest tube problems, Nursing (US) 11 (6): 62-68

GUIDELINES: MANAGEMENT OF UNDERWATER SEAL DRAINAGE

Equipment

1 Sterile chest drainage bottle
2 Sterile disposable tubing
3 Drainage bottle holder — if available
4 Suction pump, such as Robert's — if required
5 Two pairs of artery forceps — tips to be covered with rubber

Procedure

Action	Rationale
1 Attach the intrapleural drain to the drainage tube. *Note:* This should lead to the long tube whose end is under water seal.	1 Water-seal drainage provides for the escape of air, fluid and debris into a drainage bottle. The water acts as a seal and keeps the air from being drawn back into the pleural space.
2 Ensure that drainage tubing is 2.5 cm below the water level (Figure 18.3).	2 If the tube is not deep enough under the water level, there is a danger of it emerging above the water line if the bottle is moved. If the tube is too deep, a higher intrapleural pressure is required to expel air.

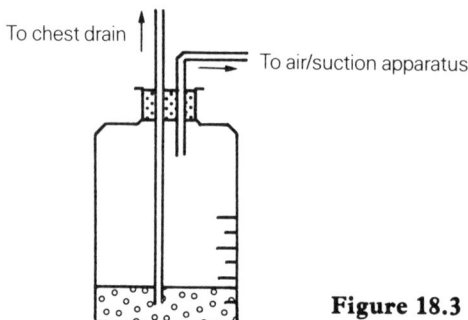

To chest drain
To air/suction apparatus

Figure 18.3 Underwater seal drainage

Action	**Rationale**
3 The other, shorter tube, is **a** Left open to the atmosphere **b** Attached to a controlled suction apparatus, e.g. Robert's pump.	**a** To allow gas to escape. **b** Although drainage of liquids and/or debris relies on gravity and the mechanics of respiration, additional controlled suction may be necessary to accelerate the process.
4 Establish the original level of fluid by **a** Marking with a piece of tape **b** Filling to a preset amount. *Note:* All bottles used should, preferably, be calibrated. 5 When recording fluid drainage: **a** Note the date and time **b** Mark hourly or daily increments by taping the level on the drainage bottles. *Note:* When using tape specify whether the upper, mid or lower border of the tape is the level to be measured at (Figure 18.4).	4 This provides a base-line for measurement of fluid drainage. **b** This marking will show the amount of fluid loss and how fast fluid is collecting in the drainage bottle. If the fluid is blood, it serves as a basis for retransfusion or reoperation, if following surgery. Inaccuracies of 100-200 ml can occur if the incorrect border is used.

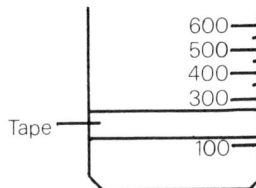

Figure 18.4 Specify whether the upper, mid or lower level of the tape is to be measured

Action	**Rationale**
6 Secure tubing to the bed clothes by the use of tape and safety pins.	6 This will prevent kinking, looping or pressure on the tubing which may cause reflux of fluid into the pleural space or impede drainage, causing blocking of the intra-pleural drain by debris.

Action	**Rationale**
7 Ensure that artery clamps are in close proximity to patient, i.e. taped to the wall, clamped to the bed clothes or on the bedside locker.	7 In the event of accidental disconnection of the drainage tubing from the intrapleural drain, the artery clamps should immediately be applied to the intrapleural drain to prevent entry of air (on inspiration) into the pleural space — leading to pneumothorax. When moving the patient, the drainage tubing is more likely to become disconnected, therefore the artery clamps should be readily available. There may be medical orders to apply the clamps, at set intervals, to delay drainage; e.g. following instillation of drugs or radioactive substances it is normal to clamp the tubing for 24 hours.
8 Ensure that the patient is sitting in a comfortable position which allows optimum drainage. Encourage the patient to change his/her position frequently. This may be enhanced by adequate pain control, using drugs which do not depress respiration.	8 Correct positioning aids drainage by gravity and by ensuring that the patient breathes freely, to promote gaseous exchange. Changing position also promotes better drainage as well as avoiding discomfort and pressure sores.
9 Ask the physiotherapist to help encourage the patient with mobility, chest and arm exercises.	9 To promote drainage and avoid the complications of pressure sores and stiffness of the arm on the side of drain insertion.
10 Ensure patency of tubing by 'milking' tubing towards the drainage bottle, if necessary. Take care not to disconnect tubing whilst executing this manoeuvre. *Note:* This is only necessary if draining fluid.	10 'Milking' the tubing prevents it from becoming clogged with clots or fibrin. Constant attention to maintaining the patency of the tube will facilitate prompt expansion of the lung and minimize complications.
11 Ensure that there is fluctuation (swinging) of the fluid level in the drainage tube under water seal.	11 Fluctuation of the water level in the tube shows that there is effective communication between the pleural cavity and the drainage bottle, provides a valuable indication of the patency of the drainage system, and is a gauge of intrapleural pressure.

Action	Rationale
12 Ensure that the drainage bottle remains at floor level, except when the patient is being helped to move. The drainage bottle should never be raised above the level of the intrapleural drain.	12 To prevent backflow of fluid into the pleural space.
13 Caution visitors and ancillary staff against handling any part of the system or displacing the drainage bottle.	13 To prevent backflow and to guard against accidental disconnection of the tubing which would allow air entry.

GUIDELINES: CHANGING DRAINAGE TUBING AND BOTTLES

Equipment

1 Sterile drainage bottle
2 Sterile water
3 Two pairs of artery clamps — tips covered with rubber
4 Suitable antiseptic solution, e.g. Hibisol
5 Sterile tubing

Procedure

Action	Rationale
1 Explain the procedure to the patient.	1 To gain the patient's consent and cooperation.
2 Wash your hands.	2 To minimize the risk of infection.
3 Prepare the drainage bottle by putting in a set amount (enough to cover the end of the long arm of the drainage tubing) of sterile water and taking note of that level. Mark this level with tape. If tubing is to be changed, attach clean tubing to the drainage bottle prepared.	3 To provide an underwater seal. Enough water should be in the bottle to ensure maintenance of the seal. Too much water creates pressure and reduces the capacity of the bottle for drainage. It is essential to note the amount of water added to the bottle for accurate measurement of drainage.
4 Take the equipment to the bedside.	
5 Clamp the intrapleural drain using both artery clamps, before changing the bottle or the tubing.	5 To avoid tension pneumothorax occurring when the water seal is broken.
6 Clean your hands with a suitable antiseptic solution, e.g. Hibisol.	6 To minimize the risk of infection.

Action	**Rationale**
7 Remove the bung with the drainage tubing from the underwater seal bottle and replace it in the clean bottle. Ensure that there is an airtight connection between the bung and bottle. If tubing is being changed, the bung will already be in place in the sterile bottle.	7 To prevent air entry and reduce the risk of infection.
8 Take the clamps off the intrapleural drainage tube.	8 To re-establish drainage.
9 Make the patient comfortable.	
10 Remove equipment.	
11 Record in appropriate documentation the amount of drainage, deducting the water originally in the bottle.	11 For accurate recording of the amount of drainage.
12 Empty and clean the bottle and return it to the central sterile supplies department.	

Note: If an underwater seal drain is established to drain air from the pleural space, there is probably no need to change either connection tubing or bottle. However, if fluid and debris are drained the bottle may need changing frequently (at least daily), depending on the amount drained. The tubing need only be changed if there is a copious amount of debris and there is a danger of it becoming blocked. Changing the tubing or the bottle breaks the closed system and provides a potential portal of entry for bacteria.

GUIDELINES: REMOVAL OF AN INTRAPLEURAL DRAIN

Equipment

1 Sterile dressing pack
2 Cleansing lotion
3 Surgical gloves
4 Stitch cutter
5 Collodion lotion
6 Adhesive tape
7 Plaster remover

Procedure

This is a procedure usually carried out by a member of the medical staff, preferably the doctor who inserted the drain. However, it may be performed by a qualified nurse if he/she has been instructed and supervised in the removal of intrapleural drains.

Action		**Rationale**
Doctor/First Nurse	*Assisting Nurse*	
1 Explain the procedure to patient and allow the patient to practise the procedure beforehand.		1 To obtain the patient's consent and co-operation. Speed and accuracy are essential in this procedure so all equipment must be at hand.
2 Wash your hands.	2 Wash your hands.	2 To minimize the risk of infection.
3 Prepare equipment using strict aseptic technique.	3 Assist in preparation of equipment without causing contamination.	
4 Remove the old dressing, using forceps.		
5 Cut the knot from the purse-string suture.		5 Allows mobility of the suture.
6 Cut the suture holding the drain in place.	6 Hold the drain in place.	6 To prevent the drain falling out.
7 Tie the purse-string suture lightly to skin level.		7 To enable rapid tightening of the suture when the drain is removed.
8 Instruct the patient to breathe in to the maximum and to hold his/her breath. This manoeuvre should have been practised beforehand.		8 To minimize the risk of tension pneumo-thorax occurring as the drain is removed. Prior preparation of the patient ensures full cooperation.
	9 Steadily pull out the drain.	9 If the drain is pulled out too quickly, tension pneumothorax may occur.
10 As the drain leaves the skin, tighten the purse-string suture and tie a firm double knot. Speed is essential. Cut the ends to 1.25 cm.		10 The purse-string suture must be tightened immediately the drain leaves the chest to avoid tension pneumothorax.
11 Place gauze with collodion over the suture.	11 Strap the gauze firmly in place.	11 To provide a tight seal.
12 Tell the patient that he/she may exhale and relax.		

Action	Rationale
13 Remove any debris from the site of the wound and ensure that the patient is comfortable.	
14 Clear equipment away.	
15 Wash your hands.	15 To prevent cross-infection.
16 Empty and clean the drainage bottles and send them to the central sterile supplies department.	
17 Record the amount of drainage in appropriate documents.	17 To provide an accurate record.

NURSING CARE PLAN

Problem	Cause	Suggested Action
1 Lack of drainage	1 Kinking, looping or pressure on the tubing may cause reflux of fluid into the intrapleural space or may impede drainage, causing blocking of the intrapleural drain.	1 Check the system and straighten tubing as required. Secure the tubing to prevent a recurrence of the problem.
2 No fluctuation of fluid in tubing from the underwater seal	2 **a** Re-expansion of the lung	2 **a** Ask medical staff if the drain may be removed following chest X-ray. The purpose of the drain has been fulfilled. Keeping the drain in any longer than necessary may lead to hazards from infection or air re-entry.
	b Tubing is obstructed by blood clots or fibrin	**b** 'Milk' the tubing towards the drainage bottle to try to dislodge the obstruction and re-establish patency.
	c Tubing is looped or kinked	**c** Straighten tubing as required. Secure the tubing to prevent a recurrence.
	d Failure of the suction apparatus.	**d** Disconnect the suction apparatus and leave this tube open to the air, allowing intrapleural air to escape.

Problem	Cause	Suggested Action
3 Constant bubbling of fluid in the drainage bottle	3 An air leak in the system	3 Clamp the intrapleural drain, momentarily, close to the chest wall and establish whether there is a leak in the rest of the system. Clamping the tubing shows whether the leak is below the level of the clamp. However, if the clamp is left on for too long, and the leak is at thoracic level, i.e. air is entering the pleura, this will increase the patient's pneumo-thorax. Inform medical staff as leaking and trapping of air in the pleural space can result in tension pneumo-thorax.
4 Patient shows signs of rapid, shallow breathing, cyanosis, pressure in the chest, subcutaneous emphysema or haemorrhage	4 Tension pneumo-thorax; mediastinal shift; postoperative haemorrhage; severe incisional pain; pulmonary embolus or cardiac tamponade	4 Observe, record and report any of these signs to a doctor immediately.
5 Incisional pain		5 Provide adequate analgesia, as prescribed, to reduce the patient's discomfort and to enable him/her to perform deep breathing exercises and mobilization to ensure adequate drainage and to avoid complications.
6 Accidental discon-nection of the drainage tubing from the intra-pleural drain		6 Apply an artery clamp to the drain immedi-ately in order to avoid air entering the pleural space; this is more of a danger if the patient is exhaling at the time. Re-establish the con-

Problem	Cause	Suggested Action
		nection as soon as possible in order to re-establish drainage. If necessary, use a clean, sterile drainage tube; tubing may have been contaminated when it became disconnected. If air entry has occurred, report this to a doctor. Record the incident in the relevant records. The patient may have been upset by the incident and will need reassurance.
7 Patient needs to be moved to another area, e.g. X-ray department		7 Place the drainage bottle below the level of the intrapleural drain, as close to the floor as possible, in order to prevent reflux of fluid into the pleural space. Do not clamp the drain unless the doctor has ordered it: this may obstruct drainage and allow clot formation if fluid is being drained. Attach clamps to the patient's gown, in case of accidental disconnection *en route.*
8 Intrapleural drain falls out		8 Pull the purse-string suture immediately to close the wound. Cover the wound with an occlusive sterile dressing. Inform a doctor. The objective is to minimize the amount of air entering the pleural space. The drain will probably need reinserting.

19

INTRAVENOUS DRUG ADMINISTRATION

REFERENCE MATERIAL

The involvement of nursing staff in the administration of intravenous drugs was formally recognized in the mid-1970s following the publication of the Breckenridge Report. A working party had been established in 1974 under the chairmanship of Lord Breckenridge as a result of the increasing use of the intravenous route for drug administration. There was concern that hazards such as microbial contamination and drug incompatibilities were not fully appreciated and that the staff participating were not adequately trained in the procedures used.

The terms of reference of the working party were as follows:

1 To identify and investigate the problems associated with this form of intravenous therapy
2 To consider the responsibilities of the various parties involved
3 To consider modification of nurse training to ensure safe practice
4 To produce guidelines for the three main professions, i.e. doctors, pharmacists and nurses
5 To assess the value of various aids, e.g. charts for reference.

The working party received evidence from a number of sources and considered pharmaceutical data. In 1976 the findings were published by the Department of Health and Social Security. The report proposed a rational approach to intravenous drug administration, established guidelines for documentation and outlined the responsibilities of health authorities and health professionals. The responsibility of medical staff was to ensure that the drug was adminstered by the most effective and safest route and that the instructions to facilitate this were clearly written.

An intravenous additive service provided by pharmacists was favoured. In situations where this was not practical, pharmacists were to act as an information source for other personnel. It was accepted that nursing staff could undertake the addition and administration of intravenous drugs. The nurse, however, should be qualified (i.e. should be a registered general nurse or an enrolled nurse) and have undergone a period of training and assessment in both the theoretical knowledge and practical procedures involved in such drug administration. He/she should be issued with a certificate of competence and fully understand the legal implications of undertaking such an extension of the role of the nurse.

In all intravenous therapy the nurse's responsibility continued to incude the following:

1 Checking the infusion fluid and container for any obvious faults or contamination
2 Ensuring the adminstration of the prescribed fluid to the correct patient
3 Observing whether the intravenous line remains patent
4 Inspecting the site of insertion and reporting abnormalities
5 Controlling the rate of flow as prescribed
6 Monitoring the condition of the patient and reporting any changes
7 Maintaining appropriate records.

Permitted methods of intravenous drug administration by nurses were identified:

1 Continuously, or intermittently, by addition to an intravenous infusion in a bottle, bag or burette. This method may include the use of a variety of equipment, e.g. a small volume syringe pump or a Y administration set.
2 Intermittently by injection into the latex rubber section of an intravenous administration set.
3 Intermittently by injection into a cannula or winged infusion device. The device's patency may be maintained by use of a stylet or by heparinization.
4 Intermittently by injection via a three-way tap or stopcock. This method is not advised, however, due to the increased risk of contamination associated with these devices. Streamlined adaptors are now available and are preferred.

Additional Guidelines

Certain guidelines were also issued in 1976 about general intravenous management related to the areas of nursing involvement. These included the following:

1 The infusion container should not hang for more than 24 hours. This was reduced to 8 hours in the case of blood or blood products.
2 The administration set must be changed every 24 hours. It is desirable to record the time and date when this is due.
3 The site of the infusion should be inspected at least daily for complications such as infiltration or inflammation.
4 The sterile dressing covering the insertion site must be changed daily, at the time of inspection or whenever it is touched, e.g. at the time of

administration of an intravenous injection.

In the light of more recent research, it is now possible to propose further recommendations. It is desirable that a closed system of infusion is maintained wherever possible, with as few connections or stopcocks as is necessary for its purpose. This reduces the risk of extrinsic bacterial contamination, especially if three-way taps or their equivalents are excluded.

Problems associated with the insertion site of the cannula have been shown to rise substantially after the device has been in position for 48 hours. Routine resiting is, therefore, advised if at all possible. Although the nurse is not normally responsible for this duty, he/she may be able to remind the doctor when this time has elapsed.

In order for the insertion site to be readily available for inspection, it may be necessary for the nurse to assume responsibility for taping the cannula in place as well as dressing the insertion site. Nonsterile tape should not cover the site, the equivalent of an open wound, and a method must be devised so that the site remains visible and the cannula is stable. The procedure illustrated in Figure 19.1 is recommended.

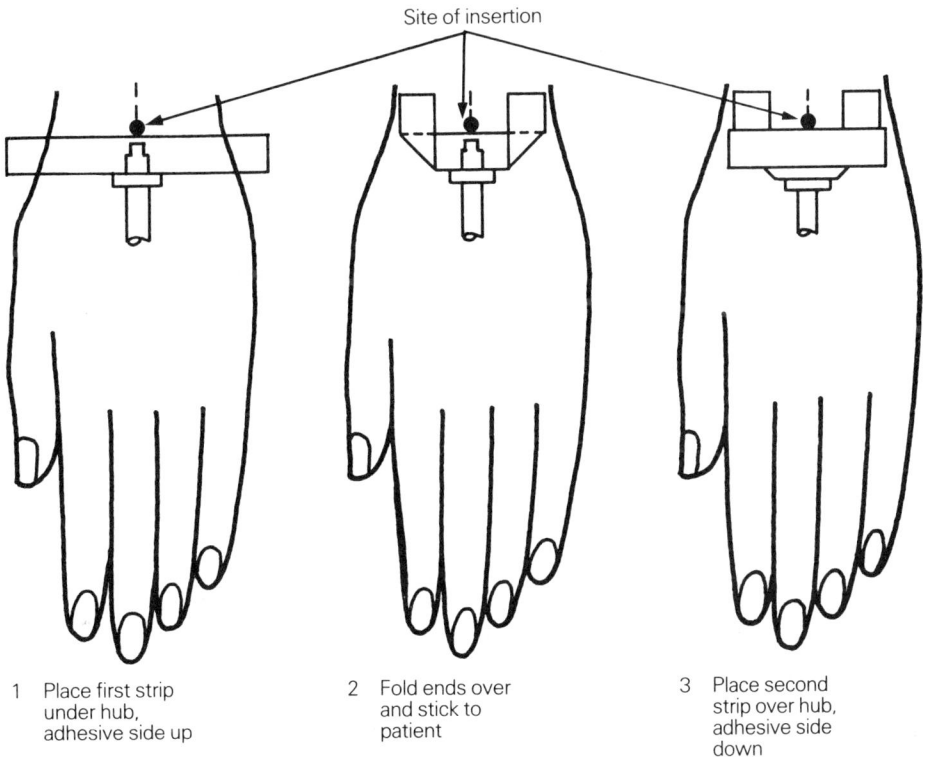

Site of insertion

1 Place first strip under hub, adhesive side up

2 Fold ends over and stick to patient

3 Place second strip over hub, adhesive side down

Figure 19.1 Site of insertion

The purpose of all recommendations is to reduce the complications, especially infection, associated with intravenous therapy. Competent, informed management and adherence to basic principles will ensure this.

Removal of the intravenous device or cannula should be an aseptic procedure. The cannula must be taken out gently in order to prevent damage to the vein and pressure should be applied immediately. This pressure should be firm and not involve any rubbing movement. A haematoma will occur if the needle is carelessly removed, causing discomfort and a focus for infection. Pressure should be applied until bleeding has stopped, then a light sterile dressing applied.

Drugs are used for three basic purposes:

1   Diagnostic purposes, e.g. assessment of liver function or diagnosis of myasthenia gravis
2   Prophylaxis, e.g. heparin to prevent thrombosis or antibiotics to prevent infection
3   Therapeutic purposes, e.g. replacement of fluids or vitamins, supportive purposes (to enable other treatments, such as anaesthesia), palliation of pain and cure (as in the case of antibiotics).

Drugs administered intravenously also fall within the above-mentioned categories.

Advantages of Using the Intravenous Route

1   An immediate therapeutic effect is achieved due to rapid delivery of the drug to its target site.
2   Total absorption allows precise dose calculation and more reliable treatment.
3   The rate of administration can be controlled and the therapeutic effect maintained or modified as required.
4   Pain and irritation caused by some substances when given intramuscularly or subcutaneously are avoided.
5   Intravenous administration is suitable for drugs which cannot be absorbed by any other route due to large molecular size and irritation to or instability in the gastrointestinal tract.

Disadvantages of Using the Intravenous Route

1   There is an inability to recall the drug and reverse the action of it. This may lead to increased toxicity or a sensitivity reaction.
2   Insufficient control of administration may lead to speed shock. This is characterized by a flushed face, headache, congestion, tightness in the chest, etc.
3   Additional complications may occur, such as the following:
    a Microbial contamination through a point of access into the circulation for a period of time

b Vascular irritation, e.g. chemical phlebitis

c Drug incompatibilities and interactions if multiple additives are prescribed.

Principles to be Applied Throughout Preparation and Administration

Asepsis

Aseptic technique must be adhered to throughout all intravenous procedures to prevent extrinsic bacterial contamination. The nurse must employ good handwashing and drying techniques or use an alcohol-based skin cleanser as an alternative. Injection sites or bungs should be cleaned using an alcohol-based antiseptic, allowing time for it to dry. A non-touch technique should be employed when changing infusion bags or bottles and these procedures should be completed as quickly as possible. If asepsis is not maintained, local infection, septic phlebitis or septicaemia may result. Any indication of infection, e.g. redness at the insertion site of the device or pyrexia, requires removal of the cannula and further investigation.

Inspection of fluids, drugs, equipment and their packaging must be undertaken to detect any points where contamination may have occurred during manufacture and/or transport. This intrinsic contamination may be detected as cloudiness, discoloration or the presence of particles.

Sterility will ensure that the patient does not receive an injection or infusion of microbes.

Safety

In order to ensure safe preparation and administration of the drug two nurses must check all details of the prescription and all calculations. The nurse must also check the compatibility of the drug with the diluent or infusion fluid. He/she should be aware of the types of incompatibilities and the factors which could influence them. These include pH, concentration, time, temperature, light and the brand of the drug. If insufficient information is available, a reference book or the pharmacy should be consulted. Stability after reconstitution must also be checked and constant monitoring of both the mixture and the patient is important. The preferred method and rate of intravenous administration must be determined.

Drugs should never be added to the following: blood; blood products, i.e. plasma or platelet concentrate; mannitol solutions; sodium bicarbonate solution. Only specially prepared additives should be used with fat emulsions or amino acid preparations.

Accurate labelling of additives and records of administration are essential.

Any protective clothing which is advised should be worn.

Comfort

Both the physical and psychological comfort of the patient must be considered.

By maintaining high standards throughout, the patient's physical comfort should be assured. Comprehensive explanation of the practical aspects of the procedure together with balanced information about the effects of treatment will contribute to reducing anxiety.

Methods of Administering Intravenous Drugs

Three methods are recommended: continuous infusion, intermittent infusion and intermittent injection.

Continuous Infusion

Continuous infusion may be defined as the administration of a large volume of fluid, i.e. 250-1000 ml, over a number of hours that may be repeated over a period of days. An exception to this may be a small volume infusion (e.g. of heparin) delivered continuously via a syringe pump.

A continuous infusion may be used when

1 The drugs to be administered must be highly diluted.
2 A maintenance of steady blood levels of the drug is required.

Preprepared infusion fluids with additives such as those containing potassium chloride should be used whenever possible. Only one addition should be made to each bottle or bag of fluid after the compatibility has been ascertained. The additive and fluid must be mixed well to prevent a layering effect which can occur with some drugs. The danger is that a bolus injection of the drug may be delivered. To safeguard this, any additions should be made to the infusion fluid before the fluid is hung on the infusion stand. The infusion container should be clearly labelled after the addition has been made. Constant monitoring of the infusion fluid mixture and the patient should occur.

Intermittent Infusion

Intermittent infusion is the administration of a small volume infusion, i.e. 50-250 ml, over a period of between 20 minutes and 2 hours. This may be given as a specific dose at one time or at repeated intervals during 24 hours.

An intermittent infusion may be used when

1 A peak plasma level is therapeutically required.
2 The pharmacology of the drug dictates this specific dilution.
3 The drug is not stable for the time required to administer a large volume infusion.
4 The patient does not require or cannot tolerate large volumes of fluid.

Delivery of the drug by intermittent infusion may utilize a system such as a Y set, if the simultaneous infusion is of a compatible fluid, or a burette set with a chamber capacity of 100 or 150 ml. A small volume infusion may also be connected to a heparinized cannula if no fluids are required between doses.

All the points considered when preparing for a continuous infusion should be taken into account here, e.g. preprepared fluids, single additions, adequate mixing, labelling and monitoring.

Calculation of Accurate Rate of Administration (Continuous or Intermittent)
The rate of administration of a continuous or intermittent infusion may be calculated from the following equation:

$$\frac{\text{No. millilitres to be infused}}{\substack{\text{No. hours over which} \\ \text{infusion is to be delivered}}} \times \frac{\text{No. drops per millilitre}}{60} = \substack{\text{No. drops to be} \\ \text{delivered per minute}}$$

In this equation, 60 is a factor for the conversion of the number of hours to the number of minutes; the number of drops per millilitre is dependent on the administration set used and the viscosity of the infusion fluid.

Direct Intermittent Injection
Direct intermittent injection is a procedure for the introduction of a small volume of drug(s) into the cannula or the injection site of the administration set using a needle and syringe. This may take a few seconds or a number of minutes.

A direct injection may be used when

1 A maximum concentration of the drug is required to vital organs. This is a 'bolus' injection which is given rapidly over seconds, as in an emergency.
2 The drug cannot be diluted due to pharmacological or therapeutic reasons. This is given as a controlled 'push' injection over a few minutes. Rapid administration could result in toxic levels and an anaphylactic-type reaction. Manufacturers' recommendations of rates of administration (i.e. millilitres or milligrams per minute) should be adhered to. In the absence of such recommendations, administration should proceed slowly.
3 A peak blood level is required and cannot be achieved by small volume infusion.

Delivery of the drug by direct injection may be via the cannula through a resealable latex bung, injection port or adaptor, or via the injection site of an administration set. Whatever method is chosen, the same procedure should be followed. This includes the following:

1 Removal of any bandage or dressing present to inspect the insertion site of the cannula
2 Confirmation of the patency of the vein and its ability to accept an extra flow of fluid or irritant chemical.

Administration into the injection site of a fast running drip may be advised if the infusion in progress is compatible. Alternatively a stop-start procedure may be employed if there is doubt about venous integrity. If the infusion fluid is incompatible with the drug, the line may be switched off and a syringe of normal saline used as a flush.

In some centres a heparin lock may be utilized. This means maintaining the patency of the cannula using a weak solution of heparin. A plug with a resealable injection cap is inserted into the end of the intravenous device. Sufficient heparin to fill the 'dead space' and of a concentration to prevent fibrin formation is injected. The cannula can then be left for a number of hours before reheparinization is required. The time is dependent on the strength of heparin used. After every use reheparinization is obviously required.

The advantages of using a heparin lock are as follows:

1 It reduces the risk of circulatory overload.
2 It reduces the risk of vascular irritation.
3 It decreases the risk of bacterial contamination as it eliminates a continuous intravenous pathway.
4 It increases patient comfort and mobility.
5 It may reduce the cost of intravenous equipment.

An alternative method of maintaining patency is the use of a stylet which can be inserted into certain cannulae.

If a number of drugs are being administered, normal saline must be used to flush in between each to prevent interactions. This flush should also be repeated at the end of the administration.

The insertion site of the device should be observed throughout for swelling or redness. Patients must be constantly consulted about any pain or discomfort they may be experiencing. Problems that arise during administration will involve the vein. Patency throughout should not be assumed. Early detection of extravasation of any drug, especially in concentrated form, is essential to meet the aims of therapy.

These aims can be summarized as the effective delivery of treatment without discomfort or tissue damage to the patient and without compromising venous access, especially if long term therapy is proposed.

Summary

The nurse is responsible for administering intravenous drugs safely by the methods listed. In order to do this he/she requires a thorough knowledge of the prinicples and their application, and a responsible attitude which ensures that he/she does not give intravenous medications without full knowledge of immediate and late effects, toxicities and nursing implications.

Knowledge of equipment and techniques for combining multiple additives is also essential.

Only by investigating these topics can the nurse develop into a confident and safe practitioner.

References and Further Reading

British Medical Association Pharmaceutical Society of Great Britain (1983) British National Formulary, British Medical Association Pharmaceutical Society of Great

Britian No 6

Department of Health and Social Security (1976) Health services development. Addition of drugs to intravenous fluids, London: HMSO HC (76) 9 (Breckenridge Report)

Maki D G et al. (1973) Infection control in intravenous therapy, Annals of Internal Medicine 79: 867-887

Marks M D (1978) Management of intravenous therapy, in Cancer Nursing — Medical, edited by R Tiffany, Faber and Faber, pp.73-112

Mehtar S (1981) A review of bacteriological observation in the care of IV cannulae, British Journal of Intravenous Therapy 2 (4): 16-22

Plumer A L (1982) Principles and Practice of Intravenous Therapy, 3rd edition, Little, Brown

Sager D Bomar S (1980) Intravenous Medications, J B Lippincott

GUIDELINES: ADMINISTRATION OF DRUGS BY CONTINUOUS INFUSION

This procedure may be carried out by the infusion of drugs from a bag, bottle or burette.

Equipment

1 Clinically clean receiver or tray containing the prepared drug to be administered
2 Patient's prescription chart
3 Recording sheet or book as required by law or hospital policy
4 Protective clothing as required by hospital policy for specific drugs
5 Container of appropriate intravenous infusion fluid
6 Swab saturated with isopropyl alcohol 70%
7 Drug additive label

Procedure

Action	Rationale
1 Explain the procedure to the patient.	1 To obtain the patient's consent and cooperation.
2 Inspect the infusion.	2 To check it is running satisfactorily and that the patient is not experiencing any discomfort at the site of insertion.
3 Wash your hands and assemble the necessary equipment.	
4 Prepare the drug for injection as per procedure.	
5 Check the name, strength and volume of intravenous fluid against the prescription chart.	5 To ensure that the correct type and quantity of fluid is administered.
6 Check the expiry date of the fluid.	6 To prevent an ineffective or toxic

Action	Rationale
	compound being administered to the patient.
7 Check that the packaging is intact.	7 To maintain asepsis.
8 Inspect the container and contents in a good light for cracks, punctures, air bubbles, discoloration, haziness, and crystalline or particulate matter.	8 To maintain asepsis. To prevent any toxic or foreign matter being infused into the patient.
9 Check the identity and amount of drug to be added with another nurse. Consider: **a** Compatibility of fluid and additive **b** Stability of mixture over the prescribed time **c** Any special directions for dilution, e.g. pH, optimum concentration, etc. **d** Sensitivity to external factors such as light **e** Any anticipated allergic reaction. If any doubts exist about the listed points, consult the pharmacist or appropriate reference works.	9 To minimize any risk of error. To ensure safe and effective administration of the drug. To enable anticipation of toxicities and the nursing implications of these.
10 Any additions must be made immediately prior to use.	10 To prevent any possible microbial growth or degradation.
11 Wash your hands thoroughly.	11 To maintain asepsis.
12 Expose the injection site on the container by removing any seal present.	
13 Clean the site with the swab and allow it to dry.	13 To maintain asepsis.
14 Inject the drug using a new sterile needle into the bag, bottle or burette. A 23g or 25g needle should be used.	14 To enable resealing of the latex or rubber injection site.
15 If the addition is made into a burette at the beside: **a** Avoid contamination of the needle and inlet port. **b** Check that the correct quantity of fluid is in the chamber. **c** Switch the infusion off briefly so that a bolus injection is not given.	**a** To maintain asepsis and prevent incompatibility, etc.

Action	Rationale
16 Invert the container a number of times, especially if adding to a flexible infusion bag.	16 To ensure adequate mixing of the drug.
17 Check again for haziness, discoloration, etc. This can occur even if the mixture is theoretically compatible, thus making vigilance essential.	17 To detect any incompatibility or degradation.
18 Complete the drug additive label and fix it on the bag, bottle or burette. Complete the patient's recording chart and other hospital and/or legally required documents.	18 To maintain accurate records. To provide a point of reference in the event of any queries. To prevent any duplication of treatment.
19 Place the container in a clinically clean receptacle. Wash your hands and proceed to the patient.	19 To maintain asepsis.
20 Check again that the infusion is running well and that the contents of the previous container have been delivered.	20 To confirm that the vein and/or cannula remain patent. To ensure that the preceding prescription has been administered.
21 Switch off the infusion and hang the new container quickly using a non-touch technique.	21 To achieve a safe and aseptic changeover.
22 Restart the infusion and adjust the rate of flow as prescribed.	22 To deliver the mixture accurately.
23 If the addition is made into a burette, the infusion can be restarted immediately following mixing and recording and the infusion rate adjusted accordingly.	
24 Ask the patient if he/she is experiencing any abnormal sensations, etc.	24 To ascertain whether there are any problems. If so, investigate.
25 Discard waste, making sure that it is placed in the correct containers, e.g. 'sharps' into a designated receptacle.	25 To ensure safe disposal and avoid injury to staff. To prevent reuse of equipment.

GUIDELINES: ADMINISTRATION OF DRUGS BY INTERMITTENT INFUSION

This procedure is carried out via a heparinized cannula or when patency is maintained by a stylet.

Equipment

Equipment for this procedure is as described for the previous procedure (i.e. items 1-7 on page 213) together with the following:

8   Intravenous administration set
9   Intravenous infusion stand
10   Clean dressing trolley
11   Clinically clean receiver or tray
12   Sterile needles and syringes
13   Normal saline 0.9%, 20 ml for injection
14   Heparin, in accordance with hospital policy, plus sterile bung or sterile stylet
15   Alcohol-based lotion for cleaning injection site
16   Alcohol-based hand wash solution
17   Sterile dressing pack
18   Hypoallergenic tape

Procedure

Action	Rationale
1 Explain the procedure to the patient.	1 To obtain the patient's consent and cooperation.
2 Prepare the intravenous infusion and additive as described previously (see items 2-11 on pages 213-214).	
3 Prime the intravenous administration set with infusion fluid mixture and hang it on the infusion stand.	
4 Draw up 10 ml of normal saline 0.9% for injection in two separate syringes, using an aseptic technique.	
5 Draw up heparin, as required by hospital policy, and check.	
6 Place the syringes in a clinically clean receiver or tray on the bottom shelf of the dressing trolley.	
7 Collect the other equipment and place it on the bottom shelf of the dressing trolley.	
8 Place a sterile dressing pack on the top of the trolley.	
9 Check that all necessary equipment is present.	9 To prevent delays and interruption of the procedure.

Action	Rationale
10 Wash your hands thoroughly before leaving the clinical room.	10 To maintain asepsis.
11 Proceed to the patient.	
12 Open the sterile dressing pack.	
13 Add lotion for cleaning the skin to the gallipot in order to wet the cotton wool balls.	
14 Wash your hands with soap and water or with an alcohol-based hand wash solution.	14 To maintain asepsis.
15 Remove the patient's bandage and dressing.	15 To observe the insertion site.
16 Inspect the insertion site of the cannula.	16 To detect any signs of inflammation, infiltration, etc. If present, take appropriate action.
17 Wash your hands or clean them with an alcohol-based hand wash solution.	17 To maintain asepsis.
18 Place a sterile towel under the patient's arm.	18 To create a sterile field.
19 Remove the injection bung or stylet from the cannula while applying digital pressure at the point within the vein where the cannula tip rests.	19 To prevent blood spillage.
20 Inject gently 10 ml of normal saline 0.9% for injection.	20 To confirm the patency of the cannula.
21 If no resistance is met, no pain or discomfort is felt by the patient, no swelling is evident, no leakage occurs around the cannula and there is a good backflow of blood on aspiration, it can be assumed that the cannula is patent.	
22 Connect to the infusion.	22 To commence treatment.
23 Open the control valve.	23 To check free flow.
24 Check the insertion site and ask the patient if he/she is comfortable.	24 To confirm that the vein can accommodate the extra fluid flow and that the patient experiences no pain, etc.
25 Adjust the flow rate as prescribed.	25 To ensure that the correct speed of administration is established.
26 Tape the administration set in a way that places no strain on the cannula.	26 To reduce the risk of mechanical phlebitis or infiltration.
27 Cover the cannula with a sterile topical swab and tape it in place.	27 To maintain asepsis.

Action	**Rationale**
28 If the infusion is to be completed within 40 minutes, bandaging is unnecessary and the patient may be instructed to keep the arm resting on the sterile field.	
29 Cover the dressing trolley and equipment with a sterile towel and leave by the bed.	29 To maintain asepsis.
30 Return at frequent intervals.	30 To check flow rate, patient comfort and for signs of infiltration.
31 If the infusion is to be in progress for longer than 40 minutes, a bandage should be applied. The equipment may be cleared away and reassembled at the end of the infusion.	31 To provide support and to promote patient comfort.
32 When the infusion is complete, wash your hands and recheck that all the equipment required is present.	32 To maintain asepsis and ensure that the procedure runs smoothly.
33 Stop the infusion when all the fluid has been delivered.	33 To ensure that all of the prescribed mixture has been delivered.
34 Wash your hands or clean them with an alcohol-based hand wash solution.	34 To maintain asepsis.
35 Disconnect the infusion set and flush the cannula with 10 ml of normal saline 0.9% for injection.	35 To flush any remaining irritating solution away from the cannula.
36 Insert a new sterile bung or stylet.	
37 If a new sterile bung is inserted, heparinization must follow.	37 To maintain the patency of the cannula for future use.
38 Clean the injection site of the bung with a swab saturated with isopropyl alcohol 70%.	38 To maintain asepsis.
39 Administer heparin, as prescribed, using a 23g or 25g needle.	39 To maintain the patency of the cannula and enable resealing of the latex injection site.
40 Cover the insertion site and cannula with a new sterile topical swab. Tape it in place.	40 To maintain asepsis.
41 Apply a bandage.	41 To provide support and increase the patient's comfort.
42 Ensure that the patient is comfortable.	

Action	**Rationale**
43 Discard waste, placing it in the correct containers, e.g. 'sharps' into a designated container.	43 To ensure safe disposal and avoid injury to staff. To prevent reuse of equipment.

GUIDELINES: ADMINISTRATION OF DRUGS BY DIRECT INJECTION, BOLUS OR PUSH

This procedure may be carried out via any one of the following:

1 The injection site of an intravenous administration set
2 An adaptor or injectable plug into a cannula or winged infusion device (patency may be maintained by stylet or by heparinization)
3 A three-way tap, stopcock or adaptor.

Equipment

1 Clinically clean receiver or tray containing the prepared drug(s) to be administered
2 Patient's prescription chart
3 Recording sheet or book as required by law or hospital policy
4 Protective clothing as required by hospital policy or specific drugs
5 Clean dressing trolley
6 Clinically clean receiver or tray
7 Sterile needles and syringes
8 Normal saline 0.9%, 20 ml for injection
9 Heparin, in accordance with hospital policy, or a sterile intravenous stylet
10 Alcohol-based lotion for cleaning injection site
11 Sterile dressing pack
12 Hypoallergenic tape

Procedure

Action	**Rationale**
1 Explain the procedure to the patient.	1 To obtain the patient's consent and cooperation.
2 Check any infusion in progress.	2 To see if it is running satisfactorily, and that the patient is not experiencing any discomfort at the site of insertion.
3 Wash your hands and assemble necessary equipment.	
4 Prepare the drug for injection as per procedure.	
5 Prepare a 20 ml syringe of normal saline 0.9% for injection, as described, using aseptic technique.	

Action	Rationale
6 Draw up heparin, as required by hospital policy, and check.	
7 Place syringes in a clinically clean receptacle on the bottom shelf of the dressing trolley, along with the receptacle containing any drug(s) to be administered.	
8 Collect the other equipment and place it on the bottom of the trolley.	
9 Place a sterile dressing pack on top of the trolley.	
10 Check that all necessary equipment is present.	10 To prevent delays and interruption of the procedure.
11 Wash your hands thoroughly.	11 To maintain asepsis.
12 Proceed to the patient.	
13 Open the sterile dressing pack. Add lotion for cleaning the skin to a gallipot in order to wet the cotton wool balls.	
14 Wash your hands or clean them with an alcohol-based hand wash solution.	14 To maintain asepsis.
15 Remove the bandage and dressing.	15 To observe the insertion site.
16 Inspect the insertion site of the cannula.	16 To detect any signs of inflammation, infiltration, etc. If present, take appropriate action.
17 Observe the infusion, if in progress, to confirm that it is running as desired. If the infusion is normal saline 0.9% with no additives, confirmation of patency and flushing with a separate syringe of normal saline is not necessary.	
18 Wash your hands or clean them with an alcohol-based hand wash solution.	18 To maintain asepsis.
19 Place a sterile towel under the patient's arm.	19 To create a sterile field.
20 Clean the injection site with a swab soaked in alcohol-based solution. Allow the site to dry.	20 To maintain asepsis.
21 Switch off the infusion or close the fluid path of a three-way tap or stopcock.	21 To prevent excessive pressure within the vein. To prevent contact with an incompatible infusion fluid. To allow the nurse

Action	Rationale
	to concentrate on the site of insertion and injection.
22 Inject normal saline 0.9% gently.	22 To confirm patency of the vein. To prevent contact with an incompatible infusion fluid.
23 Use a sterile 23g or 25g needle if the injection is made through a resealable latex site.	23 To enable resealing of the site at the end of the injection.
24 Change syringes and inject the drug smoothly in the direction of flow at the specified rate.	24 To prevent excessive pressure within the vein. To prevent speed shock.
25 Observe the insertion site of the cannula throughout.	25 To detect any complications at an early state, e.g. extravasation or local allergic reaction.
26 Blood return and/or 'flashback' must be checked frequently throughout the injection.	26 To confirm that the device is correctly placed and that the vein remains patent.
27 Consult the patient during the injection about any discomfort, etc.	27 To detect any complications at an early stage, and ensure patient comfort.
28 If more than one drug is to be administered, flush with normal saline between administrations by restarting the infusion or changing syringes.	28 To prevent drug interactions.
29 At the end of the injection, flush with normal saline by restarting the infusion or changing syringes.	29 To flush any remaining irritant solution away from the cannula site.
30 Instructions in the manufacturers' literature may specifically recommend that the drug is given into the injection site of an infusion that is running rapidly.	30 To increase dilution and reduce venous irritation.
31 Check that the infusion fluid in progress and the drug are compatible. If not, change the fluid.	31 To prevent drug interaction.
32 Open the control clamp of the giving set fully. Inject the drug at a speed sufficient to slow but not stop the infusion.	32 To prevent a backflow of drug up the tubing.
33 Observe the insertion site of the cannula carefully.	33 To detect any complications at an early stage. Extra pressure within the vein caused by both fluid flow and injection of the drug may cause rupture.

Action	Rationale
34 After the final flush of normal saline adjust the infusion rate as prescribed *or* open the fluid path of the three-way tap or stopcock *or* maintain the patency of the cannula by using heparin solution or an intravenous stylet.	34 To continue accurate delivery of therapy.
35 Cover the insertion site with new sterile topical dressing and tape it in place.	35 To maintain asepsis.
36 Apply a bandage.	36 To provide support and increase the patient's comfort.
37 Make sure that the patient is comfortable.	
38 Record the administration on appropriate sheets.	38 To maintain accurate records, provide a point of reference in the event of any queries and prevent any duplication of treatment.
39 Discard waste, making sure that it is placed in the correct containers, e.g. 'sharps' into a designated receptacle.	39 To ensure safe disposal and avoid injury to staff. To prevent reuse of equipment.

NURSING CARE PLAN

The problems associated with injection and infusion of intravenous fluids and drugs fall into two categories:

1 Local venous complications associated with the cannula insertion site
2 Systemic problems which affect the whole patient, exerting effects on vital organs and their functions.

The nurse must observe the insertion site, the infusion and the patient regularly to detect any complications at the earliest possible moment and to prevent progression to more serious conditions. Early detection also includes paying attention to the patient's comments. The patient's symptoms and physical signs both constitute reasons for a resiting of the cannula or discontinuation of the infusion. Signs and symptoms are used as problem headings.

Problem	Possible Causes	Preventive Nursing Measures	Suggested Actions
1 Infusion slows or stops	1 **a** Change in position of the following:		
	(1) Patient	(1) Check the height of the fluid container if the patient is active, as all infusions run by gravity.	(1) Adjust the height accordingly.
	(2) Limb	(2) Tape, bandage or splint the limb if infusion is sited at a point of flexion. Instruct the patient on the amount of movement permitted. Continued movement could result in mechanical phlebitis.	(2) Move the arm or hand until infusion starts again. Retape, bandage or splint the limb again carefully in the desired position.
	(3) Administration set	(3) Check for kinks and/or compression if the patient is active or restless.	(3) Correct accordingly.
	(4) Cannula	(4) Tape the cannula firmly to prevent movement. It may come into contact with the vein wall or a valve. Infusions sited in small veins are prone to this problem.	(4) Remove the bandage and dressing and manoueuvre the cannula gently until the infusion starts again. Retape carefully.
	b Technical problems:		
	(1) No air inlet in the rigid container	(1) Ensure that the container is vented.	(1) Vent if necessary.
	(2) Empty container	(2) Check fluid levels regularly.	(2) Replace the fluid container before it runs dry.
	(3) Venous spasm due to chemical irritation or coldness	(3) Dilute drugs as recommended. Remove solutions from the refrigerator a short time before use.	(3) Apply a warm compress to soothe and dilate the vein, increase blood flow and dilute the infusion mixture.

Problem	Possible Causes	Preventive Nursing Measures	Suggested Actions
	(4) Injury to the vein	(4) Detect any injury early as it is likely to progress and cause more serious conditions (see below).	(4) Stop the infusion and request a resite of the cannula.
	(5) Occlusion of the cannula due to fibrin formation	(5) Maintain a continuous, regular fluid flow *or* ensure that patency is maintained by heparinization or by placement of a stylet.	(5) Attempt to flush the cannula gently using a 1 ml syringe of normal saline. If resistance is met, stop and request a resiting of the cannula.
	(6) The cannula has become displaced either completely or partially; i.e. it has 'tissued'.	(6) Tape the cannula and the giving set so that no stress is placed on them. Instruct the patient on the amount of movement permitted.	(6) Confirm that infiltration has occurred by (i) inspecting the site for leakage, swelling, etc.; (ii) testing the temperature of the skin — it will be cooler if infiltration has occurred; (iii) comparing the size of the limb with the opposite one; (iv) applying a tourniquet above the cannula site — if the vein is patent, blood will flow back into the giving set. Once infiltration has been confirmed, stop the infusion and request a resiting of the cannula. If the infusion is allowed to progress, discomfort and tissue damage will result. Apply cold or warm compresses to provide symptomatic relief. Reassure the patient by explaining what is happening.

Problem	Possible Causes	Preventive Nursing Measures	Suggested Actions
2 Erythema or inflammation around the insertion site	2 **a** Phlebitis due to (1) Sepsis	(1) Adhere to aseptic techniques when performing all intravenous procedures.	(1) Stop the infusion and request a resiting of the cannula. Follow hospital policy about sending equipment for bacterial analysis. Clean the area and apply a sterile dressing. Check regularly.
	(2) Chemical irritation	(2) Dilute drugs according to instructions. Check compatibilities carefully to reduce the risk of particulate formation. Be aware of the factors involved, e.g. pH.	(3) Stop the infusion and request a resiting of the cannula. If the infusion is allowed to progress, tissue damage and severe pain will result. Apply cold or warm compresses to provide symptomatic relief. Encourage movement of the limb. Reassure the patient by explaining what is happening.
	(3) Mechanical irritation	(3) Tape, bandage or splint the limb if the infusion is sited at a point of flexion. Instruct the patient on the amount of movement permitted.	(3) Stop the infusion and request a resiting of the cannula. Although inflammation of this type progresses more slowly, it will cause discomfort. Provide symptomatic relief as above. Encourage movement and reassure the patient by explaining what is happening. Failure to detect and act when phlebitis is at an early stage, for whatever reason, will result in painful and incapacitating thrombophlebitis. Dislodgement of a thrombus could cause a pulmonary embolus.

Problem	Possible Causes	Preventive Nursing Measures	Suggested Actions
	b Infection with or without discharge	**b** Adhere to aseptic techniques when performing all intravenous procedures. Observe all recommendations for equipment changes, etc.	**b** Stop the infusion and request a resiting of the cannula. Follow hospital policy about sending equipment for bacterial analysis. Clean the area and apply a sterile dressing. Check regularly. Observe the patient for signs of systemic infection.
	c Cellulitis due to (1) Sepsis (2) Nonspecific sterile inflammation	(1) As above.	(1) As above. Due to the nature of the connective tissue any infection or inflammation spreads quickly, especially if the limb is oedematous.
	d Local allergic reaction	**d** Ask if the patient has any allergies before administration of any drugs or fluids, including sensitivities to topical solutions. Check whether the particular medication is commonly associated with local or venous flushing.	**d** Observe the patient for systemic reaction. Treat the local area symptomatically. Reassure the patient.
3 Local oedema	3 **a** During infusion: (1) Infiltration (2) Phlebitis	3 **a** Tape the cannula and giving set so that no stress is placed on the cannula. Instruct the patient on the amount of movement permitted. Check regularly for swelling, e.g. tightness of bandages or a wedding ring.	3 **a** Stop the infusion and request a resiting of the cannula before proceeding. Apply cold or warm compresses to provide symptomatic relief. Reassure the patient by explaining what is happening.
	b During injection: (1) Extravasation of medication	**b** Observe the patient carefully throughout drug administration.	**b** Stop the injection immediately extravasation is suspected. Act in accordance with hospital policy. Some drugs may cause inflammation

Problem	Possible Causes	Preventive Nursing Measures	Suggested Actions
			and supportive, symptomatic relief will be required. Others may have the potential to cause necrosis of tissue and further action may be necessary.
4 Oedema of the limb	4 **a** Infiltration	4 **a** Tape the cannula and giving set so that no stress is placed on the cannula. Instruct the patient on the amount of movement permitted. Check regularly for swelling, as above.	4 **a** Stop the infusion and request a resiting of the cannula. Provide symptomatic relief and support. Reassure the patient.
	b Circulatory overload	**b** Administer infusion fluids at the prescribed rate and do not make sudden alterations of flow. Be aware of the patient's renal and cardiac status. Monitor intake and output routinely.	**b** Slow the infusion. Monitor vital signs for increase in blood pressure and respirations. Place the patient in an upright position and keep him/her warm to promote peripheral circulation and relieve stress on the central veins. Reassure the patient. Notify a doctor immediately.
5 Pain at the insertion site	5 All of the previous listed conditions may be accompanied by soreness or pain.	5 As previously listed.	5 Provide local symptomatic relief as required. Administer systemic analgesia, as prescribed, if necessary.
6 Pyrexia, rigors, tachycardia	6 Septicaemia	6 Adhere to aseptic techniques when performing all intravenous procedures. Inspect all equipment, infusion fluids, etc., before use. Observe recommendations for additives, equipment changes and general management.	6 Notify a doctor immediately. Follow hospital policy about sending equipment for bacterial analysis.

Problem	Possible Causes	Preventive Nursing Measures	Suggested Actions
7 Decrease in blood pressure, tachycardia, cyanosis, unconsciousness	7 Embolism: **a** Air	**a** Check the containers and change before they run dry, especially bottles. Clear all air from tubing before commencing infusion. Check all connections regularly and make sure they are secure.	**a** Turn the patient on to his/her left side and lower the head of the bed to prevent air from entering the pulmonary artery. Notify a doctor immediately. Reassure the patient by explaining what is happening.
	b Particle	**b** Check all infusion fluids before and after any additions have been made. Check drug compatibility and stability. Observe the solution throughout the infusion for precipitate formation.	**b** As above, but also change the container and giving set. Replace with new equipment and normal saline 0.9% infusion from a different batch. Follow hospital policy about sending contaminated fluid and equipment for bacterial analysis.
8 Itching, rash, shortness of breath	8 Allergic reaction due to sensitivity to an intravenous fluid, additive or drug.	8 Ask the patient if he has any allergies *before* administration of any drugs or fluids. Check whether the particular medication is commonly associated with any allergic reactions and observe the patient more closely.	8 Stop drug infusion or injection and maintain the patency of the intravenous line using normal saline 0.9%. Notify a doctor immediately. Reassure the patient.
9 Flushed face, headache, congestion of the chest, possibly progressing to loss of consciousness	9 Speed shock due to too rapid administration of drugs.	9 Administer drugs and infusion at the correct rate. Check the flow rate frequently. Use mechanical aids if the delivery rate is crucial.	9 As above.

20

IODINE-131 PROTOCOL

Definition
Iodine-131 is an unsealed liquid radioactive source with a half-life of 8 days. It emits both gamma and beta radiation. The chief contribution to the therapeutic dose absorbed by an iodine concentrating organ is from the beta radiation.

Indications
1 The thyroid gland concentrates iodine-131 by selective absorption, causing it to receive a large radiation dose. For thyrotoxicosis a treatment of 75-400 MBq of iodine-131 can be given.
2 Iodine-131 plays an important role in the treatment of well differentiated thyroid cancers of the papillary and follicular type.
3 By the same selective absorption process, metastases that function similarly to the thyroid tissue will also concentrate iodine-131 and be destroyed.

REFERENCE MATERIAL
Treatment Programme for Carcinoma of the Thyroid

Surgical Removal of the Thyroid
Normal thyroid tissue usually concentrates iodine-131 more efficiently than the malignant tissue. Some malignant tissues only concentrate iodine-131 after normal tissues have been removed, therefore it is normal practice to remove the thyroid surgically before administration of iodine-131.

Ablation Dose of Iodine-131
Following a thyroidectomy an initial ablation dose of iodine-131 is administered. A dose of 1100 MBq is commonly given, but up to 5500 MBq may be given in older patients. This ablates residue thyroid tissue and/or residue tumour of the thyroid.

If the cancer is inoperable, a repeated treatment with iodine-131 is prescribed. The first treatment ablates normal functioning thyroid tissue and the second is used to treat malignant tissue.

Treatment Course

Once the thyroid gland has been ablated, the functioning metastases will concentrate the iodine-131 and be destroyed. To achieve this, repeated courses, commonly of 5500 MBq, are given with the aim of eventually removing

1　Deposits in local lymph nodes
2　Distant metastases.

Principles of Protection Policies

The precautions to be observed by individual hospitals and institutions should be available in written form to hospital personnel.

Film Badges

Film badges should be worn at all times when on duty.

A Yellow Radiation Warning Notice Board

Such a warning board must be displayed at the door of the treatment room:

1　It indicates what radioactive substances have been administered.
2　The permissable time allowance indicated by the warning notice is intended as a guide. Routine nursing procedures can safely be carried out but unnecessary time must not be spent in close promixity to the patients while the warning notice is displayed.
3　The time given in the table is such that a nurse remaining at a distance of approximately 60 cm from the patient for the time indicated each day would, after five consecutive days, receive the maximum permissible dose for the working week.

General Care

Whenever possible, the ward manager should organize the duties of the staff so that the nursing care of such patients is shared. No one nurse is subjected, therefore, to repeated exposure to radiation during the period when the warning notice is in operation and displaying a permissable time.

In the event of any article needing to be removed from the patient's room, the physics department should be informed so that its safe removal can be monitored; i.e. there may be a need to store the article in the physics department if levels of radioactivity are unacceptably high.

The patient must be strictly confined to the treatment area unless required for uptake measurements, scans or X-rays. These should be organized by the physics department. It is important that the patient washes, bathes and changes into clean clothes before going to these departments.

Iodine-131 has a relatively short half-life and its activity decays rapidly. Following administration the patient's body fluids will be highly radioactive, especially during the first few days (see Figure 20.1).

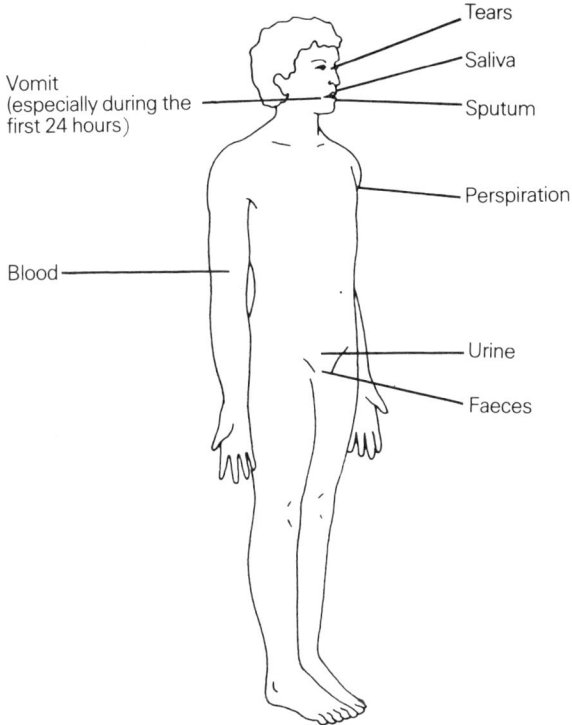

Figure 20.1 The patient's body fluids will be highly radioactive especially during the first few days after administration of iodine-131

The principles of

1 Distance
2 Shielding
3 Time minimization

are important in the safe use of all radioactive material. Since iodine-131 is in an unsealed form, however, it is important to guard against contamination both of personnel and the hospital environment by the correct use of protective gloves, gowns and overshoes, thereby preventing the transfer of active material to the individuals and areas outside the treatment area.

In the event of any accident involving contaminated material, the physics department must be advised immediately, even if the incident occurs outside normal working hours.

Contaminated bare hands must be washed thoroughly in hot, soapy, running water, special attention being given to the areas around the fingernails, between the fingers and the outer edges of the hands. If gross contamination of the hands is suspected, the physics department must be advised and the washing procedure continued until the arrival of the appropriate personnel. The applications of cosmetics, eating, drinking or smoking while there is any possibility that the hands are contaminated is absolutely contraindicated.

Preparation of an Iodine-131 Therapy Room

Equipment

Equipment should be kept to a minimum. It must be checked to ensure that it is in working order as maintenance staff will only be allowed into the room in exceptional circumstances. Such items as disposable bed linen, gloves, aprons, overshoes, cutlery and crockery should be kept separate in a utility room or anteroom along with the patient's treatment chart and a Geiger counter.

Personal Items

Patients are advised not to take their personal belongings into the room. These should be stored away from the iodine-131 treatment room. Valuables should be sent home or put in the hospital safe. If the patient wishes to have his/her own possessions, it must be clearly understood that they will not be allowed out of the iodine-131 treatment room without permission.

Protective Floor Covering

Each patient is assessed individually to decide what protective floor covering is necessary. The types available are as follows:

Absorbent Paper   This is used to retain accidental urine spills or splashes. Normally one piece is kept in place by two-sided tape immediately next to the toilet. One piece below a catheter bag is sufficient.

Polythene Sheeting   If there is the likelihood of vomiting or incontinence, polythene sheeting may be placed over the floor area and kept in place with two-sided tape. This will also be put in place should the patient not be fluent in English or if the patient is incapable of understanding the instructions given.

Cleaning of an Iodine-131 Therapy Room

During occupancy of the treatment room by the patient, cleaning of the room is kept to a minimum and should be organized by the physics department.

When the patient is discharged, decontamination of the room will be arranged by the physics department who will inform the remaining personnel when the decontamination has been completed. The domestic staff may then enter the room and clean it thoroughly.

Preparation of the Patient

Before Admission

Twenty-one Days Prior to Admission Patients taking tetraiodothyronine (T4) (thyroxine) must stop taking this medication.

Ten Days Prior to Admission Patients taking triiodothyronine (T3) must stop taking this medication.

Three Days Prior to Admission Occasionally, to enhance the uptake of iodine-131, three daily injections of thyroid stimulating hormone are administered.

On Admission

Before the administration of iodine-131, any symptoms of diarrhoea or constipation must be remedied. Diarrhoea is a hazard as it can contaminate the treatment area. Constipation not only inhibits the elimination of radioactivity, but obscures any radiological investigations, e.g. scanning.

Patients and relatives must be fully acquainted with the radiation protection procedures and agree to cooperate with them.

The patient should also agree to stay in hospital until the physics department states that the radioactivity level is at a legally permissable level for discharge.

Discharge of the Patient

A patient must not be discharged from hospital until the amount of iodine-131 activity present in his/her body has fallen below a certain legal requirement. The value for that level will depend upon

1 Mode of transport
2 Journey time involved
3 Home circumstances.

Each patient is individually assessed, usually by the physics department, as in certain cases the biological half-life of iodine-131 is relatively long. An estimate has to be made of how long it will take for the residual activity in the patient to fall to values which will require no further precautions after they leave the hospital.

Patients who are discharged with more than 138.75 MBq of iodine-131 in their bodies are given special written and verbal instructions before discharge.

Reference and Further Reading

Royal Marsden Hospital (1978) Physics Manual Protocol, Royal Marsden Hospital.

GUIDELINES: NURSING THE PATIENT BEFORE THE ADMINISTRATION OF IODINE-131

Action	Rationale
1 The patient is to be fasted for 2 hours before and after administration of a dose. Offer a light diet for the remainder of the day.	1 To reduce the risk of nausea and/or vomiting.
2 Administer a prophylactic anti-emetic.	
3 Check that the preparation of the room and the patient is complete.	
4 Ensure that any surplus items, e.g. water jug and glasses, have been removed.	4 To prevent contamination of extraneous equipment.
5 Assist the patient to remove dentures.	5 To prevent radioactive material being trapped in the mouth.
6 The patient drinks the dose through a straw supervised by physics department staff. These staff are usually responsible for preparing the dose prescribed by the doctor and for bringing it to the patient.	6 Drinking through a straw reduces the amount of radioactive material left around the mouth.
7 Offer the patient a drink of water to rinse out the mouth.	7 To remove any iodine-131 from inside the mouth.
8 Apply a wristband showing the radiation warning symbol to the patient's wrist.	8 To identify the patient as being radioactive.
9 Place a yellow radiation warning notice board at the entrance to the treatment room.	9 To identify the patient as radioactive.

GUIDELINES: NURSING THE PATIENT AFTER ADMINISTRATION OF IODINE-131

Action	Rationale

Entering the Room

Action	Rationale
1 Put on disposable gloves.	1 To prevent contamination of the hands.
2 Put on a suitable protective gown: **a** Plastic disposable apron, e.g. for presenting meals **b** Long-sleeve cotton gown, e.g. for lifting patient	**a** To have adequate protection for short procedures when contamination will not occur. **b** To be protected from small amounts of contamination, e.g. from the patient's skin.

Action	**Rationale**
c Disposable water-repellant gown, e.g. for dealing with vomit or incontinence.	c To be protected from large amounts of contamination.
3 Work quickly and efficiently, keeping within the time allowance stated on the door.	3 To prevent risk of over-exposure to radiation.

Maintaining Patient Comfort and Hygiene

1 Encourage the patient to bathe at least once a day.	1 To remove radioactive perspiration from the skin.
2 Encourage the patient to wash his/her hands thoroughly after each possible contact with body fluids, e.g. cleaning teeth, going to the toilet, etc.	2 To remove radioactive material from his/her hands.
3 The patient must remove and clean his/her dentures under running water regularly.	3 To remove radioactive saliva from around dentures.
4 The patient must remove and rinse his/her contact lenses in their usual cleaning fluid regularly.	4 To remove radioactive tears from lenses.
5 Encourage a good fluid intake.	5 To increase the urinary output and elimination of radioactivity.
6 Ensure that the patient has his/her own personal toilet facilities and flushes the toilet twice after use.	6 To prevent contamination of others and of the environment. Urine of patients treated with iodine-131 is highly radioactive.
7 If the patient is bedbound, catheterize him/her before the dose is given. Empty the catheter bag every 4-6 hours, or more frequently if necessary.	7 Catheterization reduces the nursing time spent with the patient. Frequent emptying of the bag reduces the level of radioactivity within the area.
8 If the patient requires a bedpan or urinal, this item must be kept solely for this patient's use. The bedpan or urinal must be handled carefully with gloved hands and the contents disposed of in the toilet, which is flushed twice. The bedpan or urinal may be washed in the bedpan washer. It should be sealed in a plastic bag for the journey to and from the sluice.	8 To prevent contamination of the environment and of other patients and staff.
9 If leakage occurs from injection sites, abdominal paracentesis sites, etc., the nurse should contact the	9 It must be remembered that all body fluids are potentially contaminated with radioactivity.

Action	**Rationale**
medical staff and the physics department immediately. Any contact with the dressing should be done with long-handled forceps.	
10 Gloves and a protective gown must be worn whenever handling soiled bed linen.	10 To prevent contamination of the nurse's hands or uniform.
11 All soiled linen must be deposited in a special container provided for this purpose.	11 Soiled linen must not go direct to the laundry but should be dealt with by the appropriate personnel.

Visitors

1 Visiting is discouraged during the first 24 hours following administration of iodine-131.	1 The patient is very radioactive during this period.
2 On the second and subsequent days, visiting inside the room is allowed if the physics department staff do not advise to the contrary.	
3 Visitors must adhere to the instructions for entering a room. They must sit at least 120 cm from the patient and confine their stay to the time stated on the notice board.	3 To minimize the exposure of visitors to radiation.
4 Physical contact with the patient or bed linen is not allowed.	4 To prevent contamination of the visitors.
5 Children and pregnant women must not be allowed into the room.	5 Rapidly dividing cells are at greatest risk of damage from radioactivity.

On Leaving the Room

1 Remove gloves by peeling them off your hands, taking care not to touch the outside surfaces with your bare hands.	1 To prevent transfer of contaminated material from the gloves' outer surfaces to your hands.
2 Remove your overshoes and your apron or gown and discard them in the bin provided.	2 These are removed after the gloves as they are less likely to be contaminated.
3 Wash your hands thoroughly.	3 To remove any contamination picked up from the protective clothing.
4 Using the radiation monitor or Geiger counter, monitor the activity of your hands, feet and clothes. If contamination has	4 To ensure that no active material is present on the nurse.

Action	**Rationale**
occurred, inform the physics department immediately and continue to wash the contaminated area until only background radioactivity shows on the monitor.	

GUIDELINES: EMERGENCY PROCEDURES

Action	**Rationale**

Incontinence and/or Vomiting

1 Inform the physics department immediately. Put on gloves and a gown. Remove the patient from the contaminated area.	
2 If physics department staff are not immediately available, use a Geiger counter to assess the extent of the spillage.	
3 Put some absorbent material on top of all the radioactive wet area.	3 To absorb contamination.
4 Leave the area until physics department staff arrive. Polythene sheets may be placed over all of the contaminated area.	

Contamination of Bare Hands

1 Wash your hands in hot soapy water, paying special attention to the areas around the fingernails, between the fingers and on the outer edges of the hands. Continue washing until only the background radioactivity shows on the monitor.	1 To remove radioactive material from any areas where it might be trapped.
2 If a wound is produced in a contamination accident, wash thoroughly under running water, opening the edges of the cut. This should be continued until physics department staff can demonstrate that no residual radioactivity remains in the wound.	2 To stimulate bleeding and permit thorough flushing of the cut.

Death

1 Inform the physics department	1 So that the physics department

Action	**Rationale**
immediately.	staff can begin making the necessary arrangements for removal of the body to the mortuary.
2 Two nurses wearing gloves, plastic aprons, gowns and overshoes should perform last offices. All orifices must be carefully packed. Any vomit, bleeding, faeces or urine must be cleaned from the body.	2 To avoid contamination with body fluids. Minimal handling of the body reduces the risk of contamination.
3 The body should be totally enclosed in a plastic cadaver bag.	3 To avoid contamination of the porters and the mortuary staff.
4 Transfer of the body should be arranged with the physics department.	4 The physics department will supervise the transferral of the body.

Cardiac Arrest

1 When alerting the emergency resuscitation team, the switchboard must also be told to inform the physics department.	
2 Do not use mouth to mouth resuscitation. All areas should be supplied with an Ambu bag for this purpose.	2 Mouth to mouth contact could seriously contaminate the resuscitator.
3 The physics department will supervise and provide shielding for the crash team.	
4 Overshoes, gloves and gowns must be put on as soon as is practicably possible.	4 The emergency equipment may have been contaminated by the patient.

Fire

1 Every effort should be made to contact the physics department.	1 To help in the evacuation of the patients treated with iodine-131.
2 Following evacuation the patients treated with iodine-131 should be kept at a safe distance from the other patients and staff.	2 To prevent exposure of others to radiation.

21

IRIDIUM-192 IMPLANTS

Definition

Iridium-192 is a radioisotope which can be used in the form of pins or wires as in interstitial therapy.

The half-life of iridium-192 is 74.2 days. It is an ideal choice because of the low energy of its gamma emission, which simplifies radiation protection, and because in the form of a platinum-iridium alloy it can be drawn into thin flexible wires.

The wires consist of an active platinum-iridium alloy core encased in a sheath of platinum, 0.1 mm thick, which screens out the beta radiation from the iridium-192.

Modern afterloading techniques reduce the radiation exposure to the radiotherapist and other staff involved.

Indications

Treatment with iridium-192 is indicated under the following circumstances:

1 As a primary treatment for small primary lesions, especially tongue or breast lesions
2 As a 'boost' dose after external radiotherapy for larger primary tumours or where nodes are also involved
3 To treat recurrence.

REFERENCE MATERIAL

When a patient is selected for interstitial therapy the medical staff assess the size of the tumour. The physics department is responsible for ordering the source and coordinating with the radiotherapists.

The patient is usually admitted the day before treatment. Ideally, the patient should be nursed in a cubicle or in a bed away from the main thoroughfare.

Types of Implant (see Figure 21.1)

Hair Pins and Single Pins

These types of implants are usually used intraorally. They are slotted into tissue using steel guides to get accurate alignment. Radiological examination is used to check the position of the guides before the iridium is inserted.

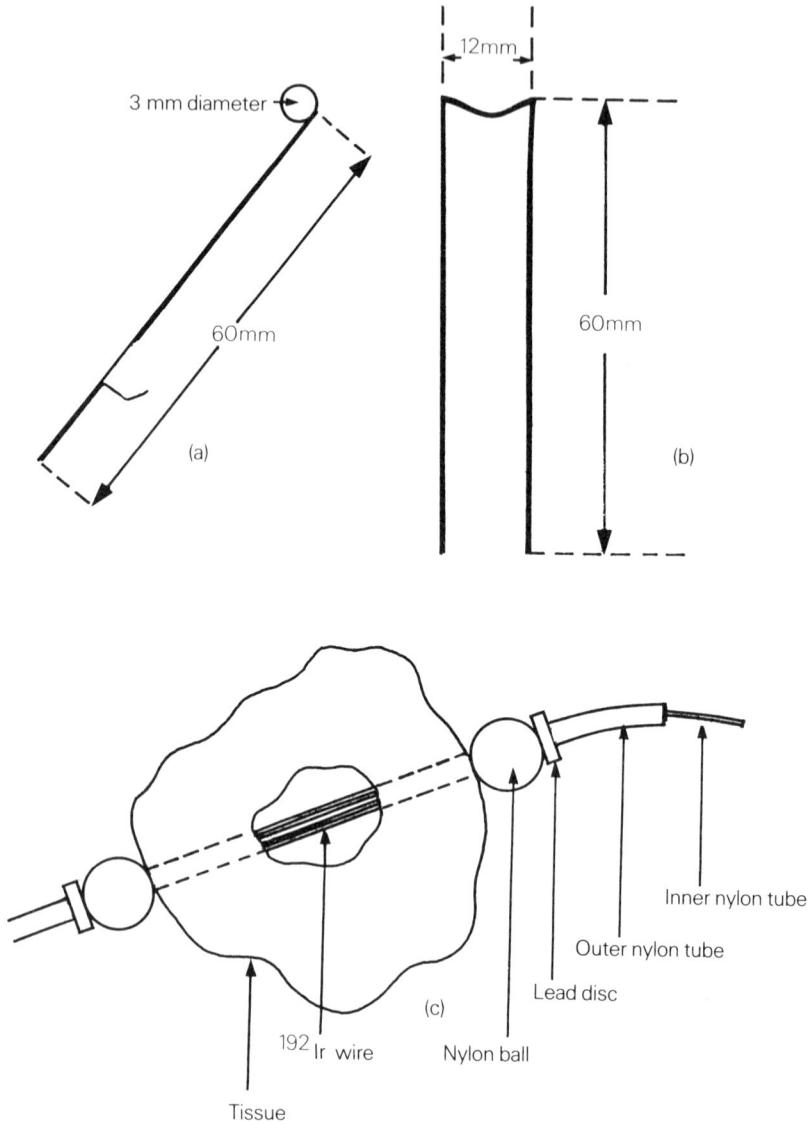

Figure 12.1 Iridium pins and wires. **a** Iridium-192 single pin. **b** Iridium-192 hair pin. **c** Iridium-192 wire in nylon cannula. Typical assembly in tissue

At the end of the procedure, further X-rays are taken to identify the exact position of the active sources so that the dosage and expected time of removal can be calculated. The pins are held in place by sutures.

Iridium Wires

Iridium wires are usually used for breast lesions and are inserted via a polythene cannula. Both ends of each tube protrude through the skin. When the correct alignment has been established, the iridium wire is afterloaded, usually on the ward. The wires are held in the cannulae with crimped lead washers.

Removal of Implants

The radiotherapist is responsible for calculating how long a radioactive implant should stay in place. This is usually for 3-6 days, depending on the size of the tumour. Removal of the implant is usually carried out on the ward by the radiotherapist.

Discharge of the Patient

The patient should normally be discharged the day after the removal of the implant. The patient should be warned about the brisk local reaction which he/she may experience due to the rapid cell breakdown induced by the radiation. In order to minimize the risk of infection or soreness, the patient should be taught how to care for the treated area, e.g. frequent oral toilet.

References and Further Reading

Amersham International Ltd (1978) Interstitial Therapy Using Iridium-192, Amersham International

Paine C H (1972) Modern afterloading methods for interstitial radiotherapy, Clinical Radiology 23: 263-272

Pierquin B et al. (1978) The Paris system in interstitial radiation therapy, Acta Radiologica: Oncology, Radiation, Physics, Biology (Stockholm) 17 (1): 33-48

Royal Marsden Hospital (1978) Physics Manual Protocol, Royal Marsden Hospital

GUIDELINES: CARE OF PATIENTS WITH INSERTIONS OF SEALED RADIOACTIVE SOURCES

Action	Rationale
1 When transferring patients from theatre to ward, the nurse and porter should remain at the head and foot of the bed and at least 120 cm from the centre of the bed in the event of any delay in the transfer. If the source is intraoral, the nurse should stand at the foot of the bed.	1 To minimize the risk of exposure to radiation.

Action	**Rationale**
2 A yellow radiation hazard board should accompany the patient back from theatre. This must remain at the bottom of the bed or outside the cubicle until the source is removed.	2 To warn everybody that the patient has a radioactive source.
3 Nursing staff must calculate the time allowed with the patient in any 24-hour period. This time should be written on the yellow hazard notice on the bed or cubicle door.	3 To minimize over-exposure to radiation.
4 A Geiger counter should be available on the ward.	4 To monitor radioactivity if a dislodged source is suspected, e.g. in the bed linen.
5 One nurse should be delegated responsibility for the nursing care of the patient. The time spent with the patient should be shared between all staff on duty and time spent in nursing procedures must be kept to a minimum.	5 To minimize the risk of over-exposure to radiation.
6 Every nurse must wear a radiation monitoring badge above the level of the lead shield.	6 To record the extent of exposure to radiation.
7 All bed linen and waste materials removed from the patient area should be monitored before being removed from the ward.	7 To prevent loss of an accidentally dislodged source.
8 If a source becomes dislodged, use the long-handled forceps provided to put the source into a lead pot. Care should be taken not to damage the source. It must never be handled directly with the fingers.	8 To minimize the dose of radiation received.
9 Visitors must remain at least 120 cm away from the patient. The visit should not last longer than the time shown on the warning notice. No children or pregnant women are allowed to visit.	9 To minimize the risk of over-exposure to radiation.

GUIDELINES: CARE OF PATIENTS WITH INTRAORAL SOURCES

Action	Rationale
1 Encourage frequent mouth care. The patient should void the solution into a bowl and not into a handbasin.	1 To reduce the risk of infection. To prevent the loss of a dislodged source.
2 Provide a soft, pureed or liquid diet.	2 To reduce the risk of the patient biting into the source or his/her tongue. Eating is often difficult when implants are present.
3 Avoid spicy and/or hot foods. Discourage the patient from smoking and/or drinking alcohol.	3 To prevent exacerbation of local reaction or soreness.
4 Encourage ingestion of carbonated drinks.	4 To alleviate dryness.
5 Provide crushed ice for the patient to suck and/or soluble aspirin as a mouthwash.	5 To minimize oral pain and discomfort.
6 Give steroids as prescribed.	6 To prevent and/or minimize swelling.
7 Provide writing equipment for the patient.	7 To reduce the need for oral communication. This is liable to increase soreness and alter the distribution of the sources.
8 Provide paper tissues and a bowl for saliva.	8 The patient may have difficulty in swallowing due to soreness and oedema.
9 The sources should be checked at regular intervals, e.g. at the beginning of a span of duty.	9 To make sure that the sources have not become dislodged.
10 The patient must be confined to the cubicle or the space around the bed. Washing is carried out in the bed area, but the general toilet facilities should be used, provided that the patient remains at a distance from other people.	10 To mimize the risk of radiation exposure to other people on the ward.

22

LAST OFFICES

'When a person dies, a number of procedures are carried out under the generic term postmortem care. *As nursing students, we learned to wash the body carefully, protect orifices, and pad certain areas to prevent bruising. The rationale for these actions was generally presented as "showing respect for the deceased". Respect is not the only reason for these procedures: there is a scientific rationale for them.'*

(Pennington, 1978)

REFERENCE MATERIAL

Little in the way of nursing reference material is available on last offices. The works listed below should be used as a basis for further reading.

References and Further Reading

Pennington E A (1978) Postmortem care: more than ritual, American Journal of Nursing 78: 846-847
Royal College of Nursing of the United Kingdom (1981) Verification of Death and Performance of Last Offices, Royal College of Nursing, Typescript BS/pn
Thomas C H (1971) Last offices — a reassessment, Nursing Mirror 132 (15):30
Williams A (1982) Procedures Following Deaths in Hospitals, Institute of Health Services Administrators

GUIDELINES: LAST OFFICES

Equipment

1 Bowl, soap, disposable towels
2 Razor, comb, scissors
3 Foam sticks for oral toilet
4 Receiver
5 Identification labels
6 Any documents required by legal requirements or hospital policy, such as notification of death cards
7 Plastic or paper shroud

8   Clean white sheet
9   Hypoallergenic tape
10 Sterile dressing pack
11 Bandages
12 Valuables or property book
13 Plastic bag for any waste

Procedure

Action	Rationale
1 Inform appropriate medical staff.	1 A registered medical practitioner who has attended the deceased person during his/her last illness is required to give a medical certificate of the cause of death. The certificate requires the doctor to state the last date on which he/she saw the deceased alive and whether or not he/she has seen the body after death.
2 Inform the appropriate senior nurse and portering staff.	2 So that relatives may be informed if they are not in the hospital at the time of death. To alert portering staff to begin arrangements for transfer of the body to the mortuary.
3 Place the patient on his/her back. Close his/her eyelids. Remove any pillows. Support the jaw by placing one pillow on the chest underneath the jaw. Remove any mechanical aids, such as foam rings, heel pads, etc. Straighten the limbs.	3 Rigor mortis occurs 2-4 hours after death.
4 Wash the patient. Clean the nostrils, ears and mouth. Replace any dentures. Trim the nails. Shave male patients.	4 For aesthetic and hygienic reasons.
5 Drain the bladder by pressing on the lower abdomen. Pack any leaking orifices.	5 Packing orifices is unnecessary unless they are leaking. All packing has to be removed either at postmortem examination or by the undertaker who will repack the orifices. Leaking orifices should be packed as they pose a health hazard to any staff coming into contact with the body.
6 Remove dressings, drainage tubes,	6 It is unnecessary to leave these in

Action	Rationale
etc., unless otherwise instructed. If tubes are left in position, cut them to just above skin level, cover them with a dressing pad and secure them with tape or a loose bandage.	position unless the patient has died within 24 hours of surgery or insertion of the drain *or* if the tube or drain is considered to have contributed to the cause of death.
7 Re-dress any wounds, secure dressings with tape or a loose bandage.	7 Loose bandages or tape should be used because as the skin cools, it loses its elasticity.
8 Remove all jewellery, in the presence of another nurse, unless requested to do otherwise.	8 To meet with legal requirements and relatives' wishes.
9 Put a plastic or paper shroud on the body unless requested to do otherwise.	9 For aesthetic reasons, particularly if relatives wish to view the body.
10 Label one wrist and one ankle with an identification label.	10 To ensure correct identification of the body.
11 Complete any documents, such as notification of death cards. Three copies of such cards are usually required. Tape one securely to the shroud.	11 To ensure identification of the body in the mortuary.
12 Wrap the body in a sheet, ensuring that the face and feet are covered and that all limbs are held securely in position.	12 To avoid possible damage to the body.
13 Secure the sheet with tape.	13 Pins, although providing more security, are contraindicated as, if they open, they pose a potential health hazard to staff. Bacterial fermentation occurs consequent to decomposition of the body.
14 If required, tape the second notification of death card to the outside of the sheet.	14 For ease of identification of the body in the mortuary.
15 Check the patient's property, with a second nurse. List this property in the valuables or property book. Lock the property in a safe place.	15 To ensure that all property can be accounted for.
16 Clear away any equipment used during this procedure.	
17 Request the portering staff to remove the body.	17 Decomposition occurs rapidly, particularly in hot weather and in overheated rooms and may create a bacterial hazard for those handling the body. Autolysis and growth of bacteria are delayed if the body is cooled.

Action	Rationale
18 If required, give the third notification of death card to the porter.	18 To be given to the head porter for identification when the undertakers remove the body from the hospital.
19 Transfer all property, etc., to the apropriate administrative department.	19 The administrative department cannot begin to process fomalities such as the death certificate or the collection of property by the next of kin until the required documents are in their possession.
20 Amend appropriate nursing documents.	

NURSING CARE PLAN

Problem	Suggested Action
1 Death occurring within 24 hours of an operation	1 All tubes and/or drains must be left in position. Spigot any cannulae or catheters. Treat stomas as open wounds. Leave any packing in position. Leave any endotrachael or tracheostomy tubes in place. Postmortem examination will be required to estabish the cause of death. Any tubes, drains, etc., may have been a major contributing factor to death.
2 Unexpected death	2 As above. Postmortem examination of the body will be required to establish the cause of death.
3 Patient with hepatitis B	3 For further information see the relevant section of procedure on hepatitis B (pages 188)
4 Patient who dies after receiving systemic radioactive iodine	4 For further information see the relevant section of procedure on iodine-131 protocol (pages 237-238).
5 Patient dies after insertion of gold grains or colloidal radioactive solution	5
6 Patient dies after insertion of caesium needles or applicators *or* iridium wires or hair pins	6 Inform the physics department as well as appropriate medical staff. Once a doctor has verified death, the sources are removed and placed in a lead container. A Geiger counter is used to check

Problem	Suggested Action
	that all sources have been removed. This reduces the radiation risk when completing the last offices procedure. Record the time and date of removal of the sources.
7 Relatives not present at the time of patient's death	7 Inform the relatives as soon as possible of the death as they may wish to view the body before last offices are completed.
8 Relatives wish to see the body after removal from the ward	8 Inform the mortuary staff, in order to allow time for them to prepare the body. The body will normally be placed in the hospital's chapel of rest. Accompany the relatives to the chapel. Seeing the dead body of the loved one can be a tremendous shock and the relatives require preparation and support for this. Ask the relatives to remain outside the chapel at first. Check that all is ready before allowing the relatives to enter the chapel. Wait outside the chapel while relatives remain with the body unless asked to stay.
9 Relatives wish the body to be placed in the hospital's chapel of rest	9 Accompany the body to the chapel and remain with it or outside the chapel according to the wishes of the relatives. When the relatives have left, contact the porters, who remove the body to the mortuary.

GUIDELINES: RELIGIOUS REQUIREMENTS FOR NON-CHRISTIANS

Jews

1 Inform the rabbi.
2 Special rites and prayers on behalf of the dying should be given whenever possible.
3 After a lapse of 1 hour, nursing staff are allowed to complete last offices.

Moslems

1 Leave the body untouched.
2 The body will be washed by another Moslem of the same sex after removal to the mortuary, and left uncovered.
3 The body should be turned to face Mecca (south-east) when in the mortuary.
4 Postmortem examinations are not usually allowed, except in the case of coroner's referrals, in which case the relatives will consult the appropriate Islamic authorities before giving consent.

Sikhs

No special arrangements are required, but postmortem examinations are not usually allowed.

Hindus

1 Inform a Hindu priest.
2 In the absence of a priest, the patient's relatives should read from the *Bhagavad Gita* before or while laying out the body.
3 Postmortem examinations are often refused.

Buddhists

No special observances are required.

23

LIFTING

The aim of successful lifting is to achieve the required results with minimal effort. In the hospital situation this must also include protecting the patient and the staff from injury.

REFERENCE MATERIAL

Potential Hazards of Lifting

When a patient has to be lifted both he/she and the nurses involved are potentially at risk of injury. The patient may experience discomfort or pain due to being held or lifted in an unsuitable fashion. For example, dragging a patient up the bed causes friction against the sheets and may create or exacerbate a sore area, especially if the patient is incontinent. Being physically lifted by others can be an unpleasant or even a frightening experience, especially if the patient has not been warned beforehand of the manoeuvre or is anxious about being dropped.

The greatest risk of injury during lifting or moving procedures is to nurses, and the occupational hazard of back pain is well known. It is estimated that 185 000 nurses (43% of the National Health Service's total nursing population of England and Wales) suffer back pain at least once a year (Northwick Park 1980). Of these episodes of back pain, 44% occur while the nurse is on duty and 84% of them are directly attributed to moving or supporting a patient. Thus one out of every six nurses is likely to suffer back pain while on duty as a result of moving or lifting a patient.

As well as the personal suffering and inconvenience caused by back pain among nurses, sick leave will reduce the staffing levels and patient care may correspondingly be affected. It is estimated that 764 000 nurse working days per year are lost in the National Health Service due to back pain.

It is, therefore, of the utmost importance that nurses are aware of the principles of safe lifting and can employ techniques which minimize the hazards of lifting both to their patients and to themselves.

Biomechanics of Lifting

The spine is capable of bearing large compression forces but is vulnerable to damage from shearing forces, along the surface of the discs, and torsional or twisting forces. Structural damage to the cartilaginous structures may occur as the result not only of one bad lifting experience, but from continual poor posture or repeated lfting of comparatively light objects in an incorrect manner.

If the trunk is nearly erect, most of the weight of the upper body and the lifted load is directed down through the vertebral column, stabilizing it and causing some compression of the discs. If, however, the trunk is horizontal, these weights produce a shearing force rather than compression on the discs.

The erector spinae muscles which provide some of the tension support of the spine during lifting are able to exert greater force for lifting a given weight when the spine is in the upright rather than the flexed position.

It is, therefore, not only safer but more efficient to lift with a straight back, utilizing the strong muscles of the legs to provide the lifting force. A crouch position is the most suitable one for lifting as this employs the quadriceps femoris muscles for the vertical movement of the lift with minimum reliance on the erector spinae.

The stress on the spine during lifting can be reduced by holding the load or the patient as close as possible to the lifter's body. A larger distance of separation will increase the muscle force on the spine and therefore increase spinal stress. For the same reasons, jerking and twisting should be avoided during lifting.

Factors Affecting Spinal Stress During Lifting

By using a pressure-sensitive radio pill it is possible to measure intra-abdominal pressure (IAP) during lifting procedures. IAP may be used as an index of spinal stress as research has shown a close correlation between the magnitude of the IAP, the size of the load and the forces acting on the spinal mechanism.

The Load

Studies have shown that the nurse's IAP increases when heavier patients are lifted. Confused, uncooperative or paralysed patients produce higher pressures than others, usually because they make the lift unpredictable or impossible to carry out in a prearranged fashion. Patient behaviour as well as weight therefore contributes to the potential hazard of lifting. Many patients, however, can assist the nurses when being lifted by pressing down with their heels, for example, or by using a hand pulley. Such cooperation is recommended not only because it reduces the load on the nurse but because it promotes the patient's comfort and reduces his/her feelings of dependence.

The Lifting Technique

The stress experienced by the spine when lifting is largely affected by the lifting technique used. The lifts most frequently used by nurses are as follows:

The Shoulder (Australian) Lift (Figure 23.1a)   The patient is sat upright and both nurses stand level with the patient's hips. The foot nearest the head of the bed points in the direction of the lift and the knees and hips are bent, keeping the back straight and the head up.

The nurses press their near shoulder against the patient's chest wall under the axillae and the patient rests his/her arms on the nurses' backs. The nurses' near arms are then placed under the patient's thighs as near the buttocks as possible so that each can grip the other's wrist. The nurses' free hands can be used to hold the head of the bed or to press down on the bed, thereby providing extra support for the lift, or they may be needed to steady the patient's back.

The nurses then simultaneously lift the patient by straightening their hips and knees and transferring their weight to their forward legs.

This lift may be used for lifting the patient up the bed or from the bed to the chair or commode, for example. Its use is contraindicated if the patient has painful ribs, is unable to sit up or cannot cooperate with the nurses.

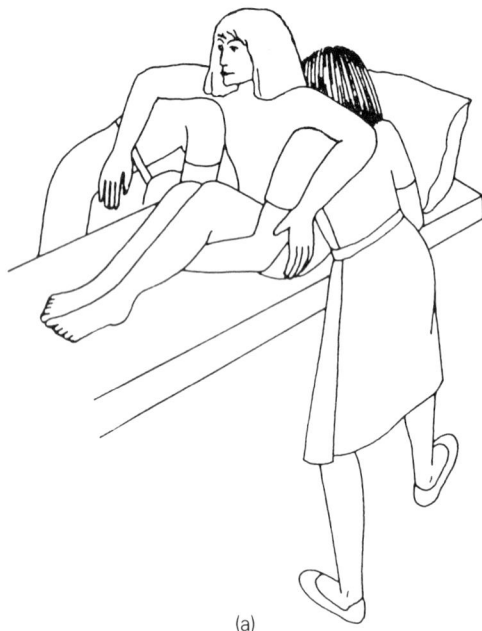

(a)

Figure 23.1a   Shoulder (Australian) lift

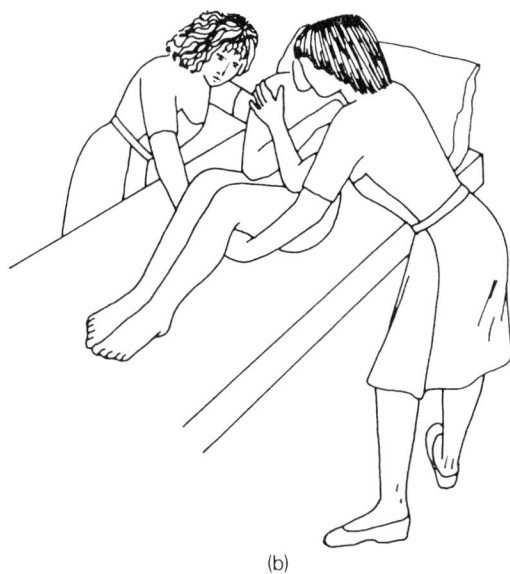

(b)

Figure 23.1b Orthodox lift

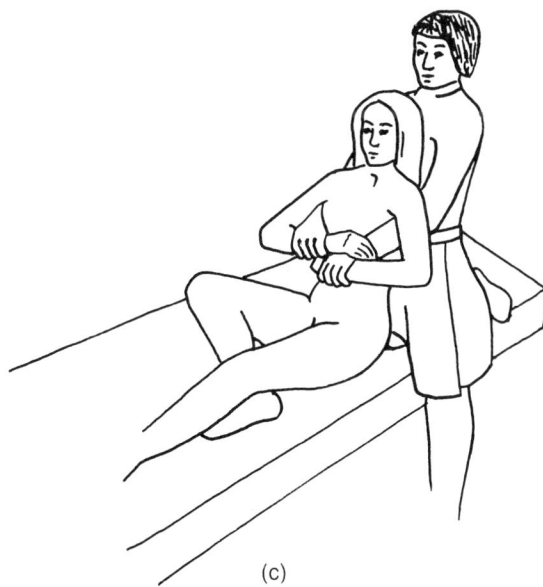

(c)

Figure 23.1c Through arm lift (second nurse not shown)

The Orthodox Lift (Figure 23.1b)   Both nurses face each other on either side of the patient. Each nurse has one foot pointing in the direction of the lift and the other foot at right angles to it. The hips and knees are bent and the spine braced.

Each nurse places his/her arm nearest the foot of the bed under the thighs of the patient — as near to the hips as possible — and grips the other nurse's hand. The other hand is placed as low as possible on the patient's back. The patient's arms are either placed over the nurses' shoulders or folded across his/her chest.

The patient is moved by the nurses straightening their legs and transferring their weight to their forward feet.

The Through Arm Lift (Figure 23.1c)   One nurse stands behind the patient, who is in the sitting position, and places his/her arms under the patient's axillae. The nurse then grips the patient's forearms as near to the wrists as possible by placing his/her hands between the patient's chest and upper arms. The patient is asked to grip one of his/her own wrists firmly.

The other nurse faces the patient and puts his/her arms under the patient's thighs from opposite sides so that the nurse can grab his/her own wrist.

The lift is performed by the nurses extending their hips and knees, while keeping their backs straight.

This lift does put unequal strain on the nurses and the one who lifts the upper part of the patient experiences higher spinal stress.

In comparing the lifting techniques mentioned above, the shoulder lift has been shown to produce significantly lower IAPs than the other two. There appears to be no significant difference between the other two manoeuvres when abdominal pressure is considered. The orthodox lift is usually considered to be as comfortable as the shoulder lift by nurses, but no difference has been observed with respect to patient comfort. The through arm lift or axilla hoist has been shown to cause patient discomfort at a level high enough positively to discourage the use of this lift.

The reason for the higher IAPs of the other lifts as compared to the shoulder lift is an outcome of the initial stooped or semistooped starting position. The shoulder lift is therefore recommended wherever this is practically possible.

Spinal stress can also be significantly reduced if the manoeuvre is done in three or four small steps as opposed to one large effort, regardless of the technique used.

Mechanical Aids

Mechanical aids should be used in situations where nurses are unable to lift a patient effectively or safely. The most frequent occurrence of such situations is in the bathroom, where two nurses lifting a patient out of the bath experience high spinal stress. In an experimental setting, Stubbs et al. (1980) stated that safety margins would be exceeded during such a manoeuvre if the patient weighted over 68 kg (10½ stones). Conversely, the stress levels were significantly reduced when the same manoeuvre was carried out using a mechanical aid. It is recommended, therefore, that when bathing heavy patients a mechanical aid, such as an Ambulift, is used.

References

Davis P R (1981) The use of intra-abdominal pressure in evaluating stresses on the lumbar spine, Spine 6 (1): 90-92

Hyde N J (1980) A comparative analysis of a lifting method commonly used by nurses versus a recommended method of lifting patients, using pressure sensitive radio pill methodology, BSc thesis, Leeds Polytechnic

Northwick Park Hospital Nursing Practice Research Unit (1980) Prevention of Back Pain in Nursing: Proceedings of the Conference . . . Held at Northwick Park Hospital . . . 26th September 1980, Nursing Practice Research Unit

Sorenson K C Luckman J (1979) Basic Nursing — A Psychophysiologic Approach, W B Saunders

GUIDELINES: LIFTING

Procedure

Action	Rationale
1 Assess the patient and the environment to establish what help or aids will be required for the lift. *Note:* A nurse should never attempt to lift a patient on his/her own.	1 To ensure that the patient is well enough to be lifted and that all necessary help and equipment can be acquired before disturbing the patient.
2 Decide how the patient is to be lifted and ensure that the other nurses(s) and the patient understand what they are going to do.	2 So that those involved in the lift can cooperate and coordinate their movements and any problems can be taken into account beforehand.
3 Prepare the area. Move equipment into a suitable position, put brakes on the bed and move any unecessary equipment out of the way. Screen the area if necessary.	3 The environment must allow safe lifting and reduce the need for the nurse to twist or be impeded in his/her movements.
4 Adopt a suitable stance for the proposed lift:	
a The feet should be apart, one foot pointing in the direction of the initial movement and the other at right angles to it.	**a** To ensure a balanced distribution of weight as the patient's weight is transferred from one foot to the other.
b Stand as close to the patient as possible.	**b** To reduce the spinal stress.
c Bend the knees and hips to allow a suitable grasp to be taken.	**c** The strong thigh and hip muscles are used to straighten the legs and thus lift the patient.
d Grasp the other lifter's hand or	**d** To enable controlled and safe

Problem	**Suggested Action**
wrist firmly, avoiding tender and painful areas. Ensure that this is comfortable for the patient.	movement of the patient without causing discomfort.
e Check that the spine is straight and that the head is in line with the trunk before lifting.	**e** To reduce spinal stress.
5 Lift the patient into the desired position. One nurse acts as leader and coordinates the moment of lifting.	5 So that the effort is exerted simultaneously by those involved and unequal strain does not fall on any one person.
6 Check that the lift was comfortable for the patient and the nurses, and note any points which could be improved upon for future use.	

Note: If something goes wrong when lifting a patient and he/she appears to be falling, it is safest to let him/her fall in a controlled fashion, i.e. by allowing him/her to slide gently to the floor or the bed. The nurse should make the patient comfortable and get assistance to lift him/her up again.

24

LIVER BIOPSY

Definition

Liver biopsy is the removal of a small piece of liver tissue by percutaneous puncture using a special needle.

Indications

Liver biopsy is a procedure performed by trained medical staff to establish a diagnosis in certain liver diseases, e.g. cirrhosis, carcinoma (primary or secondary), amyloidosis, miliary tuberculosis.

Contraindications

Liver biopsy is contraindicated in patients who

1 Are confused or uncooperative
2 Have a prolonged clotting time
3 Have an increased bleeding time
4 Have severe purpura
5 Have a coagulation defect
6 Are severely jaundiced
7 Are under the age of 3 years
8 Have a right lower lobe pneumonia or pleuritis.

REFERENCE MATERIAL

Needle biopsy of the liver was first used by Ehrlich in 1883. For varying reasons it fell out of favour as a diagnostic method until reintroduced in 1939 by Iversen and Roholm. It is now a widely practised technique for the diagnosis of certain liver diseases (see Figures 24.1 and 24.2). It has the advantage of being performed at the patient's bedside. No general anaesthetic is required and the patient suffers significantly less pain than with open biopsy.

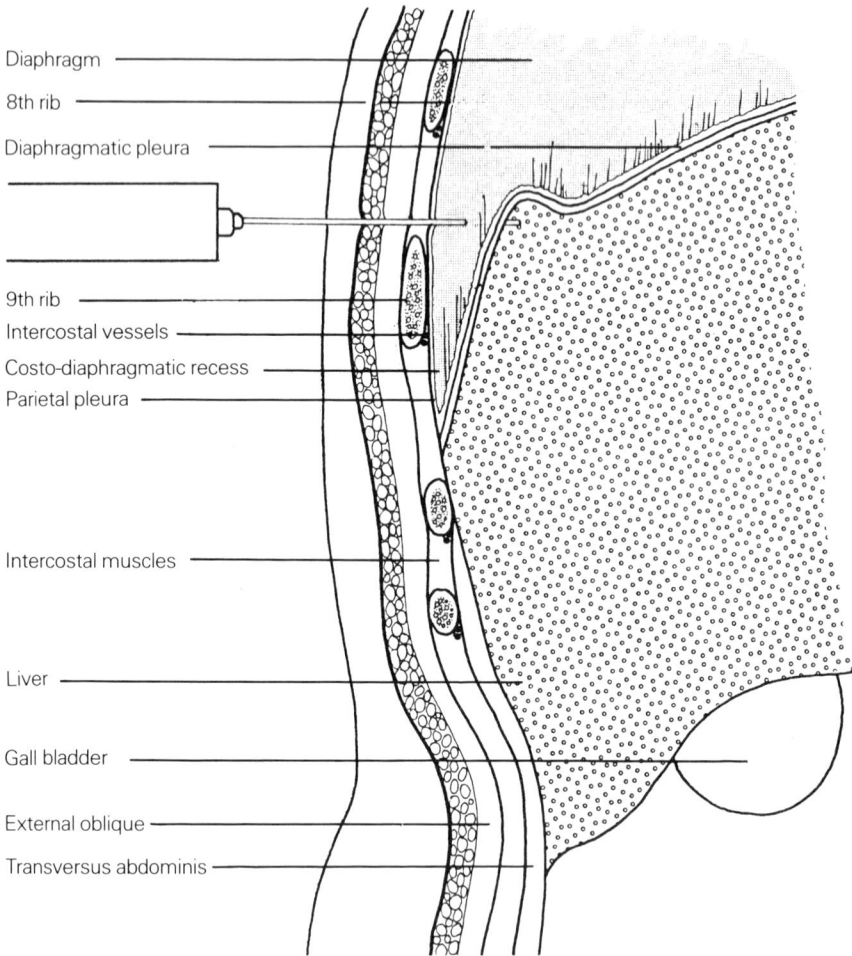

Figure 24.1   Anatomy and physiology of the liver

Anatomy and Physiology

The liver is the largest organ in the body, weighing about 1.5 kg. It is highly vascular, is situated to the right upper side of the abdomen below the diaphragm and extends vertically for 15-18 cm. Laterally it measures about 20-30 cm and its anterior posterior measurement is about 10-13 cm. The lower surface is covered with peritoneum. The liver has two lobes: a large right lobe, under which the gall bladder lies and a smaller left lobe. The hepatic flexure of the colon lies underneath the liver.

The function of the liver is sevenfold:

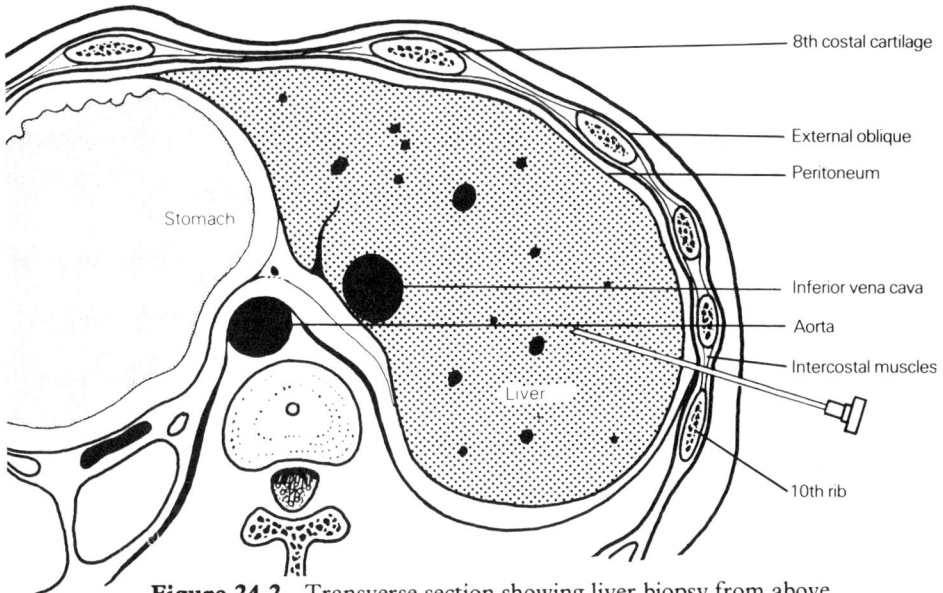

Figure 24.2 Transverse section showing liver biopsy from above

1 To process digested food and convert it into substances which the body can use
2 To store converted food substances until the body requires them
3 To produce plasma proteins — albumen, globulin and fibrinogen
4 To store vitamins A, B, D, E and K
5 To reprocess body substances, e.g. haemoglobin and amino acids
6 To detoxify poisons
7 To maintain body temperature.

Investigations Prior to Biopsy

1 Blood is taken for
   a Bleeding, clotting and prothrombin times
   b Platelet count
   c Grouping and, if necessary, cross-matching.
2 A plain abdominal X-ray is taken to ensure avoidance of colonic puncture if the patient has a small liver.

Physical Preparation of the Patient

Fasting

Fasting is required as for preoperative cases.

Sedation

For very nervous patients a mild tranquillizer such as diazepam may be ordered by the doctor.

Complications

Haemorrhage

Haemorrhage may occur as a result of inadvertent puncture of an intra- or extra-hepatic blood vessel. Signs of this will appear within 4 hours of the biopsy. (Loss of 5-10 ml of blood from the liver surface is normal following needle biopsy.)

Peritonitis

Peritonitis may be caused by inadvertent puncture of the bile duct, resulting in bile leaking into the peritoneal cavity.

Pneumothorax

Pneumothorax may result from inadvertent puncture of the pleura.

Mortality Rate

A mortality rate of 0.17% was recorded by Zamcheck and Klausenstock (1953) following needle biopsy and the incidence of complications of any significance is quoted as being below 5% (Read 1968).

References

Abrahams P Webb P (1975) Clinical Anatomy of Practical Procedures, Pitman Medical, pp. 84-86

Bevan J (1978) A Pictorial Handbook of Anatomy and Physiology, Mitchell Beazley, pp. 48-49

Booth J A (1983) Handbook of Investigations, Harper and Row, pp. 25-27

Deeley T J (1974) Needle Biopsy, Butterworth, pp. 102-109

Kilday D (1981) Assisting with liver biopsy, in Mosby's Manual of Clinical Nursing Procedures, edited by J Hirsch and I Hancock, C V Mosby, pp. 229-232

Pagnana K D Pagnana T J (1982) Diagnostic Testing and Nursing Implications, C V Mosby, pp. 80-81

Read A E (1968) Needle biopsy of the liver, in Biopsy Procedures in Clinical Medicine, edited by A E Read, John Wright and Sons, pp. 57-68

Skydell B Crowder A (1975) Diagnostic Procedures — A Reference for Health Practitioners and a Guide for Patient Counselling, Little, Brown, pp. 121-124

Zamcheck N Klausenstock O (1953) The risk of needle biopsy, New England Journal of Medicine 249: 1062-1069

GUIDELINES: LIVER BIOPSY

Equipment

1   Antiseptic skin cleansing agent
2   Syringes and needles
3   Local anaesthetic

4   Sterile normal saline
5   Disposable scalpel
6   Plaster dressing or plastic dressing spray
7   Hypoallergenic tape
8   Liver biopsy needle, usually a Menghini or disposable Trucut needle
9   Sterile dressing pack
10 Sterile gloves
11 Formal saline

Procedure

Action	Rationale
1 Explain the procedure to the patient.	1 To obtain the patient's consent and cooperation.
2 Demonstrate holding the breath on expiration and observe the patient practising the manoeuvre.	2 To minimise the risk of accidental puncture of lung tissue when the biopsy needle is inserted into the liver, the patient will be asked to hold his/her breath on expiration.
3 Administer a sedative at an appropriate time, if ordered.	3 To reduce the patient's anxiety.
4 Assist the patient to lie in supine position with his/her right side as close to the edge of the bed as possible, the left side may be supported by a pillow. His/her right hand should be placed beneath his/her head and the head turned to the left.	4 To allow the doctor ease of access to the eighth or ninth intercostal space.
5 Continue to observe and reassure the patient throughout the procedure.	
6 Assist the doctor as required. The doctor will	
a Clean the appropriate area with an antiseptic solution.	**a** To maintain asepsis throughout the procedure and thus diminish the risk of infection.
b Give a local anaesthetic intradermally and in successive layers down to the pleura. (Usually 10-20 ml is required.)	**b** To minimize pain during the procedure and ensure maximum cooperation of the patient. (No further pain should be felt once the local anaesthetic has been introduced.)
c Make a small incision in the skin over the area to be punctured.	**c** To allow ease of introduction of the borer (part of the biopsy set).

Action	**Rationale**
d Flush the biopsy apparatus with saline to check for patency of the needle. Some saline will be left in the syringe barrel.	**d** To flush out the piece of liver obtained at biopsy, which will be in the core of the needle.
e Introduce the needle through the diaphragm and inject a little of the saline.	**e** To remove any pieces of tissue caught in the needle during its introduction.
f Ask the patient to breathe in and out fully several times. The patient will then be asked to breathe out and hold his breath. The biopsy needle is then rapidly inserted and withdrawn from the liver.	**f** At this stage there is minimal risk of puncturing lung tissue as the biopsy is obtained. Delay increases the risk of a liver tear.
7 Once the doctor has indicated that the biopsy has been obtained, cover the puncture site with a sterile topical swab and apply pressure for 5 minutes.	7 To prevent infection and stop bleeding.
8 Once bleeding is minimal or has ceased, apply a small dry dressing and secure with hypoallergenic tape. (A plastic dressing spray may be used over the puncture site.)	
9 Make the patient comfortable and position him/her on his/her right side for the next 1-2 hours.	9 To compress the liver capsule against the chest wall and prevent haemorrhage.
10 Observe the patient, initially, every 15-30 minutes for the next 1-2 hours, monitoring in particular **a** Pulse rate **b** Blood pressure **c** Respiration rate **d** Pain **e** Abdominal tenderness and/or rigidity **f** Leakage from the wound site **g** Haematoma formation. Observations may be decreased according to the patient's condition.	10 To monitor any complications that may occur as a result of the procedure.
11 Remove and dispose of equipment as appropriate.	11 To prevent spread of infection.
12 Food and fluids may be recommended when observations are stable.	12 To allow adequate time for assessment of potential complications before reintroducing diet.
13 Record necessary information in the appropriate documents and	

Action	**Rationale**
ensure that the specimen obtained is sent to the appropriate laboratory with any necessary forms and labelling.	

NURSING CARE PLAN

Problem	Cause	Suggested Action
1 Patient restless and perspiring with a low blood pressure and fast pulse rate	1 Haemorrhage from biopsy site due to either a tear in the liver or inadvertent puncture of a blood vessel	1 Ensure that the patient lies on his/her right side to produce pressure over puncture site for 1-2 hours. Record the patient's pulse and blood pressure every 15-30 minutes for the first 1-2 hours and decrease the frequency as the patient's condition allows. Call a doctor if there is any alteration in observations as the patient may require blood transfusion, analgesia and sedation.
2 Patient complains of severe pain which may be accompained by signs of shock and collapse, with abdominal tenderness and rigidity	2 Leakage of bile into the peritoneal cavity from an accidentally perforated bile duct	2 Record the patient's pulse and blood pressure every 15-30 minutes for the first 1-2 hours and decrease the frequency as the patient's condition allows. Call a doctor if there is any alteration in observations as the patient may require a laparotomy to rectify biliary duct puncture.
3 Patient complains of dyspnoea	3 Pneumothorax due to a puncture of the lung tissue caused by the patient inhaling as the biopsy needle is introduced into the liver	3 Record the patient's respiration rate every 15-20 minutes for the first 1-2 hours and decrease the frequency as the patient's condition allows. Call a doctor if there is any change in observations as the patient may require intrapleural drainage and oxygen therapy.

25

LUMBAR PUNCTURE

Definition

Lumbar puncture is the withdrawal of cerebrospinal fluid by the insertion of a special needle into the lumbar subarachnoid space for diagnostic or therapeutic purposes.

Indications

Lumbar puncture is indicated for the following purposes:

1 Diagnostic purposes
2 Introducing contrast media for radiological examinations
3 Introducing chemotherapeutic agents, e.g antibiotics or cytotoxics.

Contraindications

This procedure is contraindicated in the following cases:

1 *Raised intracranial pressure*   The procedure could lead to herniation of the brainstem (coning).
2 *Suspected cord compression*
3 *Local infection*   Meningitis is a rare complication of lumbar puncture. If skin infection is present, examination should be delayed until the problem is resolved.
4 *Uncooperative patients*   Lumbar puncture is a potentially hazardous procedure which requires maximum patient cooperation.
5 *Severe degenerative spinal joint disease*   In such cases difficulty will be experienced both in positioning the patient and in access between the vertebra.

REFERENCE MATERIAL

Anatomy and Physiology

The spinal cord extends from the base of the brain down into the spinal column

(Figure 25.1). It is encased and protected by the vertebrae. Its width decreases as it descends and below the second lumbar vetebra it continues as a fine thread, the filum terminale, which is attached internally to the coccyx. Like the brain, the spinal cord is covered by the meninges — the dura, arachnoid and pia mater. The dura and arachnoid mater line the spinal canal to the level of the second sacral vertebra, the pia becomes the filum terminale.

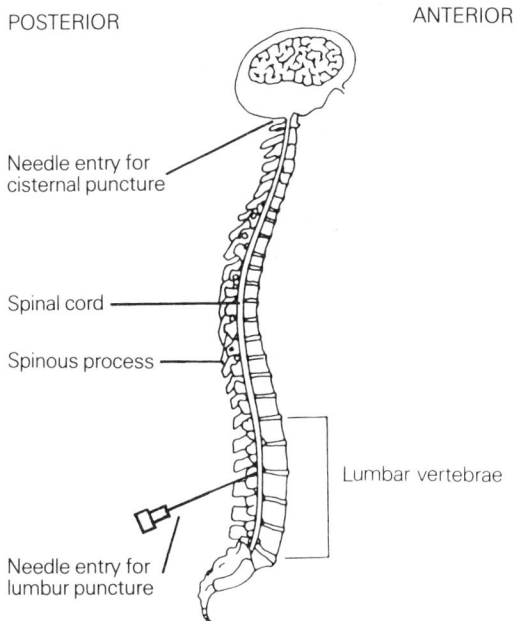

POSTERIOR

ANTERIOR

Needle entry for cisternal puncture

Spinal cord

Spinous process

Lumbar vertebrae

Needle entry for lumbur puncture

Figure 25.1 Lateral view of the spinal column and vertebrae showing the level at which the spinal cord ends, and the needle entry sites for lumbar and cisternal puncture

The subarachnoid space, which contains cerebrospinal fluid, is fairly narrow until the first lumbar vertebra, when it widens as the spinal cord terminates. Below the first lumbar vertebra the subarachnoid space contains cerebrospinal fluid, the filum terminale and the cauda equinae (the anterior and posterior roots of the lumbar and sacral nerves). This area is used to obtain specimens of cerebrospinal fluid by lumbar puncture as there is no danger of damage to the spinal cord (Figure 25.2).

The cerebrospinal fluid is secreted by the choroid plexus which is situated in the ventricles of the brain. The fluid, which is clear and colourless, fills the ventricles of the brain and the subarachnoid space. Its functions are as follows:

1   To act as a shock absorber
2   To carry nutrients to and remove metabolites from the brain.

At lumbar puncture, depending on the investigations required, about 5-10 ml of cerebrospinal fluid is removed for laboratory analysis.

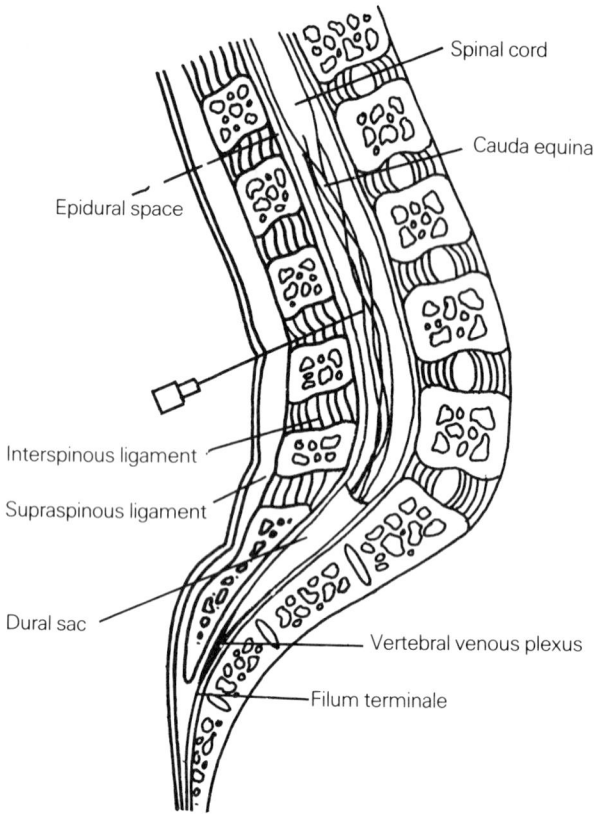

Figure 25.2 Lumbar puncture. Saggital section through lumbosacral spine

Investigations

Pressure

The pressure of the cerebrospinal fluid is investigated at the time of lumbar puncture, using a manometer. Queckenstedt's test may also be performed. The latter consists of applying pressure to the jugular vein. When normal, there is a sharp rise in pressure followed by a fall as the pressure is released. Blockage of the spinal canal will result in a sluggish rise and fall or absence of response. Queckenstedt's manoeuvre is a potentially hazardous procedure if both jugular veins are compressed at the same time. Temporal lobe or brainstem herniation may occur. Normal cerebrospinal fluid pressure is approximately 60-180 mm H_2O.

Colour

The fluid should be clear and colourless. The first 3-4 ml may be blood-stained due to local trauma at the time of insertion of the lumbar needle. In this case the blood will usually clot. The fluid clears as the procedure continues. However, if blood-staining is due to subarachnoid haemorrhage, no clotting will occur and all samples will be blood-stained.

Blood

There should not be any blood in the samples. The presence of blood indicates either a traumatic puncture or subarachnoid haemorrhage.

Blood cells

There should be no blood cells, except for a few lymphocytes, in the sample. The presence of polymorphonuclear leucocytes (white cells) is indicative of meningitis or cerebral abscess. Monocytes would indicated viral or tubercular meningitis or encephalitis.

Culture and Sensitivity

The presence of microorganisms would indicate meningitis or cerebral absess. By isolating the specific organism the appropriate antibiotic therapy may be commenced.

Protein

The total amount of the protein in the cerebrospinal fluid should be 15.45 mg/dl (=154.5 µg/ml). Proteins are large molecules which do not readily cross the blood/brain barrier. There is normally more albumen (approximately 80% of total protein) than globulin (approximately 12-20% of total protein) in cerebrospinal fluid as albumens are smaller molecules. Raised globulin levels are indicative of multiple sclerosis, neurosyphilis, degenerative cord or brain disease. Raised protein levels may indicate meningitis, encephalitis, myelitis or the presence of a tumour.

Cytology

Central nervous system tumours tend to shed cells into the cerebrospinal fluid, where they float freely. Examination of these cells after lumbar puncture will determine whether the tumour is benign or malignant.

Serology for Syphilis

If other tests are positive, the appropriate antibiotic therapy may be commenced.

Instillation of Chemotherapy

Lumbar puncture may be used as a means of introducing drugs into the central nervous system which do not cross the blood/brain barrier. This is done to treat specific infections and malignant diseases such as leukaemia, to prevent recurrence in the central nervous system when remission has been attained.

References and Further Reading

Abrahms P Webb P (1975) Clinical Anatomy of Practical Procedures, Pitman Medical, pp. 13-15

Bevan J (1978) A Pictorial Handbook of Anaotomy and Physiology, Mitchell Beazley, p.60

Booth J A (1983) Handbook of Investigations, Harper and Row, pp. 91-95

Brunner L S Suddarth D S (1982) The Lippincott Manual of Medical-Surgical Nursing, Harper and Row, Volume 3, pp 6-10

Clough C Pearce J M S (1980) Lumbar puncture, British Medical Journal 280: 297-299

Pagana K D Pagana T J (1982) Diagnostic Testing and Nursing Implications, C V Mosby, pp. 124-128

Skydell B Crowder A S (1975) Diagnostic Procedures — A Reference for Health Practioners and a Guide for Patient Counselling, Little, Brown, pp.15-19

Vannini V Pogliani G (1980) The New Atlas of the Human Body, Corgi, p.58

GUIDELINES: LUMBAR PUNCTURE

Equipment

1 Antiseptic skin-cleansing agent
2 Selection of needles and syringes
3 Local anaesthetic
4 Sterile gloves
5 Sterile dressing pack
6 Lumbar puncture needles of assorted sizes
7 Disposable manometer
8 Three sterile specimen bottles (These should be labelled 1, 2 and 3. The first specimen, which may be blood-stained due to needle trauma, should go into bottle 1. This will assist the laboratory to differentiate between blood due to procedure trauma and that due to subarachnoid haemorrhage.)
9 Plaster dressing or plastic dressing spray

Procedure

Action	Rationale
1 Explain the procedure to the patient.	1 To obtain patient's consent and cooperation.
2 Assist the patient into the required position: **a** Lying (Figure 25.3) (1) One pillow under his/her head	**a** To ensure maximum widening of the intervertebral spaces and thus easier access to the sub-arachnoid space.

Action	**Rationale**
(2) Firm surface	
(3) On side with knees drawn up to the abdomen and clasped by the hands	
(4) Support patient in this position by holding him/her behind the knees and neck.	To avoid sudden movement by the patient which would produce blood-stained fluid.

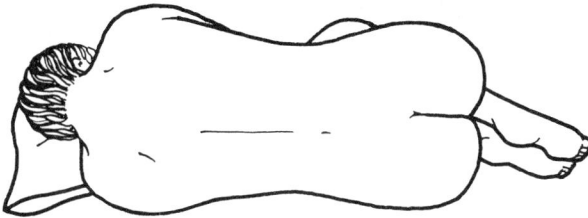

Figure 25.3 Position for lumbar puncture. Head is flexed onto chest and knees are drawn up to the abdomen

b Sitting	**b** This position may be used for those patients unable to maintain the lying position. It allows more accurate identification of the spinous processes and thus the intervertebral spaces.
(1) Patient straddles a straight-backed chair so that his/her back is facing the doctor.	
(2) Patient folds his/her arms on the back of the chair and rests his/her head on them.	
3 Continue to support, encourage and observe the patient through-out the procedure.	
4 Assist the doctor as required. The doctor will proceed as follows:	
a Clean the skin with the anti-septic cleansing agent.	**a** To maintain sterility throughout.
b Identify the area to be punctured and infiltrate the skin and subcutaneous layers with local anaesthetic.	
c Introduce a spinal puncture needle between the 3rd and 4th or 4th and 5th lumbar vertebrae and into the subarachnoid space.	**c** This is below the level of the spinal cord but still within the subarachnoid space.
d Ensure that he has entered the subarachnoid space and will probably attach the manometer to the spinal needle.	**d** To obtain a cerebrospinal fluid pressure reading (normal pressure is 60-180 mm H_2O).

Action	**Rationale**
e Decide whether Queckenstedt's manoeuvre may be performed (see Figure 25.4).	**e** To check for obstruction to cerebrospinal fluid flow in the spinal column. (Usually obstruction is caused by a tumour.)

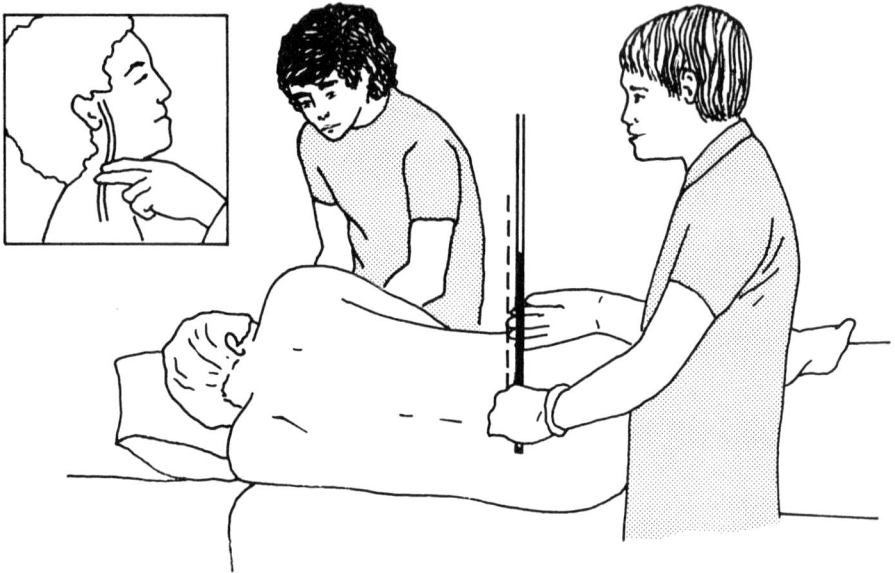

Figure 25.4 Queckenstedt's manoeuvre

f The appropriate specimens of cerebrospinal fluid (about 10 ml in total) are obtained for analysis.

g Once all specimens have been obtained and the appropriate pressure measurements made the spinal needle is withdrawn.

5 When the needle is withdrawn, apply pressure over the lumbar puncture site using a sterile topical swab.	5 To maintain asepsis and to stop blood and cerebrospinal fluid flow.
6 When all leakage from the puncture site has ceased, apply a plaster dressing or plastic dressing spray.	6 To prevent secondary infection.
7 Make the patient comfortable. He/she should lie flat or the head	7 To avoid headache and decrease the possibility of brainstem

Action	Rationale
should be tilted slightly downwards for a period of up to 24 hours (according to the doctor's instructions).	herniation (coning) due to a reduction in cerebrospinal fluid pressure.
8 Observe patient for the next 24 hours for the following:	
a Leakage from the puncture site	a There may be a small amount of blood-stained oozing. The presence of clear fluid should be reported immediately to the doctor, especially if accompanied by fluctuation of other observations, as it may be a cerebrospinal fluid leak.
b Headache	b Not unusual following lumbar puncture. Usually relieved by lying flat and, if ordered by the doctor, a mild analgesic.
c Backache	c As above.
d Neurological observations/vital signs	d These may indicate signs of a change in intracranial pressure. (For further information see procedures on neurological observations and the vital signs, pp. 301-305.)
9 Encourage a fluid intake of 2-3 litres in 24 hours.	9 To replace lost fluid and assist the patient to micturate, which may be difficult due to the supine position.
10 Remove equipment and dispose of as appropriate.	10 To prevent the spread of infection.
11 Record the procedure in the appropriate documents.	
12 Ensure that specimens are appropriately labelled and sent with the correct forms to the laboratory.	

NURSING CARE PLAN

Problem	Cause	Suggested Action
1 Pain down one leg during the procedure	1 A dorsal nerve root may have been touched by the spinal needle	1 Inform the doctor, who will probably move the needle. Reassure the patient that no permanent damage has occurred.
2 Headache following	2 Removal of the sample	2 Reassure the patient

Problem	**Cause**	**Suggested Action**
procedure (may persist for up to a week)	of cerebrospinal fluid	that it is a transient symptom. Ensure that he/she lies flat for the specified period of time. Encourage a high fluid intake to replace fluid lost during the procedure. Administer an analgesic as ordered. If the headache is severe and increasing, inform a doctor — there is a possibility of rising intracranial pressure.
3 Backache following procedure	3 **a** Removal of the sample of cerebrospinal fluid **b** Position required for puncture	3 Reassure the patient that it is a transient symptom. Ensure that he/she lies flat for the appropriate period of time. Administer an analgesic as ordered.
4 Fluctuation of neurological observations, i.e. level of consciousness, pulse, respirations, blood pressure or pupillary reaction	4 Herniation (coning) of the brainstem due to the sudden decrease of intracranial pressure. *(Raised intracranial pressure is a contra-indication to lumbar puncture.)*	4 Observe the patient every 30 minutes for the first 2 hours for signs of alteration in intracranial pressure. The frequency may be diminished to 4-hourly as the patient's condition allows. Report any fluctuations in these observations to a doctor immediately.
5 Leakage from the puncture site	5 **a** Resolution of bleeding **b** Leakage of cerebro-spinal fluid	5 **a** No further action required. **b** Report immediately to a doctor, especially if accompanied by fluctuation in neurological observations.

26

MOUTH CARE

Definition
Mouth care is the process of cleaning the contents of the buccal cavity.

Indications
Mouth care is indicated for the following reasons:

1   To achieve and maintain oral cleanliness
2   To prevent infection
3   To keep the oral mucosa moist
4   To promote patient comfort
5   To help prevent and treat stomatitis, especially in patients undergoing chemotherapy or radiotherapy.

There aims are interrelated. Cleanliness of the soft tissue is dependent on the mouth remaining moist and infection is related to the amount of debris on the teeth. This debris accumulates on the teeth irrespective of moisture. A dry mouth is uncomfortable for the patient, so comfort can only be attained when the mouth is clean, moist and infection free. The only effective way to ensure a moist mouth is by adequate systemic hydration, enabling the tissues to remain moist, and by the production of saliva.

The patients most at risk of developing mouth problems are those who become dehydrated or whose mouths produce insufficient saliva to maintain cleanliness and moisture of the soft tissue.

Inadequate intake also reduces the rate at which debris is removed. Because such patients are not totally dependent, the nursing staff may not recognize their need for mouth care or the need to supervise the oral hygiene which these patients practise.

REFERENCE MATERIAL

A Selection of Agents Used for Mouth Care
The choice of agents used for mouth care is determined by the individual needs of

the patient together with a nursing assessment of the buccal cavity. The most commonly used agents are evaluated below.

Saline

This solution is made up as required by dissolving salt in water. An isotonic solution is recommended for mouth care, i.e. 4.5 grams of salt to 500 ml of water (4.5 grams of salt is equivalent to 1 level teaspoonful). Stronger solutions may be irritating to the mucosa and will be unpleasant to the taste. Sterile sachets of normal saline are available for immunosuppressed patients. Saline is thought to aid the formation of granulation tissue and promote healing. No damaging effects are known at concentrations that are isotonic or below and the solution is cheap and easy to use. Normal saline is ineffective for removing hardened mucus, debris or crusts.

Sodium Bicarbonate

This solution is prepared as required by diluting approximately 1 teaspoonful of sodium bicarbonate in 500 ml of warm water. It has a good cleaning effect and is suitable for dissolving mucin and loosening debris even if oral ulcers are present. If the solution is made too concentrated, it will taste unpleasant and may damage the mucosa. It is recommended that sodium bicarbonate is only used in mouth care when crusts or hardened or tenacious mucous is present.

Hydrogen Peroxide

This mouthwash solution is made up immediately prior to use by diluting the preparation in the strength advised by the hospital pharmacist. Hydrogen peroxide is decomposed to water and oxygen on contact with the enzyme catalase present in blood and tissues. The vigorous release of oxygen bubbles during this reaction acts as a mechanical cleaning agent and is, therefore, useful for loosening necrotic ulcers, crusting and debris. This may also result in the breakdown of new tissue in fresh granulation surfaces. The increased oxygen concentration created by the reaction does inhibit the growth of anaerobic organisms but the foaming effect within the mouth is potentially dangerous if the cough reflex is impaired in any way. Suction should be available if this is the case. Hydrogen peroxide may act as an irritant to the tongue and buccal mucosa, especially where stomatitis is present. It is advisable, therefore, to clean the mouth after its use with water or normal saline.

Lemon Juice

Lemon juice is an effective salivary stimulant used in several mouth care preparations. Its effectiveness as a salivary stimulant may be counter-productive if the patient is unable to swallow all the saliva produced or if this stimulation leads to exhaustion of the saliva reflex resulting in severe drying of the soft tissues. Lemon juice can also decalcify the teeth and may cause pain when applied to broken or irritated mucosa such as when stomatitis or oral lesions are present.

Glycerin

Glycerin has a characteristic ability to bring relative humidities into equilibrium because of its mode of osmotic action. This means that when applied undiluted or in a strong solution to the skin or mucous membranes, it absorbs moisture from them and may lead to dehydration. If glycerin is required to moisten the mouth, it must be used in a diluted form, less than 40% concentration, so that moisture is drawn from the diluent towards the tissues.

Oraldene

Oraldene is a popular commercially available mouthwash containing 0.1% hexetidine solution. It has an antibacterial and antiprotozoal effect and the manufacturer recommends its use for patients with stomatitis, ulcers and halitosis. Its value has not been investigated in comparison with other products but it is a relatively expensive mouthwash and patients have complained of it being too strong even when diluted as recommended.

Bocasan

This product is presented in individual sachets containing sodium perborate and sodium hydrogen tartrate. The sachet contents are dissolved in 30 ml of water prior to use and, when rinsed around the mouth, they react to release bubbles of oxygen. This product compares with hydrogen peroxide in that cleaning is achieved by the mechanical action of the bubbles released and by the increased oxygen environment incompatible with anaerobic growth. The mouth should not be rinsed with anything else for half an hour after using this agent.

The effectiveness of Bocasan against hydrogen peroxide has not been evaluated but the taste is considered unpleasant and it is comparatively expensive. Because of the risk of toxicity from boric acid accumulation, the use of Bocasan is contraindicated for patients with renal insufficiency. It would appear that hydrogen peroxide should be the agent of choice here. The precautions for use include the availability of suction when the cough reflex is impaired due to the frothing action.

Synthetic Saliva

This product was designed for use by astronauts unable to produce saliva in a low gravity environment. The constituents resemble those of natural saliva and may be used as often as required for dry mouths without any detrimental effect. This is particularly useful for patients with impaired saliva production.

Chlorhexidine

An aqueous solution of chlorhexidine 0.1-0.2% is sometimes prescribed as a mouthwash. It has a disinfectant action on Gram-positive and Gram-negative bacteria and is useful in preventing the accumulation of plaque and the development of gingivitis when brushing is contraindicated. It does, however, have an unpleasant taste. An alcoholic solution of chlorhexidine may be used for soaking dentures in patients with oral infections of *Candida* species.

Thymol

Thymol is the main component of the majority of mouthwash tablets in current use. The solution has a mild disinfectant action and is easy to use, cheap and has a pleasant refreshing taste. It should be used with caution in patients with gastrointestinal disorders or imparied kidney function due to the absorption of thymol during mouth care procedures.

Vaseline

Vaseline may be used sparingly on the lips to create an occlusive oil film that prevents the loss of moisture by evaporation. Mineral oils are not recommended for this purpose due to the small risk of aspiration pneumonia.

Milton

This product may be used as a mouthwash when diluted in the ratio 2-5ml Milton: 100 ml water. The main advantage of this agent over others is its antiviral action and it should be used whenever viral invasion of the mouth is suspected.

Commercially Available Mouthwashes

Most commercially available mouthwashes, such as Listerine, are acidic in nature and may have a high alcohol content that patients with an impaired oral mucosa may find painful. Their beneficial action extends little beyond creating a pleasant taste for a short time.

Instruments Used in Mouth Care

The most commonly used instruments in mouth care are evaluated below.

Swabbing with a Gloved Finger or with a Topical Swab and Forceps

This is a useful method of cleaning debris from the soft tissue of the mouth, especially in edentulous patients. Swabbing will not remove debris from the teeth, where it is most likely to accumulate. A gloved finger can be useful for cleaning sore mouths as many nurses feel this is more sensitive than using other instruments. A topical swab wrapped around the end of a pair of forceps is not generally recommended as it is more time consuming than other methods and clumsy to use. There is also a greater risk of trauma to the gums from the pointed end of the forceps.

Foam Sticks

Foam sticks are useful for cleaning oral mucosa but will not remove debris between or from the surface of the teeth. They are easy to use and there is little risk of mechanical trauma from them. The stick should be rotated gently over the mucosa so that all of the foam surface is utilized.

Toothbrushes

Research indicates that a toothbrush is the best way of cleaning teeth as the fine hairs loosen the debris trapped between the teeth and remove plaque from the tooth surface: 'The present evidence in favour of the use of a toothbrush for the care of teeth is so outstanding that it would seem to remove all question that this is the method of choice for teeth cleaning' (Howarth 1977).

A small toothbrush with soft bristles that the patient can keep throughout his/her stay in hospital is recommended. There is some evidence for advocating the use of automatic toothbrushes, especially for patients who are unable to use an ordinary toothbrush correctly. The type with an oscillating movement is favoured as those with a purely rotational movement may damage the gums. Teeth should be brushed with firm individual strokes so that any loosened debris is directed away from the gums. The toothbrush should be rinsed and dried after use.

The Frequency of Mouth Care

The frequency of mouth care depends entirely on patient assessment and varies with the particular circumstances of the individual. Dental decay will not take place until plaque and debris have been in place for 24 hours or more. Brushing the teeth after each meal should minimize this risk. Certain factors act as stressors to the state of the oral mucosa. These include the following:

1 Mouth breathing
2 Continuous oxygen therapy
3 Intermittent suction
4 No oral intake.

After experiencing all the above for only 1 hour, a healthy young adult developed dryness of the lips and mouth together with colour changes in the oral mucosa (DeWalt and Haines 1969). It is reasonable to expect more rapid changes in a more debilitated individual. Normally the saliva lubricates and cleans the mouth and reduces the need for frequent mouth care. For patients who complain of a dry mouth, saliva production may be stimulated by the use of chewing gum or an artificial saliva preparation. Patients with poor appetites should be offered mouth care before and after a meal as a dirty mouth may inhibit the appetite.

References and Further Reading

Bruya M A Madeira N P (1975) Stomatitis after chemotherapy, American Journal of Nursing 75: 1349-1352

Daeffler R (1980) Oral hygiene measures for patients with cancer I-II, Cancer Nursing 3: 347-356, 427-432

Daeffler R (1981) Oral hygiene measures for patients with cancer III, Cancer Nursing 4: 29-35

DeWalt E M Haines A K (1969) The effects of specific stressors on healthy oral mucosa, Nursing Research 18 (1): 22-27

Ettinger R L Manderson R D (1975) Dental care of the elderly, Nursing Times 71: 1003-1006

Harris M D (1980) Tools for mouth care, Nursing Times 76: 340-342

Howarth H (1977) Mouth care procedures for the very ill, Nursing Times 73: 354-355

Lane B Forgay M (1981) Upgrading your oral hygiene protocol for the patient with cancer, Candian Nurse 77 (11): 27-29

Ostchega Y (1980) Preventing and treating cancer chemotherapy's oral complications, Nursing (US) 10 (8): 47-52

Sheperd J P (1978) The management of the oral complication of leukaemia, Oral Surgery 45: 543-548

Todd B (1982) Drugs and the elderly: dry mouth — causes and cures, Geriatric Nursing 3 (2): 122-123

Wallace J Freeman P A (1978) Mouth care in patients with blood dyscrasias, Nursing Times 74: 921-922

GUIDELINES: MOUTH CARE

Equipment

1   Clinically clean tray
2   Gallipots or plastic cups
3   Mouthwash or clean solutions
4   Foam sticks
5   Clean receiver or bowl
6   Paper tissues
7   Topical swabs
8   Wooden spatulae
9   Small soft toothbrush
10   Toothpaste
11   Disposable gloves
12   Denture pot

All the above items may be left on the patient's locker when appropriate and should be cleaned, renewed or replenished daily.

13   Small torch

Procedure

Action	Rationale
1 Explain the procedure to the patient.	1 To obtain the patient's consent and cooperation.
2 Wash and dry your hands.	2 To reduce the risk of cross-infection.
3 Prepare the solutions required.	3 Solutions must always be prepared immediately prior to use to maximize their efficacy and

Action	**Rationale**
	minimize the risk of microbial contamination.
4 Remove the patient's dentures if necessary, using paper tissues or topical swabs, and place them in a denture pot.	4 Removal of dentures is necessary for cleaning of underlying tissues. A tissue or topical swab provides a firmer grip of the dentures and prevents contact with patient's saliva.
5 Inspect the patient's mouth with the aid of a torch and spatula.	5 The mouth is examined for changes in condition with respect to moisture, cleanliness, infected or bleeding areas, ulcers, etc.
6 Using a small toothbrush and toothpaste, brush the patient's natural teeth, gums and tongue.	6 To remove adherent materials from the teeth, tongue and gum surfaces. Brushing stimulates gingival tissues to maintain tone and prevent circulatory stasis.
7 Brush the inner and outer aspects of the teeth with firm individual strokes directed outwards from the gums.	7 Brushing loosens and removes debris trapped on and between the teeth and gums. This reduces growth medium for pathogenic organisms and minimizes the risk of plaque formation and dental caries. Foam sticks are ineffective for this.
8 Give a beaker of water or mouthwash to the patient. Encourage him/her to rinse his/her mouth vigorously then void contents into a receiver. Paper tissues should be to hand.	8 Rinsing removes loosened debris and toothpaste and makes the mouth taste fresher. The glycerin content of toothpaste will have a drying effect if left in the mouth.
9 If the patient is unable to rinse and void, use a rinsed toothbrush to clean the teeth and moistened foam sticks to wipe the gums and oral mucosa. Foam sticks should be used with a rotating action so that most of the surface is utilized.	
10 Apply artificial saliva or lemon glycerin swabs to the tongue if appropriate and/or vaseline to dry lips.	10 To increase the patient's feeling of comfort and wellbeing.
11 Clean the patient's dentures on all surfaces with a denture brush or toothbrush. Rinse them well and return them to the patient.	11 Cleaning dentures removes accumulated food debris which could be broken down by salivary enzymes to products which irritate and cause inflammation of the

Action	Rationale
	adjacent mucosal tissue. Commercial denture cleaners, such as Steradent, may have an abrasive effect on the denture surface. This then attracts plaque and encourages bacterial growth.
12 Dentures should be soaked in chlorhexidine in spirit for 10 minutes if oral *Candida* species are present.	12 Soaking in chlorhexidine reduces the risk of reinfecting the mouth with dirty dentures.
13 Discard remaining mouthwash solutions.	13 To prevent the risk of contamination.
14 Wash and dry your hands.	14 To minimize the risk of cross-infection.

NURSING CARE PLAN

Problem	Cause	Suggested Action
1 Dry mouth	1 **a** Inadequate hydration	1 **a** Monitor the fluid balance and increase the fluid intake where necessary.
	b Impaired production of saliva, e.g. as a consequence of radiotherapy	**b** Apply artificial saliva to the tongue as required. Give the patient ice cubes to suck.
	c Presence of specific stressors, e.g. mouth breathing, oxygen therapy, no oral intake, intermittent oral suction	**c** Inspect the mouth frequently, e.g. half-hourly. Swab mucosa with water.
2 Dry lips	2 As above	2 Smear a thin layer of vaseline over the lips.
3 Thick mucus	3 **a** Postoperative closure of a tracheostomy	3 Use sodium bicarbonate solution in the mouth care procedure. Rinse the mouth afterwards with water or saline.
	b Radiotherapy **c** Poor swallowing mechanism	
4 Patient unable to tolerate toothbrush	4 Pain, e.g. postoperatively; stomatitis	4 Use foam sticks or a swab on a gloved finger to clean the patient's gums and mucosa. Saline is advisable. For severe pain use an anaesthetic mouth

Problem	Cause	Suggested Action
		spray or mouthwash prior to giving mouth care.
5 Toothbrush inappropriate or ineffective	5 **a** Infected stomatitis **b** Accumulation of dried mucus, blood or debris	5 Take a swab of any new lesions for culture prior to giving mouth care. Use a mechanical cleaning agent, e.g. hydrogen peroxide or Bocasan, for swabbing or rinsing around the mouth. Rinse with water or saline after using peroide but not after using Bocasan.
6 Patient at risk of developing systemic or widespread infection from oral invasion of pathogens	6 Immunosuppressive or neutropenic states	6 Use sterile water and/or sterile saline for mouthwashing and dilution of agents.

27

NASOGASTRIC FEEDING

Definition

Enteral feeding refers to any method of nutrient ingestion involving the gastrointestinal tract and includes oral and tube feeding. Tube feeding may include gastrostomy or jejunostomy, but more commonly nasogastric feeding. Nastogastric feeding can be a very useful method of providing a complete liquid diet to patients.

Indications

Patients to be considered are those who cannot or will not eat food in adequate amounts to meet their nutritional requirements. They may

1 Be unable to eat, e.g. following oral surgery or because of an oesophageal fistula
2 Be unable to eat adequately, e.g. because of swallowing difficulties or a painful mouth
3 Require higher than normal amounts of calories and protein.

All patients, however, must have a normal gastrointestinal anatomy or have partial digestive absorptive function of some small bowel.

REFERENCE MATERIAL

Nasogastric feeding can be a very successful method of nutrition for the patient. It is less costly and potentially less hazardous than intravenous feeding. If it is to be successfully implemented, however, it is important to understand the principles involved in administering nutrition by this method.

Types of Patient Suitable for Nasogastric Feeding

As mentioned above, it is essential that the patient has an intact gastrointestinal tract. Given this requirement, patients with the following problems are normally suitable for nasogastric feeding:

1 Compromised access to the normal gastrointestinal tract, e.g. facial and jaw injuries, carcinoma of the mouth and hypopharynx, oesophageal surgery, radiation therapy, chemotherapy
2 Functional abnormalities of the gastrointestinal tract, e.g. fistulae or short bowel syndrome
3 Metabolic abnormalities of the gastrointestinal tract, e.g. malabsorption, pancreatitis, radiation enteritis
4 Hypercatabolic states, e.g. burns, major sepsis, major trauma, surgery.

Assessment

Prior to initiation of nasogastric feeding, the patient must be assessed. This is vital for the subsequent selection of suitable equipment and type and quantity of food and will act as a base-line to monitor the patient's progress. If there is a nutritional team in the hospital, members should be involved in the assessment and in the development of any care plans.

Initial Assessment of the Patient

This should include a record of the following:

1 Age, sex, height and weight
2 Nutritional history, e.g. any recent weight loss
3 Presenting medical, surgical and psychiatric problems.

Further Assessment

The gathering of anthropometric, biochemical and immunological material should be carried out, preferably by a member of the nutritional team.

Estimation of the Patient's Protein Calorie Requirement

If nutritional team support is unavailable in the hospital, Table 27.1 is offered as a guideline for estimating a patient's protein calorie requirement.

Table 27.1 Guidelines for estimation of patients' protein calorie requirements

Type of patient	Protein (g)	Energy (kcal)
Medical (uncomplicated)	45-75	1500-2500
Surgical (uncomplicated)	75-105	2000-3500
Hypercatabolic, e.g. major surgery, burns	120-200	3000-4500

Other Requirements

It is also important to estimate the patient's electrolyte and fluid requirements and to ensure that these will be met by the feed. If long term feeding is necessary, the patient's mineral and vitamin requirements must be assessed.

Types of Nasogastric Feeds

Many different feeds have been developed over the years. These range from liquidized hospital food to commercially prepared feeds that are ready for use. The latter type are those most commonly used in hospitals in the United Kingdom. These feeds, however, must

1 Meet the nutritional requirements of the patient
2 Flow easily in the nasogastric tube
3 Be easy to prepare and sterile.

Table 27.2 lists the properties of three such feeds.

Table 27.2 The properties of three commercially prepared nasogastric feeds

	Fortison	Clinifeed ISO	Isocal
Manufacturer	Cow & Gate	Rousell	Mead Johnson
Basis of feed	Milk or soya	Milk	Soya and milk
Volume in can or Bottle	500 ml	375 ml	237 ml
per can or bottle			
calories (kcal)	500	375	251
protein (g)	20	10.5	8
carbohydrate (g)	60	49	31.5
Other properties	Low osmolarity Lactose free	Low osmolarity	Low osmolarity Lactose free
Cost of can or bottle (1983 prices)	£1.06	93p	60p
Cost per 100 calories (1983 prices)	21p	24.8p	24.0p

The fixed composition of ready for use feeds may at times limit them in conditions that require modification of a particular nutrient or electrolyte. In these instances it might be more appropriate to use a hospital-prepared feed as the composition may be altered more easily to meet the requirements of the patient.

Equipment

Tubes

A variety of nasogastric tubes are available. They vary in the material from which they are made, the internal diameter and the length. Soft plastic tubes with a narrow bore, such as Clinifeed tubes, are the most suitable as they are more comfortable than the large, stiff tubes and are less likely to cause ulceration. Silicone tubes are even softer but are expensive. PVC tubes are also recommended.

Reservoir

There are two types of reservoir available:

1 PVC bags with a capacity of 500-1500 ml
2 Rigid glass or plastic bottles.

Bags have an advantage in that they require less storage space. Among their disadvantages are that they are unsatisfactory to wash and reuse and filling the bags and reusing the calibrations may be difficult because of their flexible nature. Bottles require the use of an airway and larger storage space. They are easy to wash and reuse and calculation of fluid is more accurate. Reservoirs should be discarded after 24 hours.

Administration of the Feed

Temperature

The temperatures at which tube feeds are administered range from cold to hot. The reasons for administration at a particular temperature are various. Using cold tube feeds has been associated with diarrhoea (Gormican 1970) but Holt et al. (1964) reported no such difficulty in giving cold formula to infants. Faron (1967) found no ill effects after giving feeds from the refrigerator. A study on primates (Williams and Walike 1975) showed that cold tube feeds had only a minimal effect on gastric emptying and motility. On this basis, it is recommended that tube feeds are given at room temperature unless the patient states a preference for warmed feeds.

Rate

The feed must be given over a period of time that suits the patient. In normal subjects, forced or rapid feedings were related to an increased incidence of accelerated heart rate, nausea, gagging and regurgitation (Hanson et al. 1975). Gregg and Rees (1970) recommend that rapid adminstration is avoided to prevent distension and nausea.

Quantity

The volume of feed given will depend on the patient's daily nutrient requirements and the number of feeds given. For the average patient existing solely on a nasogastric diet, the recommended intake would be in the region of 2625 kcal per day.

Frequency

The ideal way to feed a patient by the nasogastric route would be to administer the feed continuously, thereby minimizing undesirable side effects and maximizing the absorption. This can be achieved by using a pump that regulates the flow of the feed and reduces the danger of the tube becoming blocked. Most patients, however, find 24 hour feeding too restrictive, especially if they are mobile. This method is, therefore, only employed for patients who are unable to tolerate intermittent feeding.

The frequency of intermittent feeding is usually determined by the total daily intake, duration and volume of each feed. Usually feeds are administered every 2-4 hours and the duration is normally 1-2 hours, depending on volume and the individual patient's tolerance. Some patients may prefer to have feeds during the night, especially if they cannot tolerate the entire prescribed feed during the day.

Patient Monitoring

Several complications affecting the fluid and electrolyte balance of the body and associated with tube feedings have been identified. These occur particularly in unconscious patients or in those who cannot communicate or alleviate their thirst. Hypernatraemia, uraemia and dehydration are potential complications, especially when fluid losses are increased as in the presence of diarrhoea. Day and Buckell (1977) and Ohlson (1962) advise monitoring the patient's urine solute concentration, blood urea, electrolytes and haemoglobin. Ideally, monitoring nutritional status requires measurement of 24-hour urea nitrogen excretion, weight and serum albumen. Mid upper arm circumference and triceps skinfold thickness are also a useful measure of somatic protein and fat stores, provided that these are measured accurately by one or two observers only. Nitrogen balance should be carried out to determine the efficacy of the feed. Such monitoring should be carried out by a member of the nutritional team.

Attitudes to Tube Feeding

Eating is not only a physiological necessity but also a social and emotional experience. Nasogastric feeding dramatically alters the patient's attitude to food. The nurse plays a vital role in helping patients to understand and accept this method of feeding. The nurse can make it pleasant and relaxed or it can become a distressing affair, guaranteed to destory the patient's confidence. The outcome is, therefore, dependent on the nurse's attitude and clinical knowledge.

References and Further Reading

Day S Buckell M (1977) Feeding the unconscious patient, Proceedings of the Nutrition Society 30: 184-190

Faron M F (1967) Controlling bacterial growth in tube feeding, American Journal of Nursing 67: 1246-1247

Gault H M et al. (1968) Hypernatraemia, azotaemia and dehydration due to high protein tube feeding, Annals of Internal Medicine 68: 778-791

Gormican A (1970) Prepackaged tube feedings, Hospital 44: 58-60

Gregg S H Rees O M (1970) Scientific Principles in Nursing, C V Mosby

Hanson R L (1973) Effects of administration of cold and warmed tube feedings, in Communicating Nursing Research 6, edited by M V Batey, WICHE, pp. 136-140

Hanson R L et al. (1975) Patient responses and problems associated with tube feeding, Washington State Journal of Nursing 47 (1): 9-13

Holt E et al. (1964) A study of premature infants fed cold formulas, Journal of Paediatrics 61: 556-561

Lee H A (1979) Why enteral nutrition? Research and Clinical Forums 1 (1): 15-24

Mitchell H S et al. (1968) Cooper's Nutrition in Health and Disease, 15th edition, J B Lippincott

Ohlson M (1962) Handbook of Experimental and Therapeutic Diets, Burgess

Pareina M D (1959) Therapeutic Nutrition with Tube Feeding, Charles C Thomas

Walike B C et al. (1975) Patient problems related to tube feeding, in Communicating Nursing Research 7, edited by M V Batey, WICHE, pp. 89-112

White D T et al. (1972) Fundamentals: The Foundation of Nursing, Prentice Hall

Williams K R Walike B C (1975) Effect of temperature of tube feeding on gastric motility of monkeys, Nursing Research 24: 4-9

GUIDELINES: NASOGASTRIC INTUBATION WITH CLINIFEED TUBE

Equipment

1 Clinically clean tray
2 Clinifeed tube
3 Guide wire for tube
4 Sterile receiver
5 Sterile water or normal saline
6 Hypoallergenic tape
7 Adhesive patch or Clinifeed comfort patch
8 Glass of water
9 Antiseptic solution, such as Savlodil

Procedure

Action	Rationale
1 Explain the procedure to the patient.	1 To obtain the patient's consent and cooperation.
2 Arrange a signal by which the patient can communicate if he/she wants the nurse to stop, e.g. by	2 The patient is often less frightened if he/she feels able to have some control over the procedure.

Action	**Rationale**
raising his/her hand.	
3 Assist the patient to sit in a semiupright position in the bed or chair. Support the patient's head with pillows.	3 To allow for easy passage of the tube. This position enables easy swallowing and ensures that the epiglottis is not obstructing the oesophagus.
4 Wash your hands and assemble the equipment needed. Pour normal saline into the receiver and check that the guide wire is free from kinks. Pass the wire through the normal saline and insert it into the tube as far as the plastic safety stopper will allow (see Figure 27.1).	4 Lubrication of the wire promotes easy insertion and removal of the wire from the tube. The safety stopper prevents protrusion of the wire from the tube end, a potential source of trauma to the nasopharynx and oesophagus.

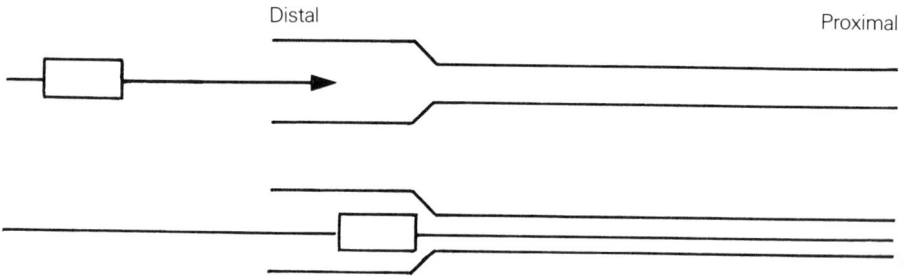

Figure 27.1 Passing a nasogastric tube

5 Check that the nostrils are patent by asking the patient to sniff with one nostril closed. Repeat with the other nostril.	5 To identify any obstructions liable to prevent intubation.
6 Insert the proximal end of the tube into the clearest nostril and slide it backwards and inwards along the floor of the nose to the nasopharynx. If any obstruction is felt, withdraw the tube and try again in a slightly different direction or use the other nostril.	6 To facilitate the passage of the tube by following the natural anatomy of the nose.
7 As the tube passes down into the nasopharynx, ask the patient to start swallowing and sipping water.	7 To focus the patient's attention on something other than the tube. A swallowing action closes the glottis, enabling the tube to pass into the oesophagus.

Action	**Rationale**
8 Advance the tube through the pharynx as the patient swallows until approximately 10-15 cm of tube remain visible.	
9 Remove the guide wire by using gentle traction. If the wire is difficult to remove, then remove the tube as well. Do not discard the wire.	9 If the wire sticks in the tube, it may be indicative that the tube is in the bronchus. After use the guide wire should be cleaned carefully with an antiseptic solution, such as Savlodil, and dried thoroughly. Each wire may be used up to a maximum of five times.
10 Secure the tube to the nostril with hypoallergenic tape and to the cheek with an adhesive patch or a Clinifeed comfort clip. Do not spigot the end of the tube.	10 To maintain the tube in place. To ensure patient comfort. Feeding via the tube must not begin until a doctor confirms the correct position of the tube by X-ray.

GUIDELINES: NASOGASTRIC INTUBATION WITH TUBES OTHER THAN CLINIFEED

Equipment

1 Clinically clean tray
2 Nasogastric tube that has been stored in a deep freeze for at least half an hour before the procedure is to begin, to ensure a rigid tube that will allow for easy passage
3 Topical gauze
4 Lubricating jelly
5 Hypoallergenic tape
6 20 ml syringe
7 Blue litmus paper
8 Receiver
9 Spigot
10 Glass of water
11 Stethoscope

Procedure

Action	**Rationale**
1 Explain the procedure to the patient.	1 To obtain the patient's consent and cooperation.
2 Arrange a signal by which the	2 The patient is often less frightened

Action	**Rationale**
patient can communicate if he/she wants the nurse to stop, e.g. by raising his/her hand.	if he/she feels able to have some control over the procedure.
3 Assist the patient to sit in a semi-upright position in the bed or chair. Support the patient's head with pillows.	3 To allow for easy passage of the tube. This position enables easy swallowing and ensures that the epiglottis is not obstructing the oesophagus.
4 Mark the distance which the tube is to be passed by measuring the distance on the tube from the patient's ear lobe to the bridge of the nose plus the distance from the bridge of the nose to the bottom of the xiphisternum. Mark this distance with tape.	4 To indicate the length of tube required for entry into the stomach.
5 Wash your hands and assemble the equipment needed.	
6 Check that the patient's nostrils are patent by asking him/her to sniff with one nostril closed. Repeat with the other nostril.	6 To identify any obstructions liable to prevent intubation.
7 Lubricate the tube for about 15-20 cm with a thin coat of lubricating jelly that has been placed on a topical swab.	7 To reduce the friction between the mucous membranes and the tube.
8 Insert the proximal end of the tube into the clearest nostril and slide it backwards and inwards along the floor of the nose to the nasopharynx. If an obstruction is felt, withdraw the tube and try again in a slightly different direction or use the other nostril.	8 To facilitate the passage of the tube by following the natural anatomy of the nose.
9 As the tube passes down into the nasopharynx, ask the patient to start swallowing and sipping water.	9 To focus the patient's attention on something other than the tube. The swallowing action closes the glottis, enabling the tube to pass into the oesophagus.
10 Advance the tube through the pharynx as the patient swallows until the tape-marked tube reaches the point of entry into the external nares. If the patient shows signs of distress, e.g. gasping or cyanosis, remove the tube immediately.	10 Distress may indicate that the tube is in the bronchus.

Action	Rationale
11 Ascertain whether the tube is in the stomach by	
a Aspirating the contents of the stomach with a syringe. The aspirate should turn blue litmus paper red.	**a** The appearance of stomach contents verifies the position of the tube.
b Placing a stethoscope over the epigastrium and injecting 2-5 ml of air into the tube.	**b** Air can be detected by a 'whooshing' sound when entering the stomach.
12 Tape the tube to the patient's nose and secure the distal end in a suitable position. Spigot the tube.	12 To maintain the tube in place. To ensure patient comfort.

GUIDELINES: ADMINISTRATION OF A NASOGASTRIC FEED

Equipment

1 Prescribed feed
2 Reservoir and airway
3 Giving set
4 Small tapered connection or Clinifeed comfort clip
5 Three-way tap, if required
6 2 and 10 ml syringes
7 Stethoscope
8 Glass of water
9 Clean jug
10 Suitable stand for holding reservoir

The reservoir and airway, giving set and connections should be kept in a tank containing a solution such as Milton by the patient's bedside.

Procedure

Action	Rationale
1 Explain the procedure to the patient.	1 To obtain the patient's consent and cooperation.
2 Wash your hands.	2 To minimize cross-infection.
3 Take the feed and necessary equipment to the patient's bedside. If the patient is capable of doing so, he/she should assist in the procedure.	3 To encourage feelings of independence.
4 Remove the reservoir from the tank and drain the fluid back into the tank. Do not rinse before use.	4 Rinsing may introduce infection and counteracts the cleansing effect of a solution such as Milton.
5 Remove the cap of the reservoir,	

Action	Rationale
and pour the prescribed feed into it.	
6　Replace the cap and insert the giving set. Close the airway. Hang the reservoir on the stand beside the patient. Run the feed through to the end of the tubing, collecting the waste from a solution such as Milton in a jug. Clamp the tubing firmly.	6　To prevent the feed escaping from the reservoir via the airway. Running the feed through the tubing removes excess solutions, such as Milton, and any air bubbles from the system and prevents them from reaching the stomach.
7　Check the position of the nasogastric tube by ascultation or aspiration. (See the procedure on non-Clinifeed intubation above.)	7　To ensure that the tube is in the stomach before feeding begins.
8　Connect the giving set to the nasogastric tube using a three-way tap, if required.	8　The three-way tap allows addition of drugs or water for flushing without having to disconnect the system.
9　Open the airway and set the flow of feed at the required rate. Pumps are commercially available for administering very slow rates of feeding.	9　The rate of feed must be regulated to meet the patient's need. If possible, the patient should control his/her own feeding rate.
10　Return periodically to check the patient's comfort and the rate of flow of the feed.	10　The rate of flow of the feed may alter suddenly, especially if the patient is not immobile.
11　On completion of a feed, disconnect the giving set from the distal end of the nasogatric tube and flush the tube with 10 ml of water.	11　To remove particles of feed likely to block the tube.
12　Wash the reservoir and the giving set in hot water and a suitable detergent. Rinse well.	12　Washing with detergent removes any feed left in the equipment. Thorough rinsing is required to prevent inactivation of solutions such as Milton by the detergent.
13　Submerge the syringes, giving set and reservoir in a solution such as Milton in a suitable tank. Leave them submerged until the next feed.	13　To sterilize this equipment. The solution and equipment should be discarded every 24 hours.

NURSING CARE PLAN

Problem	Cause	Suggested Action
1　Abdominal distension,	1　**a** Feed given too	1　**a** Reduce the rate of

Problem	Cause	Suggested Action
nausea or diarrhoea	rapidly **b** Oral antibiotics	feed. **b** Administer any medication prescribed for nausea or diarrhoea.
	c Malabsorption due to enzyme depletion, villous atrophy following periods of starvation or inadequate nutrition	**c** Dilute the feed and decrease the rate of feed. Inform the nutritional team.
	d Hyperosmolar feeds	**d** As for **c** above.
	e Lactose intolerance, especially in patients of African and Asian origin or severely debilitated patients	**e** Use a lactose-free feed, e.g. Fortisan or Isocal.
	f Contaminated feed and/or equipment	**f** Obtain a stool for bacteriological investigation. Take swabs from the equipment and any solutions used.
2 Weight gain is unsatisfactory and/or urea output high	2 Inadequate nutrition for patient's needs.	2 Inform the nutritional team.
3 Dehydration		3 Offer fluids. Inform the nutritional team.

APPENDIX: SUGGESTED MANAGEMENT OF A NASOGASTRIC FEEDING REGIME

	Action	Rationale
Starting the regime This will vary depending on the following: 1 Nutritional requirements of patient 2 Condition of the patient, e.g. has the patient been starved prior to starting the regime? 3 Type of feed being used.	Gradual build up, over 4 5 days, of volume and rate of feed to meet nutritional requirements.	Building up of the regime allows the gastrointestinal tract to adjust to a liquid diet, thus reducing the risk of intolerance.
Timing of feed	Four or five feeds daily. Timing determined by convenience to patient and staff.	Patients seem to prefer intermittent feeds given throughout the day. It is believed that intermittent feeding

Action	**Rationale**
Continuous feeding on a slow drip rate.	allows normal hormonal change associated with regular meals to take place. Patients find this restrictive, but it has the advantage of allowing a large volume of feed to be dripped in slowly over a long period of time; thus giving a high level of nutrition to those who cannot tolerate feed given at normal rates.

Duration of feed

Depends on volume of feed required and drip rate used.	The number of feeds and the drip rate should be decided in the light of patient requirements, condition and personal preference. Too rapid an administration may lead to nausea, distention and diarrhoea.

Monitoring the patient

1 Fluid balance	Measure daily input and output.	To monitor state of hydration.
2 Weight	Weigh twice weekly (in same clothing and at same time of day) using sitting scales.	To monitor weight changes which may be associated with a tube-feeding regimen.
3 Urine	Daily urine analysis for glucose during first week of feeding. If glucose is detected, check the urine throughout the whole period of tube feeding. An hour after the 6 p.m. feed has finished is the best time for this. Ask the patient to empty his/her bladder prior to commencing the feed.	To ensure that the urine glucose level relates to the feed just given.
4 Bowels	Check daily, by observation or by asking the patient, about the frequency	To detect and combat diarrhoea or constipation related to tube feeding.

		Action	**Rationale**
		and nature of stools.	
5	Haematological investigations	Test for urea and electrolytes and glucose levels once or twice weekly.	To monitor the patient's state of hydration. Nitrogen balance may be of value in some patients.
6	General condition	Observe daily for thirst, lethargy, glycosuria and polyuria — all symptoms of dehydration.	To prevent the complication of end state dehydration.

28

NEUROLOGICAL OBSERVATIONS

Definition

Neurological observations relate to the evaluation of the integrity of an individual's nervous system by obtaining specific information about it.

Indications

Neurological observations are required to monitor and evaluate changes in the nervous system by indicating trends, thus aiding diagnosis and treatment, which in turn may affect prognosis and rehabilitation.

REFERENCE MATERIAL

The main emphasis is on assessing five critical areas:

1 Level of consciousness
2 Pupillary activity
3 Motor function
4 Sensory function
5 Vital signs.

Level of Consciousness

Level of consciousness is the single most important indicator of a patient's brain function. It ranges from alert wakefulness to deep coma with no apparent responsiveness. Categories of impaired consciousness, in order of deteriorating condition, include the following:

1   *Full consciousness*   The patient is fully aware of his/her surroundings and is orientated to time, place and person. The patient responds appropriately to auditory, visual and somatosensory stimuli.
2   *Lethargy*   The patient is inactive and indifferent. The patient responds slowly or incompletely to stimuli. Although capable of verbal responses, the

patient may ignore some stimuli completely.

3   *Obtundation*   The patient is very drowsy and indifferent, although capable of remaining awake.

4   *Confusion and delirium*   Thinking and behaviour aberrations occur due to cortex dysfunction. The confused patient is disorientated and appears dazed. The delirious patient is uncooperative and easily agitated.

5   *Stupor*   The patient can be aroused only by painful stimuli.

6   *Coma*   Response to painful stimuli may be rudimentary or absent.

Specific diseases and injuries can impair level of consciousness since they depress or destroy the brainstem's reticular activating mechanism or the conduction pathways leading to and from the cerebral cortex.

Assessment of level of consciousness involves two phases:

1   Evaluation of verbal responses
2   Evaluation of motor responses.

Changes in blood pressure and pulse normally occur late, after the patient's level of consciousness has begun to deteriorate. Call for medical assistance at the first sign of neurological deterioration.

Verbal Responses   Assess the ability of the patient to respond verbally and note any evidence of disorientation as to time, place and person. Note also the clarity with which the patient responds.

Motor Responses   In the first instance these should be elicited by noting whether the patient responds to simple verbal commands, e.g. 'Open your eyes', 'Squeeze and release my fingers'. Test both sides of the patient's body.

Painful Stimuli   Painful stimuli should only be employed if the patient does not respond to commands. Use the least amount of pressure to elicit a response. Suggested methods will be found in the guidelines below. As the ability to localize pain is lost, various responses may be observed when painful stimuli are applied:

1   *Decorticate posturing*   One or both arms are in full flexion on the chest. The legs may be stiffly extended.

2   *Decerebrate posturing*   One or both arms are stiffly extended. There is possible extension of the legs. The head may also be arched backwards.

3   *Flaccid*   No motor response is observed in any extremity.

Pupillary Activity

Pupillary constriction and dilatation are controlled by the third cranial nerve (oculomotor). Any changes may indicate third cranial nerve involvement and/or brainstem damage. (Note that pupillary changes may also be the result of drug treatment or trauma to the eye.)

Assessment of the pupils must include an evaluation of size, shape, whether or not they are equal and their reaction to light.

Motor Function

Damage to any part of the motor nervous system can affect the ability to move. Motor function assessment involves evaluation of the following:

1 Muscle strength
2 Muscle tone
3 Posture
4 Muscle coordination
5 Reflexes
6 Abnormal movements.

Muscle Strength

This involves testing the patient's muscle strength against one's own muscle resistance and then against the pull of gravity.

Muscle Tone

This involves flexing and extending the patient's limbs on both sides and noting how well such movements are resisted. Increased resistance would denote increased muscle tone and vice versa.

Posture

The posture of a patient is frequently an ominous sign and may occur spontaneously or in response to painful stimuli. Some such postures have been outlined above.

Coordination

Any disease or injury that involves the cerebellum or basal ganglia will affect coordination. Assessment of hand and arm and leg coordination can be achieved by testing the rapidity and rhythm of alternating movements and of point to point movements. Such tests are outlined in the procedural guidelines below.

Reflexes

Among the four most important reflexes are the following: blink, gag and swallow, plantar and oculocephalic, the last-mentioned being a reflect ocular movement that occurs only in patients with a severely decreased level of consciousness. When the reflex is present the patient's eyes will move in the opposite direction from the side to which his/her head is turned. If the reflex is impaired, the eyes may not move at all or only one eye may move. Blink and gag and swallow are protective reflexes. Fifth and seventh cranial nerve involvement will affect the blink reflex. Ninth and tenth cranial nerve involvement may affect the gag reflex. Plantar and oculocephalic reflexes help to determine the site of a lesion.

Abnormal Movements

When carrying out neurological observations any abnormal movements, e.g. seizures and tremors, must be noted.

Sensory Function

Constant sensory input enables an individual to alter his/her responses and behaviour to suit his/her environment. When disease or injury damages the sensory pathways, the sensory responses are always affected. Any assessment of sensory function should include evaluation of the following:

1   Central and peripheral vision
2   Hearing and ability to understand verbal communication
3   Superficial sensations (light, touch, pain) and deep sensations (muscles and joint pain, muscle and joint position).

Vital Signs

It is recommended that assessments of vital signs should be made in the following order:

1   Respirations
2   Temperature
3   Blood pressure
4   Pulse.

Respirations

Of these four vital signs, respiratory patterns give the clearest indication of how the brain is functioning since respirations are controlled by different areas of the brain. Any disease or injury that affects these areas may produce respiratory changes. The rate, quality and pattern of a patient's respirations must be noted. Abnormal respiratory patterns are listed in Table 28.1

Temperature

Damage to the hypothalamus, the temperature regulating centre, may result in grossly fluctuating temperatures.

Blood Pressure and Pulse

Observations of blood pressure and pulse will provide evidence of increased intracranial pressure. Hypertension together with bradycardia need to be monitored closely. Abnormalities of blood pressure and pulse usually occur late, after the patient's level of consciousness has begun to deteriorate.

Table 28.1 Abnormal respiration patterns

Type	Pattern	Significance
Cheyne — Stokes	Rhythmic waxing and waning of both rate and depth of respirations, alternating regularly with briefer periods of apnoea	May indicate deep cerebral or cerebellar lesions, usually bilateral. May occur with upper brainstem involvement.
Central neurogenic hyperventilation	Sustained, regular, rapid respirations, with forced inspiration and expiration	May indicate a lesion of the low midbrain, or upper pons areas of the brainstem.
Apnoeustic	Prolonged inspiratory cramp with a pause at full inspiration. There may also be expiratory pauses.	May indicate a lesion of the of the low pons or upper medulla.
Cluster breathing	Clusters of irregular respirations alternating with longer periods of apnoea	May indicate a lesion of low pons or upper medulla.
Ataxic breathing	A completely irregular pattern with random deep and shallow respirations. Irregular pauses may also appear.	May indicate a lesion of the medulla.

Recording Observations

There is no universally accepted method for recording nursing neurological observations. The Glasgow Coma Scale attempts to assess the integrity of the central nervous system on the basis of behavioural responses that denote the patient's motor activity, verbal performance and eye-opening ability. Useful summaries of this scale may be found in Abelson (1982) and Jones (1979).

References

Abelson M M (1982) Observations of the neurosurgical patient, Curationis 5 (3): 27-32

Erickson R (1980) Neurological checkpoints, in Assessing Vital Functions Accurately, Intermed Communications, pp. 131-142

Jones C (1979) Glasgow Coma Scale, American Journal of Nursing 79 (9): 1551-1553

Ricci M M (1979) Neurological assessment: keeping it ongoing, in Coping with Neurological Problems Proficiently, Intermed Communications, pp. 30-49

GUIDELINES: NEUROLOGICAL OBSERVATIONS

Equipment

1 Pencil torch
2 Thermometer
3 Sphygmomanometer
4 Tongue depressor
5 Cotton wool balls
6 Patella hammer
7 Safety pin
8 Two test tubes

Procedure

Action	Rationale
1 Inform the patient, whether conscious or not, and explain the observations.	1 **a** Sense of hearing is frequently unimpaired even in unconscious patients. **b** To ensure, as far as is possible, that the patient consents to and understand the procedure.
2 Talk to the patient. Note whether he/she is alert and is giving full attention or whether he/she is restless or lethargic and drowsy. Ask the patient who he/she is, the correct day, month and year, where he/she is, and to give details about his/her family.	2 To establish whether the patient's level of consciousness is deteriorating. If the patient is becoming disorientated, changes will occur in this order: **a** Disorientation as to time **b** Disorientation as to place **c** Disorientation as to person.
3 Ask the patient to squeeze and release your fingers and then to stick out his/her tongue. (Include both sides of the body.)	3 To evaluate motor responses.
4 If the patient does not respond, apply painful stimuli. Suggested methods are as follows: **a** Exerting pressure on the patient's fingernail bed with a pen or pencil **b** Applying pressure to the ridge under the eyebrow (the supraorbital notch).	4 Responses grow less purposeful as the patient's level of consciousness deteriorates. As the condition worsens, the patient may no longer localize pain and respond to it in a purposeful way.
5 Record, precisely, the findings.	5 Vague terms, e.g. semicomatose,

Action	**Rationale**
Write exactly what stimulus was used, where it was applied, how much pressure was needed to elicit a response, and how the patient responded.	are too vague and can be easily misinterpreted.
6 Hold the eyelids open and note the size, shape and equality of the pupils.	6 To assess the size, shape and equality of the pupils as an indication of brain damage. Normal pupils are spherical, usually at mid-position and have a diameter ranging from 1.5 to 6 mm.
7 Darken the room.	7 To enable a better view of the eye.
8 Hold each eyelid open in turn. Move a pupil torch towards the patient from the side. Shine it directly into the eye. This should cause the pupil to constrict promptly.	8 To assess the reaction of the pupils to light. Indicates no lesions in the area of the brain stem regulating pupil constriction.
9 Hold both eyelids open but shine the light into one eye only. The eye into which the light is not shone should also constrict.	9 To assess consensual light reflex. Prompt constriction indicates intact connections between the brainstem areas regulating pupil constriction.
10 Record unusual eye movements.	10 To assess cranial nerve damage.
11 Extend your hands and ask the patient to squeeze your fingers as hard as possible. Compare grip and strength.	11 To test grip.
12 Ask the patient to close his/her eyes and hold his/her arms straight out in front of him/her, with palms upwards, for 20-30 seconds.	12 To test arm strength. If one arm drifts downwards or turns inwards, it may indicate hemiparesis.
a Stand in front of the patient and extend your hands. Ask the patient to push and pull against your hands.	To test flexion and extension strength in the patient's extremities by having him/her push and pull against your resistance.
b Ask the patient to lie on his/her back in bed. Place the patient's leg with knee flexed and foot resting on the bed. Instruct the patient to keep his/her foot down as you attempt to extend his/her leg. Flex the knee and place your hand in the flexion. Instruct the patient to straighten his/her leg while you offer resistance.	

Note: If a patient cannot follow the instruction due to a language barrier or unconsciousness, observe spontaneous movements and note how strong they appear. Then, if necessary, apply painful stimuli.

Action	**Rationale**
13 Flex and extend all the patient's limbs. Note how well he/she resists the movements.	13 To test muscle tone.
14 Ask the patient to pat his/her thigh as fast as possible. Note whether the movements seem slow or clumsy. Ask the patient to turn his/her hand over and back several times in succession. Evaluate his/her coordination. Ask the patient to touch the back of his/her fingers with his/her thumb in sequence rapidly.	14 To assess hand and arm co-ordination. The dominant hand should perform better.
15 Extend one of your hands towards the patient. Ask the patient to touch your index finger, then his/her nose, several times in succession. Repeat the test with the patient's eyes closed.	
16 Ask the patient to place a heel on his/her opposite knee and slide it down his/her shin to his/her foot. Check each leg separately.	16 To assess leg coordination.
17 Ask the patient to look up or hold his/her eyelid open. With your hand, approach his/her eye unexpectedly or brush his/her eye-lashes.	17 To test the blink reflex.
18 Ask the patient to open his/her mouth and hold down his/her tongue with a tongue depressor. Touch the back of the pharynx, on each side, with a cotton wool swab.	18 To test the gag reflex.
19 Ask the patient to lie on his/her back in bed. Place your hand under his/her knee. Raise and flex it. Tap the patellar tendon. Note whether the leg responds.	19 To assess the deep tendon reflex.
20 Stroke the lateral aspect of the sole of the patient's foot. If the response	20 To assess for upper motor neurone lesion.

Action	**Rationale**
is abnormal (Babinski response), the big toe will dorsiflex and the remaining toes will fan out.	
21 Ask the patient to read something aloud. Check each eye separately. If vision is so poor that the patient is unable to read, ask the patient to count your upraised fingers or distinguish light from dark.	21 To test the visual activity.
22 Occlude the ear with a cotton wool swab. Stand a short way from the patient. Whisper numbers into the open ear. Ask for feedback. Repeat for both ears.	22 To test aural activity and comprehension.
23 Ask the patient to close his/her eyes. Using the point of an open safety pin, stroke his/her skin. Use the blunt end occasionally. Ask him/her to tell you what he/she feels. See if the patient can distinguish between sharp and dull sensations.	23 To test superficial sensations to pain.
24 Ask the patient to close his/her eyes. Fill two test tubes with water: one warm, one cold. Touch the patient's skin with each test tube and ask him/her to distinguish between them.	24 To test superficial sensations to temperature.
25 Stroke a cotton wool swab lightly over the patient's skin. Ask the patient to tell you what he/she feels.	25 To test superficial sensations to touch.
26 Ask the patient to close his/her eyes. Hold the tip of one of the patient's fingers between your thumb and index finger. Move it up and down and ask the patient to say in which direction it is moving. Repeat with the other hand. For the legs, hold the big toe.	26 To test proprioception.
27 Note the rate, quality and pattern of the patient's respirations.	27 Respirations are controlled by different areas of the brain. When disease or injury affects these areas, respiratory changes may occur.
28 Take and record the patient's temperature at specified intervals.	28 Damage to the hypothalamus, the temperature regulating centre in the brain, will be reflected in grossly abnormal temperatures.

Action	**Rationale**
28 Take and record the patient's blood pressure and pulse at specified intervals.	29 To monitor signs of increased intracranial pressure. Hypertension and bradycardia usually occur late, after the patient's level of consciousness has begun to deteriorate. Call for medical assistance as soon as it is evident that there is a deterioration in the patient's level of consciousness.

NURSING CARE PLAN

Category	**Frequency**	**Rationale**
1 All patients diagnosed as suffering from neurological or neurosurgical conditions	1 At least 4-hourly. Frequency is affected by the patient's condition.	1 To monitor the condition of the patient so that any necessary action can be instigated.
2 Unconscious patients (including ventilated and anaesthetized patients)	2 At least half-hourly; quarter-hourly if the condition is critical.	2 To monitor the condition closely and to detect trends so that appropriate action may be taken.

Chapter 29

OXYGEN THERAPY

Definition

Oxygen therapy is the provision of an atmosphere of increased oxygenation and humidity by the use of specialized equipment.

Indications

The absolute indication for supplementary inspired oxygen is inadequate tissue oxygenation. Clinical signs such as cyanosis are imprecise and misleading. The only accurate assessment of respiratory failure is the measurement of blood gases and pH. Oxygen therapy is generally indicated in the following cases:

1 Acute lower respiratory infections
2 Acute pulmonary oedema
3 Asthma
4 Carbon monoxide poisoning
5 Long term therapy in chronic obstructive pulmonary disease. *(The Lancet (1981)* has a useful reappraisal of the acute use of oxygen therapy in this instance.)

REFERENCE MATERIAL

The modern concept of oxygen therapy began during World War I, when it was used to treat soldiers suffering from respiratory failure due to exposure to poisonous gas.

Physiology

The amount of oxygen entering the blood from the lungs depends, among other things, on its pressure in the alveoli. In turn, this depends on the percentage of oxygen in the alveoli and on the atmospheric pressure. There is approximately 21% oxygen in inspired air and at sea level the pressure is about 150 mm Hg (20 kPa), whereas in the alveoli it is about 100 mm Hg (13.3 kPa). If the atmospheric pressure is reduced, the oxygen pressure in the alveoli will be reduced. Oxygen diffuses through the alveolar membrane and capillary wall, dissolves in the blood plasma and combines with haemoglobin in the red cells to form oxyhaemoglobin. The oxygen is transported from the pulmonary capillaries through the arterial system to the tissues. The amount of oxygen combined with haemoglobin varies — the oxyhaemoglobin dissociation curve. At a pO_2 of 100 mm Hg blood is 97% saturated. At lower pressures, e.g. 80 mm Hg, the saturation has scarcely altered. Between 0 and 40 mm Hg, the saturation falls rapidly. This mechanism provides a safety margin in the early stages of a fall in arterial pO_2 caused by disease, but where pO_2 is initially low, as in chronic pulmonary disease, a further fall could cause a dangerous drop in arterial pO_2. Among the causes of a low arterial pO_2 are the following:

1 *Ventilatory failure* When an inadequate volume of air is breathed in a given time.
2 *Impairment of diffusion/gas transfer*
3 *Ventilation perfusion imbalance* Some alveoli receive insufficient oxygen and carbon dioxide from the air and blood respectively, with the result that the blood entering the arteries from these alveoli contains too much carbon dioxide and too little oxygen.
4 *Shunting of blood* The passage of blood from the right side of the heart to the left without an opportunity for exchange of gases in the alveoli.
5 *Carbon dioxide narcosis* In patients with chronic respiratory diseases much of the respiratory centre's stimulus comes from lack of oxygen. If hypoxia is relieved by administering oxygen, the main stimulus to breathing is lost. The patient hypoventilates and the pCO_2 rises to anything from 80 to 100 mm Hg. This has a toxic effect on the brain resulting in stupor or coma.

General Considerations

1 Oxygen is an odourless, tasteless, colourless, transparent gas that is slightly heavier than air.
2 Oxygen supports combustion, so there is always a danger of fire when oxygen is being used. It is necessary, therefore, to
 a Avoid using oil or grease around oxygen connections
 b Eliminate antiseptic tinctures, alcohol and ether in the immediate oxygen environment
 c Prohibit the use of any electrical device in or near an oxygen tent
 d Keep any oxygen cylinders secured in an upright position away from heat
 e Place a NO SMOKING sign on the patient's door and in view of other patients and the patient's visitors
 f Have fire extinguishers available.
3 Oxygen is dispensed from a cylinder or piped system and requires
 a A reduction gauge to reduce the pressure to that of the atmosphere
 b A flow meter to regulate the control of oxygen in litres per minute.

4   Oxygen is given to relieve hypoxia, either locally or generalized.

Hypoxia is a state in which there is an insufficient amount of oxygen available in the tissue cells to meet the requirements of an organ or tissue at that moment. The aim of oxygen administration is to treat the hypoxia while decreasing the work of breathing and stress on the myocardium.

Supply of Oxygen

The British Oxygen Company (BOC) has a monopoly in the supply of 100% oxygen in the United Kingdom. It is available in compressed form in cylinders and as liquid oxygen. In hospitals it is available to the patient either piped from a central supply or direct from a cylinder by the patient's bedside. There are six cylinder capacities. The most popular sizes for hospital use are G and F. G is for static use at the bedside. At a flow rate of 4 litres per minute, this cylinder will empty in about 14 hours. F is used on wheeled stands for mobility and is convenient for emergency use. Oxygen cylinders are black with white shoulders and upper part. They are marked with the symbol O_2 and/or the word OXYGEN.

Oxygen Giving Sets

The equipment used to convey oxygen from the cylinder head or pipeline to the patient consists of a pressure gauge, regulator (optional), flow meter, tubing, mask or nasal cannulae and humidifier, if required. The pressure gauge indicates how much gas is in the cylinder and the regulator is used to reduce gas pressure in tubing and equipment distally to 60 lbf/in² (414 kPa). A regulator also ensures a steady flow rate until the cylinder is nearly empty. The flow meter indicates the oxygen flow rate in litres per minute. The majority of regulators are light bobbins or spheres that ride up and down in the bore of a transparent vertical graduated tube. As the tube is tapered and wider above, the bobbin rises to a level corresponding to the flow rate.

Methods of Administration

Venturi Masks

In Venturi masks, e.g. the Mixomask (Figure 29.1) and the Venti Mask (Figure 29.2), oxygen is blown under pressure into the mask at a given flow rate, indicated by the flow meter. Oxygen is forced through a small hole in the nozzle and comes out at high speed. This high speed jet sucks in surrounding air that travels along the wide tube towards the face mask. Provided that this type of mask is fed with oxygen at the required flow rate, only the stated percentage of oxygen will be available for the patient to breathe.

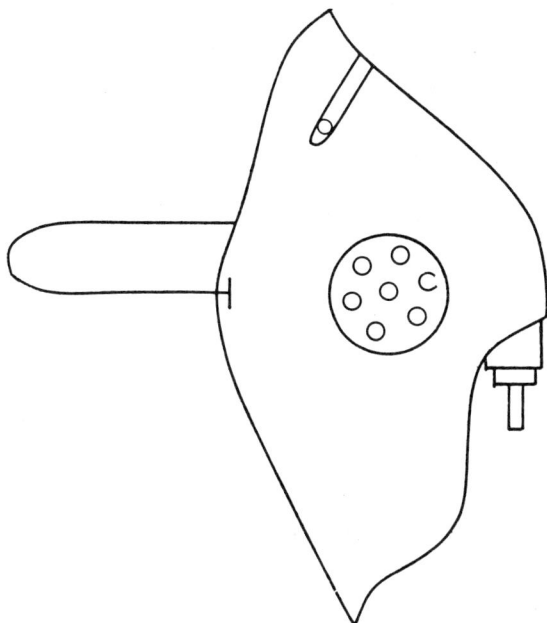

Figure 29.1 Mixomask

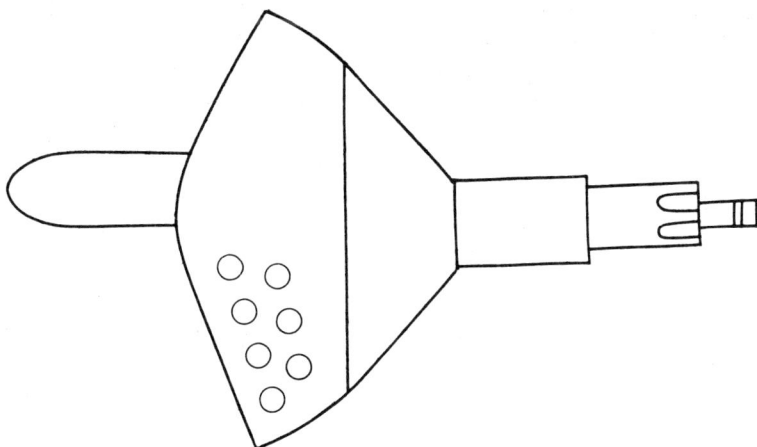

Figure 29.2 Ventimask

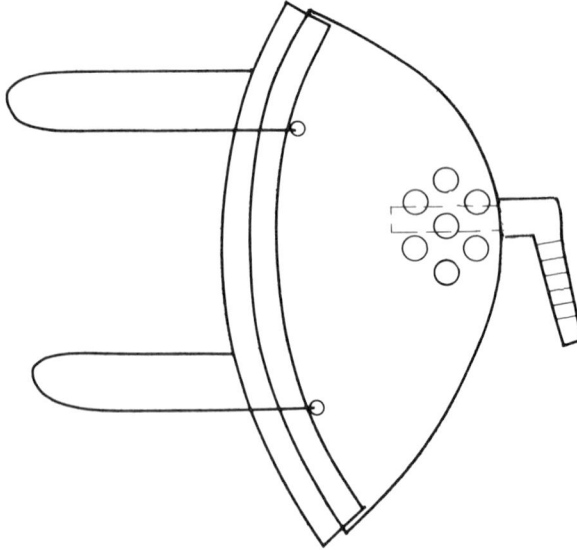

Figure 29.3   MC mask

MC Masks

Masks of this type (Figure 29.3) may be used when high concentrations of oxygen are required but when the actual percentage is not critical. Oxygen concentrations vary from 24 to 81% depending on the flow rate (1-10 litres per minute) and tidal volume. The mask consists of a soft plastic facepiece with a large central bore tube connected directly to the oxygen supply. Vent holes are provided to allow clearance of expired air and escape of unused high pressure gas. If a patient breathes at an inspiration rate of 10 litres per minute and 100% oxygen is being supplied at a rate of 2 litres per minute, then the inspired mixture comprises 8 litres of air containing 21% oxygen and 2 litres of 100% oxygen. Thus 20% of the inspired gas is pure oxygen and the remaining 80% already contains 21% oxygen. After mixing, the patient will be receiving

$$\left[\frac{80}{100} \times 21 \right] + 20 = 16.8 + 20 = 36.8\% \text{ oxygen.}$$

This demonstrates that the actual percentage delivered will not be obvious simply by regarding the flow meter on the supply. If the patient's inspiration rate alters, the delivered percentage of oxygen will also change.

Nasal Cannulae

Nasal cannulae consist of a pair of tubes about 2 cm long, each projecting into the nostril and stemming from a tube which encircles the head and which is thus self-retaining (see Figure 29.4). Oxygen is delivered in a similar way as when given via an MC mask. Cannulae have the advantage of not interfering with feeding and are not as inconvenient as masks during coughing and sneezing. Oxygen needs to be humidified if cannulae are used, as dry gas impinges directly on the nasal mucosa, which may become damaged.

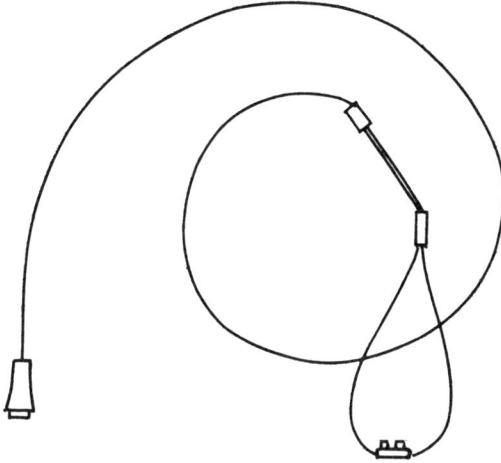

Figure 29.4 Nasal cannulae

Ambu Bag

An Ambu bag is a self-inflating rubber bag, one end of which is fitted with a one-way air valve and gas supply tube, while the other end is connected directly to a sterile tube in the trachea or to a face mask. This bag is usually used during cardiopulmonary resuscitation procedures when oxygen is fed into the supply tube. The percentage of oxygen delivered into the trachea will depend on the rate of pumping of the bag, the bag volume and also the flow rate of oxygen from the supply.

Mechanical Ventilation

Here the amount of oxygen delivered is directly controlled by a ventilator. Ventilators vary in their methods of oxygen delivery, but the same basic principles apply as in the above-mentioned types. The input oxygen is mixed with a quantity of air drawn in before or during each respiratory phase, the total volume then being delivered into the trachea.

Oxygen Tent

Oxygen tents have almost entirely been superceded in the treatment of adults by masks and cannulae (Freedman 1978). However, they are still useful when oxygen needs to be administered to restless and confused patients and children.

Hyperbaric Oxygen Therapy

Hyperbaric oxygen therapy is the administration of 100% oxygen at greater than normal atmospheric pressure. It is administered in a hyperbaric chamber. It can be used effectively in the primary treatment of acute carbon monoxide poisoning, acute gas embolism and decompression sickness. It is used as adjunctive treatment for compromised skin grafts, gas gangrene, acute cyanide poisoning and ulcers caused by microaerophilic streptococci. Evidence is also accumulating to support its use in the treatment of osteomyelitis, osteo-adiponecrosis and soft tissue injury. It may be used to administer high concentrations of oxygen systemically or locally, to promote neovascularization and to produce vasoconstriction with subsequent reduction in oedema. Increasing oxygen concentration to 100% is one method of increasing arterial oxygen content. Further increases may be achieved by increasing barometric pressure. The greater the pressure at which a gas is administered, the denser the gas and the greater the number of molecules of gas that can be delivered for a set volume. With hyperbaric oxygenation, sufficient oxygen can be dissolved in the plasma to maintain life. Applied topically, oxygen acts to increase superficial oxygen tension sufficiently to prevent tissue death from anoxia and inhibit the growth of superfical aerobic organisms.

Two types of chambers are commonly in use:

1 *Monoplace chambers* The patient is placed in an individual capsule with a transparent canopy.
2 *Multiplace chambers* A large, airtight chamber constructed to accommodate either an operating team and/or a multiplicity of patients.

Treatments are carried out over a period of days or weeks.

Humidification

Oxygen supplied from cylinders or piped sources is dry. It has a potential, therefore, for drying mucuous membranes of the air passages. Ambient air, which mixes with the oxygen during inspiration, contains enough water vapour to prevent drying of the air passages in most circumstances. Humidification is essential when oxygen is administered via a tracheostomy and desirable when nasal cannulae are used. (For further information, see the procedure on humidification, p. 191.)

References

Bolton M E (1981) Hyperbaric oxygen therapy, American Journal of Nursing 81: 1199-1201

Coady T J Bennett A (1978) Technology in nursing. Respiratory function 1. Oxygen administration, Nursing Times 74: Scann 1-4

Freedman B J (1978) Oxygen therapy in hospital practice. The indications for oxygen therapy and its safe application, Nursing Times 74: 2072-2076

Lancet (1981) Acute oxygen therapy, Lancet i: 980-981
Scottish Health Services Council Standing Medical Advisory Committee (1969) Uses and Dangers of Oxygen Therapy: Report of a Subcommittee, HMSO

GUIDELINES: ADMINISTRATION OF OXYGEN BY VENTURI MASK

Equipment

1 Oxygen source
2 Mask
3 Flow meter
4 Connecting tubing
5 'No Smoking' sign

Procedure

Action	Rationale
1 Place the NO SMOKING sign on the patient's door and in view of other patients and visitors.	1 Oxygen supports combustion.
2 Explain the procedure to the patient.	2 To obtain the patient's consent and cooperation.
3 Connect the mask, disposable tubing and flow meter to the oxygen.	3 To ensure that equipment functions as intended.
4 Turn on the oxygen.	4 To check that oxygen is flowing out of the vent holes in the flexible face mask.
5 Place the Venturi mask over the patient's nose and mouth and under his/her chin. Mould the mask to fit the patient's face (Figure 29.5).	5 To ensure that oxygen is delivered as prescribed. A correctly fitting mask is more comfortable.
6 Adjust the elastic strap around the patient's head and position the strap below the ears and around the neck.	6 Prevents leakage of oxygen. If oxygen leaks into the patient's eyes it causes extreme distress.
7 If high humidity is used, attach large bore tubing to a nebulizer and connect it to the fitting for high humidity at the base of the Venturi mask.	
8 Assess the patient's condition at frequent intervals.	
9 Change the mask and tubing daily.	9 Contaminated equipment may cause virulent infections in debilitated patients.

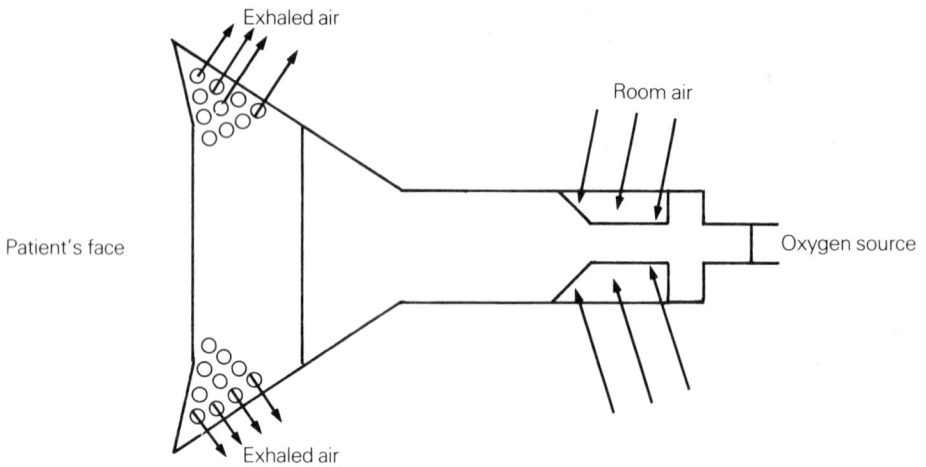

Figure 29.5   Administration of oxygen via a Venturi mask

GUIDELINES: ADMINISTRATION OF OXYGEN BY MC MASK

Equipment

1   Oxygen source
2   Mask
3   Large bore connection tubing
4   Flow meter
5   'No Smoking' sign

Procedure

Action	Rationale
1 Place the NO SMOKING sign on the patient's door and in view of other patients and visitors.	1 Oxygen supports combustion.
2 Explain the procedure to the patient.	2 To obtain the patient's consent and cooperation.
3 Attach the large bore tubing to the mask and oxygen flow meter. Set the oxygen flow at the desired level.	3 To ensure that oxygen will be delivered as prescribed.
4 Place the mask to the patient's face and adjust the straps so that the mask fits securely and there are no leaks.	4 If the mask is comfortable, the patient is more likely to tolerate it.
5 Change the mask and tubing daily.	5 Contaminated equipment may cause virulent infections in debilitated patients.

GUIDELINES: ADMINISTRATION OF OXYGEN BY NASAL CANNULAE

Equipment

1 Oxygen source
2 Plastic nasal cannulae
3 Disposable connecting tubing
4 Humidifier filled with sterile distilled water to indicated level
5 Flow meter
6 'No Smoking' sign

Procedure

Action	Rationale
1 Place the NO SMOKING sign on the patient's door in view of other patients and visitors.	1 Oxygen supports combustion.
2 Show the patient the nasal cannulae and explain the procedure.	2 To obtain the patient's consent and cooperation.
3 Prepare the nasal cannulae, connecting tubing, humidifier and flow meter to the oxygen source.	3 To ensure that oxygen is administered as prescribed.
4 Turn on the oxygen.	4 To determine whether oxygen is flowing through the nasal tips of the cannulae.
5 Turn off the oxygen.	5 Usually the patient accepts cannulae better if they are fitted with the oxygen turned off.
6 Position the tips of the cannulae in the patient's nose so that the tips do not extend more than 2.5 cm into the nares.	6 Over-long tubing is uncomfortable, which may make the patient reject the procedure. Sore nasal mucosa can result from pressure or friction of tubing that is too long.
7 Adjust the oxygen flow to the prescribed rate.	7 Inadequate flow rates may result in administration of an inaccurate oxygen concentration to the patient.
8 Fasten tubing securely.	8 Correctly secured tubing is comfortable and prevents displacement of cannulae.
9 Assess the patient's condition and the functioning of the equipment at regular intervals.	9 To ensure that oxygen is being administered as prescribed.
10 Change cannulae and humidifier tubing daily.	10 Contaminated equipment may cause virulent infections in debilitated patients.

NURSING CARE PLAN

Oxygen Delivery by Face Mask

Problem	Cause	Suggested Action
1 Noise	1 The constant oxygen flow, particularly if a nebulizer is incorporated in the system, can be irritating	1 Give further explanation to the patient.
2 Difficulty in talking	2 Mask restricts talking	2 Conversation should be reduced to a minimum. A paper and pencil will prove useful.
3 Difficulty in eating and drinking	3 Impossible to eat or drink with mask in position	3 Highly nourishing soft foods should be offered, which reduces the time the mask is not in position.
4 Feeling of claustrophobia	4 Tight fitting mask	4 Refit the mask.
5 Dry, sore mouth	5 Insufficient fluid intake; oxygen has a drying effect	5 Offer oral toilet frequently. Encourage the patient to take fluids.

Oxygen Delivery by Nasal Cannulae

Problem	Cause	Suggested Action
1 Humidifier water overflowing into gauge	1 Overfilled humidifier	1 Only fill the humidifier to the required level.
2 Air swallowing	2 Excessive flow of oxygen	2 Reduce the rate of oxygen delivery.
3 Irritation of nasal and pharyngeal mucosa	3 Excessive flow of oxygen	3 Reduce the rate of oxygen delivery.
4 Changes in patient's mental state, disturbed consciousness, abnormal colour of perspiration	4 Excessive or inadequate flow of oxygen	4 Check that the equipment and the rate of flow of oxygen are satisfactory.
5 Changes in blood pressure increasing heart and respiratory rates		5 Seek medical advice.

30

PERITONEAL DIALYSIS

Definition
Peritoneal dialysis is a procedure used for patients with inadequate renal function to rid the body of waste products, such as urea, using the peritoneum as a dialysing membrane.

Indications
Peritoneal dialysis is indicated for the following:

1 To aid in the removal of toxic substances and metabolic waste
2 To assist in regulating fluid and electrolyte balance
3 To remove excessive body fluid
4 To control blood pressure.

The use of peritoneal dialysis in chronic renal failure is now regarded as controversial (*Lancet* 1978).

REFERENCE MATERIAL
In 1926 Rosenak, basing his work on that of Ganter, conceived the possibility of using the peritoneum of humans as a dialysing membrane. The use of peritoneal dialysis reached a peak in 1959 with the introduction of commercial dialysis solutions and tubing. With the advent of haemodialysis, however, in the 1960s, peritoneal dialysis assumed a secondary role as a form of treatment for chronic renal failure. In recent years, due to improvements in equipment and technique, peritoneal dialysis has been again used in treating patients for whom haemodialysis is contraindicated.

Anatomy and Physiology
The peritoneum is the largest serous membrane of the body. In adults it has a surface area of approximately 2.2 m^2. It is a closed unit consisting of two parts:

1 The parietal peritoneum that lines the inside of the abdominal wall
2 The visceral peritoneum that is reflected over the viscera.

The space between the two parts is the peritoneal cavity. This cavity is normally a potential space containing only a small amount of serous fluid. The serous fluid lubricates the viscera and allows them to move freely upon one another and the parietal peritoneum.

The visceral peritoneum consists of five layers of fibrous and elastic connective tissue and a sixth layer called the mesothelium. Blood and lymphatic capillaries are found only in the deepest layer of tissue in adults. A substance that passes from the bloodstream into the peritoneal cavity must pass through the capillary endothelium, the mesothelium and the five layers of the visceral peritoneum. The mesothelium represents the major barrier to mass transfer for most substances.

Diffusion and osmosis are the physical processes involved in the exchange of substances across the peritoneal membrane. Diffusion is the force acting on gaseous, solid or liquid molecules to spread them from a region of high to a region of lower concentration. Osmosis is the passage of a solvent through a semipermeable membrane that separates solutions of different concentrations. The force that causes this movement of solvents is osmotic pressure and this varies directly with the concentration of the solution. As the solvent moves across the membrane, it tends to pull certain amounts of solute with it. This is known as the solvent drag effect. Solvent drag enhances the efficiency of peritoneal dialysis. Equilibration is the achievement of equalization of solute and solvent concentrations on both sides of the membrane. As equilibration is achieved, dialysis ceases and solvents and solutes can be absorbed back into the bloodstream. For peritoneal dialysis to achieve maximum effectiveness, fresh solutions must be instilled at the point of equilibration to prevent reabsorption of water and uraemic toxins.

Solution Concentrations

The osmotic pressure of dextrose is utilized in peritoneal dialysis to remove water from the patient. Commercially available dialysis solutions vary in dextrose concentrations. A dextrose concentration above 1.5% will increase the osmotic effect and thus increase the movement of water away from the patient. Hypertonic dextrose solutions enhance the removal of water; hypotonic solutions are used when removal of water is not the primary aim of dialysis.

Dialysis Cycles

Normally a cycle consists of three stages.

Stage I (Inflow)

The dialysis solution is infused into the peritoneal cavity to initiate the dialysis. The fluid infuses by gravity and its rate can be controlled by lowering or raising the container in relation to the patient's abdomen or by releasing or compressing the occluding clamp on the tubing.

Stage II (Dwell Time)

The dwell time is the time the fluid remains in the peritoneal cavity to allow for equilibration. Different dwell times may be established to remove substances of differing molecular weights. The dwell time is relevant to the type of solute and the amount of solvent removed.

Stage III (Drainage)

The drainage stage is that of the emptying of the equilibrated solution from the peritoneal cavity to complete dialysis or to prepare for the infusion of fresh solution. Drainage is also dependent on gravity.

Types of Peritoneal Dialysis

Intermittent

For acute peritoneal dialysis, a manual system is usually used to effect a quick and gentle dialysis. Optimal dialysis is achieved with short dialysis cycles of about an hour each, with a dwell time of 30 minutes. Specific numbers of exchanges are prescribed and dialysis is then discontinued temporarily, with initiation recurring as uraemia increases.

Continuous Ambulatory Peritoneal Dialysis (CAPD)

CAPD was first reported by Moncrief and Popovich in 1976. It is a closed, continuous system of peritoneal dialysis and allows the patient the independence of a life free from dialysis machines. Training in its use takes up to 3 weeks on average. Clear outlines of CAPD can be found in Ainge (1981), Sorrels (1981) and Arenz (1982).

References and Further Reading

Ainge R M (1981) Continuous ambulatory peritoneal dialysis, Nursing Times 77: 1636-1638

Arenz R (1982) Continuous ambulatory peritoneal dialysis, Association of Operating Room Nurses Journal 35 (5): 946, 948, 950, 952, 954

Brunner L S Suddarth D S (1982) The Lippincott Manual of Medical-Surgical Nursing, Harper and Row, Volume 3, pp. 253-258

Lancet (1978) Peritoneal dialysis in chronic renal failure, Lancet ii: 303

Nursing (US) (1982) Fear of floating to a renal unit: nurses' guide to peritoneal dialysis complications, Nursing (US) 12 (12): 42-43

Sorrels A J (1981) Peritoneal dialysis: a rediscovery, Nursing Clinics of North America 16 (3): 515-529

GUIDELINES: PERITONEAL DIALYSIS

Equipment

1   Dialysis administration set
2   Sterile peritoneal set containing forceps, blade and holder, topical swabs, towels, suturing equipment
3   Sterile gown, gloves
4   Peritoneal catheter and drainage bag
5   Local anaesthetic
6   Syringe, needle
7   Skin antiseptic
8   Supplementary drugs as ordered
9   Peritoneal dialysis fluid, as ordered, warmed to 37 °C

Procedure

Action	Rationale
1 Explain the procedure to the patient. An acutely ill patient may be confused and restless but every effort should be made to inform him/her of what is about to happen.	1 To obtain the patient's consent and cooperation. Some hospitals require a patient to sign a consent form before the procedure can be carried out.
2 Weigh the patient before the procedure begins and then daily.	2 To obtain a base-line. Daily weighing is helpful in assessing the state of hydration.
3 Record the patient's vital signs before the procedure begins.	3 To obtain a base-line.
4 Ask the patient to micturate and defecate before the procedure begins.	4 To avoid perforation of the bladder and/or rectum when the trocar is introduced into the peritoneum.
5 Assist the patient to lie in the supine position.	5 To ensure that the patient is in the best position for the procedure's requirements.
6 Continue to observe and reassure the patient throughout the procedure.	
7 Assist the doctor as required.	

Insertion of Catheter

1 Using aseptic technique, the doctor prepares the abdomen surgically and injects the skin and subcutaneous tissues with a local anaesthetic.	1 To prevent the possibility of contamination and infection.

Action	**Rationale**
2 A small incision is made in the abdominal wall 3-5 cm below the umbilicus. The trocar is inserted through the incision. The patient is asked to raise his/her head from the pillow after the trocar is introduced.	2 This tightens the abdominal muscles and permits easier penetration of the trocar without danger of injury to the internal organs.
3 When the peritoneum is punctured, the trocar is directed to the left side of the pelvis. The stylet is removed and the catheter is inserted through the trocar and gently maneouvred into position. Dialysis fluid is allowed to run through the catheter while it is being positioned.	3 To prevent the omentum from adhering to the catheter or occluding its opening.
4 Once the trocar is removed, the skin may be sutured and a sterile dressing placed around the catheter.	4 To prevent the loss of the catheter in the abdomen.
5 The tubing is flushed with the dialysis fluid.	5 To prevent air from entering the peritoneal cavity.

Preparation of Dialysis Fluid

1 Wash your hands. Proceed using aseptic technique.	1 To reduce risk of infection.
2 The dialysis fluid should have been warmed to body temperature (37 °C).	2 For the patient's comfort. To prevent abdominal pain. Heating causes dilation of the peritoneal vessels and increases clearance of urea.
3 Add any drugs, e.g. heparin, to the dialysis fluid if prescribed.	3 Heparin prevents fibrin clots from occluding the catheter.
4 Attach the dialysis fluid to the giving set.	
5 Attach the catheter connector to the giving set.	
6 Allow the dialysis fluid to flow freely into the peritoneal cavity. (This normally takes from 5 to 10 minutes.)	6 To ascertain whether the catheter is in the required position. The flow should be steady and brisk. If not, the tip of the catheter may be buried in the omentum or it may have been occluded by a blood clot.

Action	**Rationale**
7 Allow fluid to remain in the peritoneal cavity for the prescribed time. Prepare the next exchange while the first container of fluid is in the peritoneal cavity.	7 The fluid must remain in the peritoneal cavity for the prescribed dwell time so that potassium, urea and other waste products may be removed. The maximum concentration gradient takes place in the first 5-10 minutes. This is the most effective dwell time.
8 Unclamp the drainage tube. Drainage time will vary with each patient but, on average, should be completed in about 10 minutes.	8 To rid the body of the required products. The abdomen is drained by a siphon effect through the closed system. Drainage is normally straw coloured.
9 Clamp off the drainage tube when outflow ceases and begin infusing the next exchange, again using aseptic technique.	9 **a** To enable the next cycle to begin. **b** To prevent local and/or systemic infection.
10 Record the following **a** Time of commencement and completion of each exchange and the start and finish of the drainage stage **b** Amount of fluid infused and recovered **c** Fluid balance after each complete exchange **d** Any medication added to the dialysis fluid.	10 To detect and monitor trends and fluctuations.
11 Take and record the vital signs: **a** Blood pressure and pulse every 15 minutes during the first exchange and hourly thereafter, depending on the patient's condition **b** Temperature every 4 hours, or more frequently if condition demands.	**a** Hypotension may be indicative of excessive fluid loss due to the glucose concentration of the dialysis fluid. Changes in pulse may indicate impending shock or overhydration. **b** To monitor any signs of infection. Infection is more likely to become evident after dialysis has been discontinued.
12 Record fluid balance accurately.	12 To prevent complications such as circulatory overload and hyper-tension that may occur if most of the fluid is not recovered during the drainage stage. The fluid balance should be about even or show slight fluid loss.

Umbilicus

Peritoneal catheter is introduced through a trocar puncture

Evaluate status of fluid balance by measuring and recording

1. Intake
2. Output
   a. Urine
   b. Vomitus
   c. Stool
   d. Drainage

Keep dialysis flow sheet

Encourage deep breathing and coughing

Take vital signs

Ensure intake of therapeutic diet

Offer sweetened fluids at prescribed intervals

Assist with oral hygiene

Support peritoneal catheter when turning patient

Weigh patient daily

Assess patient's behaviour and symptoms

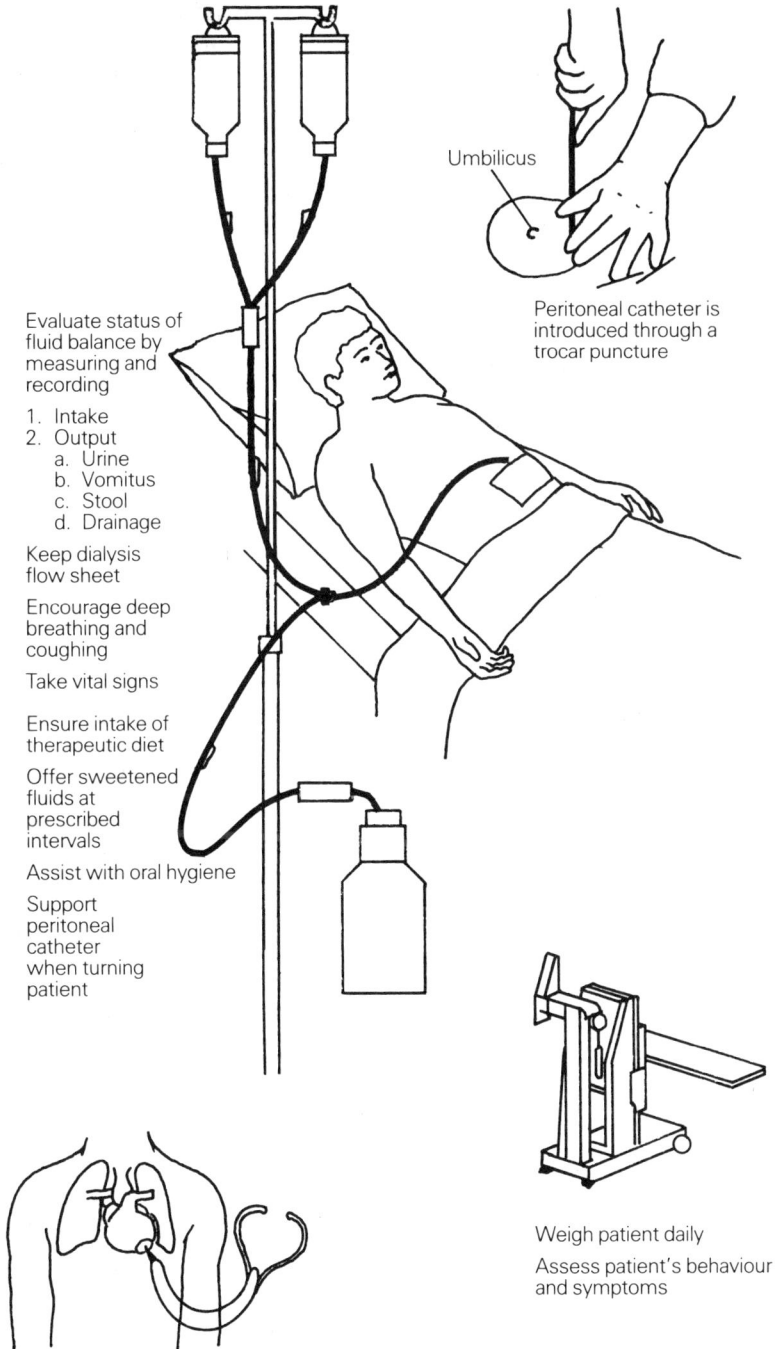

Figure 30.1 Nursing management of patient undergoing peritoneal dialysis

Action	Rationale
13 Dialysis is usually continued until blood chemistry levels are satisfactory.	13 The duration of dialysis is related to the severity of the condition and the size and weight of the patient. The usual time is about 12-36 hours, giving between 24-48 exchanges.
14 Ensure that the patient is comfortable during dialysis by attending to pressure area care and altering the patient's position as required. Assist the patient to sit in a chair for short periods as his/her condition allows.	14 The period of dialysis is lengthy and often exhausts the patient.
15 Send a specimen of peritoneal fluid for investigations daily.	15 To monitor any infections, etc.

NURSING CARE PLAN

Problem	Cause	Suggested Action
1 Peritonitis, indicated by fever, persistent abdominal pain and cramping, abdominal fullness, abdominal rigidity, slow dialysis drainage, inability to obtain a predialysis ascitic fluid specimen, cloudy drainage, swelling and tenderness around the catheter, and increased white blood cell count	1 Poor aseptic technique during catheter insertion or dialysis	1 Aseptic technique should be used throughout the entire dialysis procedure. If peritonitis is suspected, notify the doctor immediately. Send a peritoneal fluid sample to the laboratory for fluid analysis, culture and sensitivity testing, Gram staining and cell count.
2 Infection at site of entry, indicated by redness, swelling, rigidity, tenderness and purulent drainage around the catheter	2 Poor aseptic technique during catheter insertion or dialysis *or* incomplete healing around the site of entry	2 Aseptic technique should be used throughout the entire dialysis procedure. Notify a doctor. Obtain a specimen of the drainage fluid and send it to the laboratory.
3 Subcutaneous tunnel infection with cuffed catheter indicated by	3 Poor aseptic technique during catheter insertion or dialysis *or*	3 Aseptic technique should be used throughout the entire

Problem	**Cause**	**Suggested Action**
redness, rigidity and tenderness over subcutaneous tunnel	incomplete healing in subcutaneous tunnel	dialysis procedure. Notify a doctor.
4 Perforation of the bladder or the bowel, indicated by signs and symptoms of peritonitis, bright yellow dialysis fluid drainage (if bladder is perforated) or faeces in drainage (if bowel is perforated)	4 Catheter inserted when the patient had full bladder or bowel	4 Ask the patient to empty his /her bowels before the procedure begins. If perforation suspected, notify a doctor immediately.
5 Bleeding through catheter	5 Minor trauma to the abdomen *or* minor trauma to the subcutaneous tunnel (with a cuffed catheter) *or* perforation of a major abdominal blood vessel during surgery	5 Bleeding usually stops spontaneously. If it does not, notify the doctor, who may order blood transfusions. One litre hourly dialysis exchanges may be ordered until the drainage fluid is clear.
6 Dialysis fluid leakage around catheter.	6 **a** Excessive instillation of dialysis fluid *or* incomplete healing	6 **a** Instill less dialysis fluid at exchanges. Drain the patient's abdomen completely during outflow.
	b Incomplete healing around cuff of catheter	**b** Bed rest may be ordered to permit healing. Use small volumes of dialysis fluid in exchanges through a new catheter. Also drain the patient's abdomen completely during outflow.
	c Catheter obstruction	**c** Irrigate the catheter with sterile normal saline solution.
	d Catheter dislodged or improperly positioned	**d** Inform a doctor, who will replace catheter or revise its position surgically.
7 Kinking of cuffed catheter	7 Subcutaneous tunnel too short *or* scarring in the subcutaneous tunnel	7 Inform a doctor, who will remove the catheter and implant a new one.
8 Lower back pain	8 Pressure and weight of dialysis fluid in abdomen (particularly	8 Doctor may order analgesics. Exercises to strengthen patient's

Problem	**Cause**	**Suggested Action**
	so in continuous ambulatory peritoneal dialysis (CAPD) patients)	muscles and improve his/her posture may also be ordered.
9 Abdominal or rectal pain (with possible referred pain in shoulder)	9 **a** Improperly positioned catheter tip causing irritation	9 **a** Catheter position to be revised surgically.
	b Dialysis fluid accumulating under diaphragm	**b** Drain the abdomen completely during outflow.
	c Dialysis fluid not at 37°C	**c** Ensure that fluid is infused at the correct temperature.
	d If hypertonic dialysis fluid is used, only one container should be used per cycle. With 2 litres of 6.36% solution, severe shoulder pain can occur.	
	e If air enters the peritoneal cavity, pain may occur	**e** Maintain a closed system.
10 Ileus indicated by sharp pain in abdomen, constipation, abdominal distention, nausea and vomiting, and diarrohea	10 Catheter manipulated excessively during insertion.	10 Notify the doctor immediately as signs and symptoms may indicate peritonitis. A nasogastric tube to suction the stomach may be ordered. Cholinergic medication such as neostigmine may be ordered. Administer fluids and electrolytes as ordered. Encourage the patient to walk, unless ordered otherwise by the doctor. Prepare the patient for surgery, if the doctor orders. The condition may disappear spontaneously after 12 hours.

Problem	Cause	Suggested Action
11 Cramping	11 **a** Dialysis fluid warmer or cooler than 37°C	11 **a** Adjust the temperature of the dialysis fluid to 37°C before infusion.
	b Rapid infusion or drainage	**b** Decrease the infusion or drainage rate.
	c Pressure from excess dialysis fluid in abdomen	**c** Infuse less dialysis fluid at exchanges.
	d Chemical irritation	**d** Use a dialysis fluid with a dextrose concentration lower than 7%.
	e Air in abdomen	**e** Clamp off the dialysis tubing before the dialysis fluid empties completely into the abdomen.
12 Excessive fluid loss	12 Use of dialysis fluid with incorrect dextrose concentration *or* inadequate sodium intake *or* inadequate fluid intake	12 Monitor the patient's weight and blood pressure. Ensure that the patient is receiving dialysis fluid with the correct dextrose concentration. The doctor may order a reduced dextrose concentration.
13 Fluid overload	13 Use of dialysis fluid with incorrect dextrose concentration *or* excessive sodium intake *or* excessive fluid intake	13 Monitor the patient's weight and blood pressure. The doctor will order a reduced fluid and sodium intake. The doctor may also order increased use of dialysis fluid with a 4.25% dextrose concentration.
14 Hyperglycaemia	14 Use of a dialysis fluid with a dextrose concentration (the dextrose is absorbed systemically)	14 Check plasma glucose levels after dialysis. Monitor the patient (especially if he/she has diabetes mellitus or insulin deficiency) for signs and

Problem	Cause	Suggested Action
		symptoms of hyper-glycaemia. The patient's insulin dose may have to be adjusted.
15 Respiratory difficulties	15 Pressure from the fluid in the peritoneal cavity and upward displacement of the diaphragm resulting in shallow breathing	15 Elevate the head of the bed. Encourage breathing exercises and coughing.

31

PRE- AND POSTOPERATIVE CARE

Definitions

Preoperative Care

Preoperative care is the physical and psychological preparation of a patient prior to surgery.

Postoperative Care

Postoperative care consists of ensuring that the patient is nursed in the greatest possible comfort, is kept free from hazards and complications during the postoperative period, and is encouraged to take an increasing responsibility for his/her care until complete recovery is effected.

Indications

Preoperative Care

1 *Psychological*
  a To assist the patient to understand and accept the proposed surgery
  b To assess and then control levels of anxiety.
2 *Physical*
  a To teach the patient the necessary exercises, such as deep breathing exercises, leg exercises and support of wound exercises, to reduce or prevent postoperative complications
  b To ensure that the patient is in an optimum physical condition prior to surgery.

Postoperative Care

1 *Psychological* To consolidate any psychological care offered pre-operatively.
2 *Physical* To maintain life postoperatively.

REFERENCE MATERIAL

Patient Education and Postoperative Pain

The cause, nature and experience of pain is constantly being reviewed. Lazarus (1966) and Janis (1971) showed that the provision of information creates some anticipatory fear about a future event. It is suggested that this provides an opportunity for mental rehearsal of the stressful event that is to be experienced and results in less emotional disturbance for the subject when the event occurs. In the light of this research it has been argued that there is a need for a patient to experience and work through his/her anxiety, with support from health care professionals, preoperatively. Egbert et al. (1964) demonstrated how the provision of information, such as length of operation, the process of regaining consciousness, and the location and intensity of postoperative pain, could affect the recovery period. Of the two groups studied, the informed group demonstrated less postoperative pain, required less analgesia, recovered more quickly and left hospital, on average, 2.5 days earlier than the control group. This concept, referred to in psychology as locus of control, is based on the theory that if an individual feels he/she has some control over the outcome of his/her fate, he/she will function more efficiently than if he/she feels totally helpless. Zborowski (1969) has shown that cultural and racial considerations also need to be examined. Hayward (1975) suggests that nursing time spent in explanation and teaching can significantly reduce the postoperative workload.

Shaving

This is a common preoperative procedure. Alexander et al. (1983) suggest that shaving produces skin damage, invisable to the naked eye, which provides entry points for microorganisms which become focus points of infection prior to surgery. The timing of the shave is also significant; the later the shave the less incidence there is of infection postoperatively. *The Lancet* (1983) advocates the use of depilatory creams, the cost of which is phenomenally less than the cost of treating an infection.

Preoperative Fasting

It has been common practice to fast patients prior to the administration of a general anaesthetic. However, Hamilton Smith (1972) has shown that the fasting rule may vary from 4 to 12 hours or more. The majority of nurses involved in the studies did not seem to grasp the essential reasons for the fast and preferred to err by prolonging the period if they were unsure. The study also revealed that in general nurses seemed unbothered by this, saw little danger to the patient and frequently operated on a routine system to withhold food and drink from 12 midnight from all patients who were scheduled for theatre the following morning. Opinions among anaesthetists and surgeons also varied in the interpretation of 'nil by mouth'. While it is commonly accepted that the contents of the stomach may be vomitted or regurgitated during some period of general anaesthesia and inadvertently inhaled by the patient while the cough reflex is still absent, it is not always appreciated what factors affect gastric motility, and hence the gastric contents, at any period of time. A meal with a high fat content may take up to 20 hours to be processed in the stomach, whereas a glass of water takes little more than half an hour to pass into the duodenum. Anxiety and fear exhibit a delaying effect on peristaltic action, as do some anaesthetic agents and morphia. Furthermore, the stomach is never completely empty since gastric secretions continue to be produced at the rate of 30 ml per hour even in the absence of food, and it is not unusual for 200 ml to be present in the stomach of a fasting patient. It appeared from the study that not only were food and drink withheld from patients for significantly longer than was necessary, but often such a decision was left entirely to the whim of nurses whose level of understanding for this need varied considerably. The author concluded that there was a need for the nurse to acquire knowledge and experience that would enable him/her to evaluate the patient's nutritional needs as part of a more holistic approach.

References

Alexander J W et al. (1983) The influence of hair removal methods on wound infections, Archives of Surgery, 118: 347-352

Burns R B (1980) Essential Psychology, MTP

Egbert L D et al. (1964) Reduction of postoperative pain by encouragement and instruction of patients, New England Journal of Medicine 270: 825

Hamilton Smith S (1972) Nil by Mouth? Royal College of Nursing

Hayward J (1975) Information — A Prescription Against Pain, Royal College of Nursing

Janis I (1971) Stress and Frustration, Harcourt Brace

Lancet (1983) Preoperative depilation, Lancet i: 1311

Lazarus R S (1966) Some principles of psychological stress and their relation to dentistry, Journal of Dental Research 45: 1620

Phipps W J et al. (1979) Shafer's Medical-Surgical Nursing, 6th edition, C V Mosby

Zborowski M (1969) People in Pain, Jossey Bass.

GUIDELINES: PREOPERATIVE CARE

Equipment

1 Theatre gown
2 Theatre hat
3 Hypoallergenic tape for taping rings, if necessary
4 Denture container, if necessary
5 Valuables book to record valuables the patient wishes to be kept in hospital custody during surgery
6 Any equipment and documents required by law or hospital policy if a premedication is prescribed.

Procedure

Action	Rationale
1 Ensure that the patient is wearing an identification bracelet with the correct information.	1 To prevent misidentification and possible harm.
2 Ascertain whether preoperative education has been assimilated by the patient.	2 To determine whether the patient understands the reasons for surgery and how to minimize postoperative discomfort and reduce possible postoperative complications.
3 Record the patient's vital signs. Weigh the patient. Obtain a specimen of the patient's urine for analysis.	3 To establish a preoperative base-line and record any preoperative abnormalities.
4 Check that the patient has undergone any preoperative examinations, e.g. X-rays, group and cross-matching of blood, and that the results are included in the patient's notes.	4 To ensure that all relevant material is available to the surgical team if required.
5 Perform skin preparations, if necessary.	5 Shaving or the removal of hairs using a depilatory cream lessens the likelihood of wound infection. Thorough skin cleansing decreases the chances of bacteria entering the skin surface at time of surgery. (For fuller information see the reference material above.)
6 Assist the patient to change into the theatre gown and theatre hat.	6 To minimize the risk of infection.
7 Check, by asking the patient, that **a** Preoperative fasting has been observed.	**a** To prevent inhalation of undigested or semidigested food while under anaesthesia.

Action	Rationale
b Urine has been passed prior to premedication.	**b** To prevent urinary incontinence due to muscle relaxation during operation. To permit a better view of the abdominal cavity in abdominal and pelvic surgery. To decrease the chance of inadvertent injury to the bladder in the above type of surgery.
c A good bowel motion has been achieved.	**c** To ensure a clear bowel before abdominal and pelvic surgery.
d Any protheses have been removed or noted, e.g. dental crowns or bridges. Hearing aids should be left in position until the patient has been anaesthetized.	**d** To prevent trauma to the patient.
e Jewellery and cosmetics have been removed.	**e** Metal jewellery or hairpins may be lost accidentally, may cause damage to the patient, either directly or indirectly, and may cause diathermy burns. Cosmetics, including facial makeup and nail varnish, obscure the true colour of the patient's skin, thus camouflaging early signs of hypoxia.
8 Any valuables that the patient has not been permitted to retain during surgery should be recorded and maintained in hospital custody according to hospital policy.	8 To ensure their safekeeping. Wedding rings may be worn if they do not interfere with the surgery to be performed. If retained they should be taped to prevent diathermy burns.
9 Check that the form consenting to the operation has been completed and correctly signed by doctor and patient.	9 To comply with any legal requirements and hospital policy.
10 Conforming to legal requirements and hospital policy, check and administer any premedication prescribed.	
11 Advise the patient not to get up once premedication has been administered but to use the nurse call system to attend to any of his/her needs.	11 To prevent trauma to the patient as premedications, generally sedatives, may make the patient drowsy and uncoordinated.
12 Ensure that any relevant information, e.g. case notes and X-rays, accompany the patient to theatre.	12 To enable the surgical team to have full access to the patient's history.

GUIDELINES: POSTOPERATIVE CARE

Equipment

1 Airway
2 Oxygen supply
3 Disposable oxygen mask and tubing
4 Suction equipment
5 Selection of suction catheters
6 Disposable gloves
7 Disposable tissues
8 Receiver
9 Sphygmomanometer
10 Stethoscope
11 Intravenous infusion stand
12 Observation charts
13 Space blanket
14 Cotsides

Emergency cardiopulmonary resucitation equipment should also be available.

Procedure

Action	Rationale
1 Ensure that the patient is in the left lateral position if the nature of the surgery allows this. Otherwise ensure that an airway is inserted.	1 To ensure a clear airway.
2 Obtain full information about the nature of the surgery performed and any immediate postoperative instructions.	2 To ensure that the patient receives the prescribed treatment.
3 Remain with the patient until full consciousness is achieved. Orientate the patient as to time and place at frequent intervals.	3 To reassure the patient by informing him/her of the reality of his/her situation.
4 Record the patient's vital signs according to the anaesthetist's instructions or until the patient's condition is stable.	4 To establish a base-line post-operatively. To detect and monitor any fluctuations and trends in the patient's condition.
5 Note the patient's pallor.	5 To monitor any respiratory dysfunction.
6 Administer oxygen as prescribed.	
7 Check that intravenous fluids are infusing as prescribed and record this.	

Action	Rationale
8 Observe wound for **a** Type(s) of dressing(s) **b** Signs of oozing or oedema, which should be noted and recorded **c** Any drains, in which case record the amount of drainage if appropriate, e.g. Redivac bottles.	8 To establish a base-line post-operatively.
9 Suspend any drainage containers where they may be visible.	9 To prevent accidental trauma to the drains and to the patient. To observe whether drainage becomes excessive.
10 Record the patient's urinary output accurately.	10 To monitor renal function.
11 Offer the patient, if fully conscious, postoperative analgesia and/or antiemetics if prescribed.	11 To alleviate any postoperative pain and/or nausea.
12 Offer mouth care.	12 To maintain oral cleanliness. To promote patient comfort.
13 Ensure that the patient is as comfortable as possible. If it is not too painful for the patient, carry out pressure area care.	13 To promote patient comfort.
14 Introduce postoperative exercises slowly, e.g. passive limb movements, if appropriate.	14 To prevent postoperative complications.
15 Escort the patient back to the ward when the surgical team considers that his/her condition warrants it.	

NURSING CARE PLAN

Problem	Cause	Suggested Action
1 Partial or total respiratory dysfunction	1 **a** Incorrect positioning	1 **a** Readjust the patient's position.
	b Vomitus *or* oral and pharyngeal secretions	**b** Remove any oral secretions using suction.
	c Respiratory depression following prolonged general anaesthesia	**c** Call the patient to arouse him/her. Maintain oxygen therapy as prescribed. Inform a doctor.
2 Primary haemorrhage and subsequent hypo-	2 Excessive blood and fluid loss during	2 Increase the rate of intravenous infusion,

Problem	**Cause**	**Suggested Action**
tension leading to cerebral anoxia and renal underperfusion.	surgery	if allowed. Elevate the foot of the bed. Locate the bleeding point and apply pressure. Inform a doctor.
3 Postoperative pain	3 **a** Tension, anxiety and disorientation	3 **a** Explain to patient where he/she is and the nature of his/her operation. Reinforce the preoperative teaching. Explain and demonstrate how the patient can support his/her wound and move with the minimum of discomfort.
	b Surgical trauma	**b** Give regular analgesia, providing that the patient's condition allows this, and evaluate the effects.
4 Nausea	4 **a** Side effect of anaesthesia	4 **a** Maintain intravenous fluids as prescribed. Offer prescribed antiemetics and evaluate their effect. Offer mouth care.
	b Temporary ileus	**b** If the patient has a nasogastric tube in position, check the position of the tube and maintain the nasogastric tube on free drainage. Aspirate the tube hourly in the presence of nausea. Give antiemetics as prescribed and evaluate their effect. Instruct the patient not to eat or drink. Note when bowel sounds occur and flatus is passed.
5 Low urinary output	5 **a** If a catheter is in position check for kinking or blockage.	5 **a** Readjust the position of the catheter. Irrigate the patient's bladder if appropriate.

Problem	Cause	Suggested Action
	b Renal dysfunction as a result of surgery	**b** Record the patient's fluid balance and report this to a doctor.
6 Hypovolaemia	6 Inadequate hydration following major surgery	6 Increase intravenous fluids flow rate if this is allowed and inform a doctor.
7 Hypervolaemia and pulmonary oedema	7 Overhydration via intravenous route *or* cardiac failure.	7 Assist the patient into an upright or Fowler's position, if appropriate, to facilitate breathing. Decrease intravenous fluids flow rate if this is allowed and inform a doctor.
8 Patients with a high risk of deep vein thrombosis and pulmonary embolus	8 Previous history *or* position of patient during, and duration of, surgery *or* major abdominal or pelvic surgery *or* abdominal or pelvic mass *or* obesity	8 Reinforce preoperative teaching about deep breathing and hourly leg exercises. On the first postoperative day, sit the patient out of bed in a comfortable chair with his/her feet supported on a stool for short periods. The amount of time which the patient remains out of bed should be increased daily, if his/her condition allows this. Check the patient's calves daily for colour, tenderness, oedema and any complaints of pain. Record the patient's temperature 4-hourly and report any abnormalities to a doctor. Antiembolic stockings should be worn as appropriate. Administer the prescribed anticoagulant therapy.
9 Wound infection	9 Large open wound *or* bowel opened during surgery *or* orthopaedic surgery *or* obesity	9 Maintain aseptic technique when changing the dressing. Take down the dressing only when necessary. Observe the wound for signs of infection,

Problem	Cause	Suggested Action
		haematoma and pain. Report all such signs to a doctor. Record the patient's temperature and pulse 4-hourly. If signs of infection are present, take swabs for bacteriological investigation. Administer the prescribed antibiotic.
10 Chest infection	10 Painful suture line (thoracotomy and large abdominal wounds) *or* patient is a chronic smoker *or* chronic bronchitis or other respiratory condition *or* artificial ventilation	10 Reinforce preoperative teaching about deep breathing and coughing. Alter the patient's position regularly. Observe and report the nature and amount of sputum. Send a specimen of sputum for bacteriological investigation. Record the patient's temperature, pulse and respirations 4-hourly and report any abnormalities to a doctor. Administer the prescribed antibiotics. Administer regular analgesia to ease and therefore facilitate pain.
11 Septicaemia	11 Preoperative toxicity *or* perforated bowel *or* neutropenia *or* central venous line in position	11 Record the patient's temperature, pulse and blood pressure 4-hourly. Report any abnormalities to a doctor. When administering intravenous drugs, take down the dressing each time and observe the cannula site for signs of infection. Change intravenous giving sets daily. Administer any prescribed antibiotics.

32

PRESSURE SORES

Definition

Pressure sores appear as circumscribed red areas located over bony prominences or pressure points and occur when an area of the body surface is subjected to prolonged pressure.

REFERENCE MATERIAL

The Effect of Pressure on Body Tissues

As capillary pressure is about 32 mm Hg, any external pressures exceeding this will cause capillary obstruction. Most healthy people experience pressures in excess of 32 mm Hg, while lying or sitting down. In a supine position the highest points of pressure are over the sacrum, the buttocks and the heels (40-60 mm Hg for a healthy person with a reasonable body weight : height ratio). If external pressure is intermittent, however, capillary damage does not occur. Kosiak (1958, 1976) demonstrated that with constant pressure, even in denervated tissues, a critical period of 1-2 hours exists before pathological changes occur.

Localized pressure does not directly harm living tissue. It is compression of the capillaries that deprives the tissue of oxygen and nutrients and allows a build up of metabolic waste, resulting in death of tissue. Death is from anoxia and not from mechanical cell disruption (Husian 1953). Reactive hyperaemia is the normal body response to pressure ischaemia. After pressure is relieved the area shows a bright red flush as capillary dilatation occurs to return oxygen supply and remove wastes. The triggering mechanism for this is not known. After lengthy periods of unrelieved pressure, however, irreversible pathological changes occur and reactive hyperaemia becomes an insufficient compensatory system.

Relief of pressure from a body surface is the single most important factor in treating or preventing the occurrence of a pressure sore. Of prime consideration in nursing care is the positioning and regular repositioning of the patient.

Identification of Patients at Risk

Many predisposing factors are involved in the development of pressure sores:

1 *Continuous pressure* See above.
2 *Shearing* When a patient slides down a bed or a chair, unless he/she is re-positioned correctly the skin often remains in contact with the supporting surface, whereas the skeleton moves over it. Usually only epidermal tissue is lost and a superficial sore develops. As the skin's integrity has been broken, the patient is left at risk from infection.
3 *Immobility* In health, numerous spontaneous readjustments are made to relieve pressure. In illness, this defence may be lost due to lethargy, brain or nerve damage, sedation, operative techniques, loss of consciousness, etc.
4 *Vascular factors* Any disruption of the flow or volume of blood will lower the skin's resistance. Shock, involving peripheral vascular failure, creates a serious danger to pressure sore formation. Venous engorgement, anterios-clerotic changes and the vascular damage caused by smoking (Barton 1977) are all contributory factors. Anaemia impedes the effects of reactive hyperaemia.
5 *Diet* Poor nutrition increases the risk of pressure sore formation. Hypoproteinaemia, low vitamin C levels and zinc deficiencies are among the most crucial factors (Tweedle 1978).
6 *Body weight* Any deviation from ideal weight can increase risk. Thin individuals, with little subcutaneous fat, run a higher risk of sustaining relatively high local pressures over bony prominences. Obese individuals are at risk from immobility, lifting and positioning problems.
7 *Incontinence* Damp linen adds to the shearing problem. Strong acids and alkalis, present in faeces or urine, damage the surface epithelium, causing a chemical burn. When skin integrity is lost, infection and further wound breakdown are likely to occur. Incontinence tends to macerate the skin, leading to tearing. Extensive washing, as occurs with incontinent patients, tends to remove most of the skin's natural lubricants, thereby causing friction between the skin and the support device. The skin becomes dry and brittle and cracks easily.
8 *Medical condition* Medical conditions, such as diabetes mellitus, that have an effect on blood vessels as well as blood sugar, render a patient more susceptible to infection.
9 *Immunosuppression* This may occur in the malnourished, particularly the hypoproteinaemic patient, following injury or in patients with malignant disease. Immunosuppression renders the patient more likely to wound infection and delays the healing process.

Patients should be assessed on admission so that appropriate precautions can be taken. Norton et al. (1975) developed an 'at risk' scale which is shown in Table 32.1. Patients with scores of 14 or below are considered to run the greatest risk of developing pressure sores. Scores of 18-20 are achieved by people who are at minimal risk. Patients having scores of 14-18 are not considered to be at risk but they should be reassessed immediately any deterioration in their condition is observed.

Table 32.1 The Norton scale

Physical condition		Mental condition		Activity		Mobility		Incontinent	
Good	4	Alert	4	Ambulant	4	Full	4	Not	4
Fair	3	Apathetic	3	Walk/help	3	Slightly limited	3	Occasionally	3
Poor	2	Confused	2	Chairbound	2	Very limited	2	Usually/urine	2
Very bad	1	Stuporous	1	Bedfast	1	Immobile	1	Doubly	1

Devices Used for the Relief of Pressure

The most effective way of preventing or relieving pressure on an area is to minimize the pressure in that area. Usually it is sufficient for the patient to be nursed on alternating aspects of the body surface, provided that they are repositioned regularly, e.g. 2-hourly. Sometimes this is inappropriate or impossible due to the circumstances of individual patients, e.g. surgical intervention, body deformities, etc.

A wide variety of devices are available to help relieve pressure over susceptible areas. These devices differ in function and complexity and choice must be based on meeting the patent's individual needs (see Table 32.2).

Treatment of Pressure Sores

The treatment of pressure sores is usually the responsibility of the nurse and, despite an increasing amount of research, it remains one of the most controversial issues in nursing.

The variety of materials commercially available, together with the preferences of the individual nurse, makes the formulation of a comprehensive policy difficult. The following information should assist the nurse to make informed decisions about the individual types of wounds based on clinical judgement.

Relief of Pressure

A pressure sore will not heal unless the source of the pressure is removed. Correct positioning and regular repositioning of the patient are the most effective ways of relieving pressure but mechanical devices may be used as appropriate.

Table 32.2 A selection of mechanical methods for relieving pressure

Aid	Use	Advantages	Disadvantages
Sheepskin	Low risk patients. Norton score 14 or above. Good for under heels.	Warm and comfortable. Machine washable. Decreases friction.	Does NOT relieve pressure. Hardens and matts with washing. Increases heat over pressure points. Needs to be changed frequently. NOT RECOMMENDED for regularly incontinent patients.
Sorbo ring	Low risk patients. Norton score 14 or above.	At first makes patient feel comfortable.	Tends to cause oedema of skin inside the hole of the ring due to pressure of the rim of the ring on surrounding tissue. Can cause venous thrombosis. NOT RECOMMENDED for patients with known vascular complications.
Heel and elbow pads (sheepskins)	Norton scale 14 or less or patients on prolonged bed rest.	Reduce friction and shearing over the elbow and heel.	Often have inadequate methods of keeping them on. Become hardened and matted with washing.
Spenco mattress	Norton scale 14 or less or patients on prolonged bed rest.	Relieves pressure by distributing it over a greater area. Comfortable. Machine (industrial) washable. Acceptable in community settings as well as in hospital. Can be used for incontinent patients. Relatively cheap purchase price.	If patient is very incontinent of urine, even if plastic side is uppermost, there is seepage into the core material. Stitching comes undone after several launderings. Reduces self-motivated movements in very debilitated patients.
Waterbed	Moderate to high risk patients. Norton score 14 or less.	Equalizes pressure and distributes weight. Heated.	Expensive to buy, run and maintain. Makes some patients feel 'sea-sick'. Reduces self-motivated movement. Heavy to move. If not filled correctly can create more pressure than conventional bed.

Cube mattress (air blown through foam mattress by motor)	Norton score 14 or less or patient on prolonged bed rest.	Good waterproofing if patient incontinent. Cool because of air circulation. Good weight distribution. Allows self-motivated movements. Must go straight on to base of bed, not on top of mattress.	Needs electrical supply. Motor tends to be noisy. Requires space to set up motor, trunking can get caught in cot sides. Very poor connection between trunking and under-mattress. Tends to kink as well as disconnect. Removable section is useful.
Aztec bed (double air-filled mattress)	Medium risk — Norton scale 12-16.	Top mattress has intermittent inflating sections which massage patient and allow circulation of air via release holes. Superior to conventional ripple bed. Even weight distribution. Comfortable.	Source of infection if not regularly cleaned. Can puncture easily. Takes time to inflate both mattresses.
Clinitron bed	High risk patients, Norton score 10 or less or indicated because of medical condition.	As near to levitation as possible. Warm, sterile air produces beneficial environment for healing wounds. One nurse can manage even very heavy or debilitated patients on his/her own. Can be used for incontinent patients or those with heavy wound exudate.	Expensive to purchase, run and maintain. Need to reinforce floors before it can be installed. Minimizes self-motivated movements. Can be difficult for patient to get in and out of bed even with help.
Mechanaid netbed	Moderate risk patients. Norton score 14 or less.	Fits any bed. Easy to assemble and dismantle. Easy to store. No servicing, maintenance or laundry difficulties. Patient can be repositioned by one nurse. Appears to encourage relaxation and sleep. Can be lowered on to bed surface when a firm base is required.	Patients do not always like it. Wedge of pillows needed to sit patient up. Patients may lose heat. Reduces self-motivated movement. Not always easy for patients to communicate with people sitting by bed.

Hygeine

A pressure sore is an open wound and should be treated as such. Cleaning and dressing the wound must be carried out using an aseptic techinique to minimize the risk of its becoming infected.

The most commonly used cleaning solutions for non-infected wounds are normal saline and Savlodil and their advantages and disadvantages are shown in Table 32.3.

There are many commercially available products and materials suitable for dressing pressure sores. Selection should be made according to the individual needs of the patient and the nature of the sore (see Table 32.4).

Table 32.3 The advantages and disadvantages of two commonly used cleaning solutions for infected wounds

	Advantages	Disadvantages
Normal saline	Isotonic, nontoxic, nonirritant	Not an antiseptic
Savlodil	Antiseptic	Can be irritant; grows bacteria under certain conditions

The skin around the pressure sore should be treated with care and washed only as necessary for comfort and hygiene, e.g. following incontinence, sweating, etc. Frequent washing of the area is not recommended as

1 Soap may cause excessive drying of the skin.
2 The growth of microorganisms will be encouraged if the area is left moist.
3 Friction caused by washing and drying the skin may result in tissue damage.

Preliminary trials (Willington 1977) have indicated that the use of a nonionic detergent is simpler and more effective than soap for cleaning the skin.

The affected area should not be rubbed as this causes maceration and degeneration of the subcutaneous tissues, especially in the elderly, thus disposing to ulcer formation (Dyson 1978).

Promotion of Wound Healing

The treatment of pressure sores should aim at creating the ideal microenvironment for wound healing and eliminating or minimizing any factor which might delay this. Factors that tend to delay wound healing include the following:

1 *Infection* This causes further tissue breakdown.
2 *Necrotic tissue and debris* These predispose to infection.
3 *Dryness* Destruction of the epidermis exposes the dermis to dehydration, which in turn destroys epidermal remnants and delays epithelialization. Allowing oxygen to blow over a wound causes drying. There also appears to be more scarring in a dry wound, due to perhaps the problems of new cells having to bury beneath the scab (Winter 1971).
4 *Excessive heat or cold*
5 *Scab (eschar) formation* Epidermal regeneration occurs after about 18 hours. Under a suitable occlusive dressing this happens in about 6 hours (Winter 1971).

As with dressings, many agents are commercially available for the treatment of pressure sores (see Table 32.5).

References and Further Reading

Barton A A (1977) Prevention of pressure sores, Nursing Times 73: 1593-1595
Dyson R (1978) Bed sores — the injuries hospital staff inflict on patients, Nursing Mirror 146 (24): 30-32
Forrest R D (1980) The treatment of pressure sores, Journal of International Medical Research 8: 430-435
Guttman L (1976) The prevention and treatment of pressure sores, in Bed Sore Biomechanics, edited by R M Kenedi et al., MacMillan, p. 157
Husian T (1953) An experimental study of some pressure effects on tissues, with reference to the bed-sore problem, Journal of Pathology and Bacteriology 66: 347-358.
Kosiak M (1958) Evaluation of pressure as a factor in the production of ischial ulcers, Archives of Physical Medicine and Rehabilitation 40: 62-69
Kosiak M (1976) A mechanical resting surface: its effect on pressure distribution, Archives of Physical Medicine and Rehabilitation 57: 481-484
Norton D et al. (1975) An Investigation of Geriatric Nursing Problems in Hospital, Churchill Livingstone
Tweedle D (1978) How the metabolism reacts to injury, Nursing Mirror 147 (21): 34-36
Willington F L (1977) The use of non-ionic detergents in sanitary cleansing: a report of a preliminary trial, Journal of Advanced Nursing 3: 373-382
Winter G D (1971) Some factors affecting the skin and wound healing, in Bed Sore Biomechanics, edited by R M Kenedi et al., MacMillan, pp. 47-54

Table 32.4 A selection of dressings used in the treatment of pressure sores

Dressing	Use	Advantages	Disadvantages
Topical swabs	1 Directly on to clean, dry wounds. 2 As a padding over a nonadherent-type dressing.	Excellent absorbency. Sometimes air-permeable. Generally good thermal insulator.	Does not provide moist interface. No barrier to infection. Can traumatize wound when removed due to exudate adherence and capillary loop insertion.
Dressing pads	As a padding over a nonadherent-type dressing.	Superior absorbency. Partially air-permeable. Thermal insulator.	No moist interface. No barrier to infection. Exudate often seeps through, providing a fluid pathway for infection.
Lyofoam	Nonadherent dressing. Tracheostomy dressing.	Absorption of excess fluid without dehydration. Conformable. Nonfibrous.	May adhere in presence of dry serum and become hard.
Melolin	Nonadherent dressing.	Absorbent. Air-permeable. Thermal insulator. Minimum trauma when removed.	No moist interface. No barrier to infection. Non adherent part of dressing tends to adhere to wound surface and separate from rest of dressing.
Release	Nonadherent dressing.	Absorbent. Air-permeable. Thermal insulator. Minimum trauma at change. Moist interface.	
Silastic foam	Nonadherent dressing. Can be tailor-made to wound. Best used on 'clean' wounds.	Absorbent. Moist interface. Air-permeable. Thermal insulator. Barrier to infection. Minimum trauma at change. Easy to clean.	Needs skill to mix and mould. Need to make two moulds each time (one to wear and one to clean). Stability and sterility problem.
OpSite	Cover for ulcerating wounds.	Air-permeable. Barrier to infection. Impermeable to water. High elasticity and conformability. Moist interface. Reduces frequency of dressings. Wounds readily visible.	Needs considerable skill to apply due to its elasticity. Retention of fluid exudate causes bulging of dressing. Adhesive trauma on removal.

Synthaderm	Cover for ulcerating wounds.	Excellent for varicose ulcers. Air-permeable. Impermeable to water. Provides moist interface. Barrier to infection. Thermal insulator. Nonadhesive. Reduces frequency of dressings.	Tends to curl away from a wound when first applied. Some adherence occurs when it is dry. Very expensive.
Stoma care products	Cover for ulcerating wounds.	Air-permeable. Water-impermeable. Provide moist interface. Barrier to infection. Thermal insulator. Reduce frequency of dressings.	Adhesive trauma may occur on removal. Disliked by many nurses as they are not able to observe the wound continuously. Tend to crumble after a while.
Grafted skin	Cover for ulcerating wounds.	Ideal cover. Conforms to specifications to create optimum microenvironment for wound healing.	High risk of graft not 'taking', particularly in severely debilitated and malnourished patients. Requires skilled surgical and nursing care.

Table 32.5 A selection of agents used in the treatment of pressure sores

Agent	Use	Advantages	Disadvantages
Half-strength Eusol	Infected or necrotic ulcerating wounds.	Moderately good debriding agent. Relatively cheap to purchase. Easy to use. Some antiseptic properties.	Short shelf life (approximately 2 weeks). Relatively long healing times. Caustic to surrounding skin.
Hydrogen peroxide solution	Infected or necrotic ulcerating wounds.	Good debriding agent. Decomposes to liberate oxygen into wound. Antiseptic agent.	Caustic to surrounding skin. Considerable skill needed to judge when to discontinue its use.
Varidase Topical (streptokinase/streptodornase)	Infected or necrotic ulcerating wounds.	Excellent debriding agent. Promotes vascularization. Rapid healing times. Does not need an aseptic technique for dressings. Reduces frequency of dressings. Reduces odour from wound.	Relatively expensive to purchase. Has to be reconstituted using syringe and needle, therefore only available on prescription. Initially increases exudate. CONTRAINDICATED for use near major vessels (due to potential effects of streptokinase).
Povidone iodine spray	Shallow or superficial clean wounds.	Quick to apply. Good antiseptic.	Potential adverse reactions.

GUIDELINES: PREVENTION OF PRESSURE SORES

Action	Rationale
1 Assess every patient on admission using a recognized scale, such as the Norton scale.	1 To identify patient at risk of developing pressure sores.
2 Reassess every patient on a regular basis.	2 To maintain consistency in treatment.
3 Do not rub any area at risk.	3 Rubbing causes maceration and degeneration of subcutaneous tissues, especially in the elderly.
4 Wash areas at risk only if the patient is incontinent or sweating profusely. Use mild soap or a liquid detergent. Ensure that all detergent or soap is rinsed off and that the area is patted dry.	4 To maintain skin integrity and to prevent the formation of sores. Excessive use of soap can be harmful to the skin. Thorough, gentle drying of the skin promotes comfort and discourages the growth of microorganisms.
5 Use barrier creams only when indicated.	5 Barrier creams prevent damage to the epidermis. They are, however, occlusive and prevent correct moisture and oxygen exchange from the skin.
6 Encourage the patient to eat a nutritious diet, rich in protein and vitamin C.	6 Deficiencies of protein and vitamin C have been shown to render an individual more prone to pressure sores.
7 Use appropriate pressure relief devices.	7 Use of inappropriate aids may increase pressure to that area.

GUIDELINES: TREATMENT OF PRESSURE SORES

Equipment

1 Sterile dressing pack
2 Cleaning lotion of choice
3 Hypoallergenic tape
4 Sterile semiocclusive nonadherent dressing
5 Wound swab or sterile syringe

Procedure

Action	Rationale
Superficial Sores	
1 Where possible relieve the pressure on the affected area. Reposition the	1 To promote circulation and healing.

Action	Rationale
patient at least 2-hourly and record the position on the relevant chart.	To ensure consistency in the pattern of positions used.
2 Clean the wound using an aseptic technique.	2 To prevent infection. The wound should be disturbed as little as possible to allow healing to occur.
3 If necessary cover the wound with the dressing of choice.	3 To prevent leakage of exudate. To provide the optimum micro-environment for wound healing.
4 Record any changes in the appropriate documents and amend the care plan accordingly.	4 For accurate evaluation of the progress of wound healing.

Deep Sores

1 Where possible relieve the pressure over the area. Reposition the patient at least 2-hourly and record the position on the relevant chart.	1 To promote circulation and healing. To ensure consistency in the pattern of positions used.
2 Obtain a specimen of discharge with a wound swab or syringe, as required.	2 To exclude or identify any infection.
3 Clean the wound using an aseptic technique.	3 To prevent infection.
4 Infected wounds should be debrided using suitable topical agents.	4 To allow epithelialization to take place.
5 Cover the wound with an appropriate dressing.	5 To prevent leakage of exudate. To create the optimum micro-environment for healing.
6 Do not use topical swabs directly on raw wounds.	6 Revascularization and epithelialization occurs into the matrix of the topical swabs. Each time the dressing is removed the new tissue is lifted with it and bleeding occurs. Frequent dressings reduce the wound surface temperature and delay healing.
7 Fix the dressing with hypoallergenic tape.	7 Further damage will occur to broken skin if there is an allergic reaction or if tape cannot be removed easily.
8 Encourage the patient to eat a nutritious diet, rich in vitamin C and trace elements.	8 If exudate is excessive, substantial protein loss can occur. Vitamin C and trace elements promote healing.
9 Record any changes in the appropriate documents and amend the care plan accordingly.	9 For accurate evaluation of the progress of wound healing.

33

PULSE

Definition

The pulse is a rhythmic throbbing caused by regular expansion and contraction of an artery as blood is forced into it by the contraction of the left ventricle of the heart.

Indications

The pulse is taken for the following reasons:

1   To establish a base-line pulse
2   To monitor fluctuations in pulse.

REFERENCE MATERIAL

The pulse is measured at the following sites (Figure 33.1):

1	Temporal	6	Ulnar
2	Jugular	7	Femoral
3	Carotid	8	Popliteal
4	Brachial	9	Tibial
5	Radial	10	Pedal.

The heart beats about 70 times every minute normally in the adult, sending 5 litres of blood through the body. This cardiac content equals the volume of blood in each systole (the stroke volume) times the rate per minute. This may be represented as an equation:

$$\text{Cardiac output} = \text{Stroke volume} \times \text{Rate}$$

When the stroke volume decreases, as in shock, the rate increases, maintaining a constant cardiac output.

The pulse is palpated to note the following:

1	Rate	4	Quality
2	Rhythm	5	Elasticity.
3	Force or amplitude		

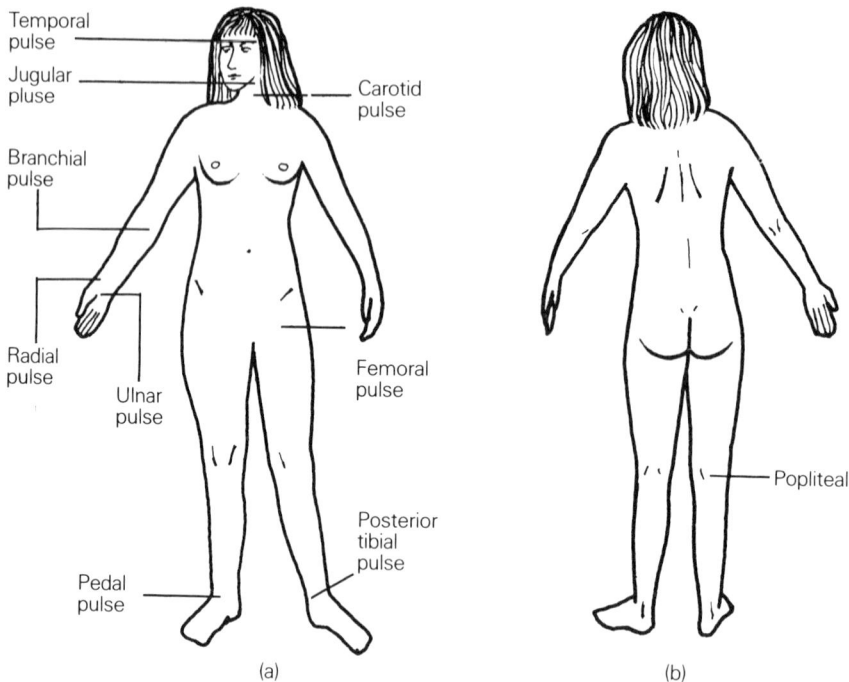

Temporal pulse

Jugular pluse

Carotid pulse

Branchial pulse

Radial pulse

Ulnar pulse

Femoral pulse

Pedal pulse

Posterior tibial pulse

Popliteal

(a)

(b)

Figure 33.1 Pulse sites

Rate

The rate is what is palpated at some peripheral artery as the pulse count. The resting adult will normally have a pulse of between 60 and 100 beats per minute. It is slightly faster in women than men and even more rapid in infants and children. There is also a mild increase in old age.

Tachycardia (rapid pulse rate) occurs as a consequence of

1	Pain	5	Anaemia
2	Anger, fear, anxiety	6	Hypoxia
3	Exercise	7	Shock
4	Fever	8	Congestive cardiac failure.

Pain, anger, fear and anxiety all stimulate the sympathetic nervous system. Congestive cardiac failure, anaemia, exercise and fever all require greater oxygenation and, therefore, greater cardiac output.

Bradycardia (slow pulse rate) occurs in all conditions that cause stimulation of the functional parasympathetic nervous system. It is also found in fit athletes.

Rhythm

The rhythm should be regular. There are two normal exceptions:

Sinus Arrhythmia

Sinus arrhythmia is an irregular pulse that increases at the peak of inspiration and decreases on expiration. It is common in children and young adults.

Premature Beat or Bigeminal Pulse

This condition occurs occasionally when some other pacemaker fires ahead of the sinoatrial node. Doing so prematurely, it causes an early systole. Because of the reduced filling time, the stroke volume is decreased enough for a pause in rhythm to be felt. Frequent premature ventricular contractions may indicate cardiac irritability, hypoxia, digitalis overdose, potassium imbalance, or are signs of more serious arrhythmias.

Force or Amplitude

The pulse pressure is the difference between systolic and diastolic pressure. Amplitude is a reflection of pulse strength. A full, throbbing pulse may indicate such conditions as complete heart block, anaemia or heart failure. Anxiety, alcohol or exercise may produce the same result.

Quality

The character of the pulse may be noted on a scale such as the following:

3+	bounding pulse
2+	normal pulse
1+	weak, thready pulse
0	absent pulse.

Paradoxical pulse is a pulse that markedly decreases in size during inspiration. On inspiration more blood is pooled in the lungs and so decreases the return to the left side of the heart; this affects the consequent stroke volume. A paradoxical pulse is usually regarded as normal, although in conjunction with such features as hypotension and dyspnoea it may indicate cardiac tamponade.

Elasticity

This refers to the elastic recoil of the arterial wall. The flexibility of the artery should be noted. The supple artery of the young adult feels very different from the hard artery of the patient suffering from arteriosclerosis.

Assessing Gross Pulse Irregularity

When there is gross pulse irregularity, it may be useful to use a stethoscope to assess the apical heart beat. This is done by placing the bell of the stethoscope over the apex of the heart and counting the beats for 60 seconds. A second nurse should record, for example, the radial pulse at the same time. The deficit between the two should be noted using, for example, different colours on the patient's chart to indicate the apex and radial rates.

References and Further Reading

Jarvis C M (1980) Vital signs: a preview of problems, in Assessing Vital Functions Accurately, Intermed Communications, pp. 20-25

King E M (1981) Illustrated Manual of Nursing Techniques, 2nd edition, J B Lippincott, pp. 466

GUIDELINES: PULSE

Procedure

Action	Rationale
1 Explain the procedure to the patient.	1 To obtain the patient's consent and cooperation.
2 Ensure that the patient is in a comfortable, but also the required position.	2 To ensure that the patient is comfortable and relaxed. To ensure an accurate reading.
3 Palpate whichever peripheral artery is being used to record the pulse.	3 For routine signs the radial artery is usually used as being the most readily available.
4 Place the second or third fingers along the appropriate artery and press gently.	4 The fingertips are sensitive to touch. The thumb and forefinger have pulses of their own that may be mistaken for the patient's pulse.
5 The pulse should be counted for 60 seconds.	5 Sufficient time is required to detect irregularities or other defects. The normal ranges are **a** About 72 beats per minute for men **b** 72-84 beats per minute for women.
6 Record the pulse rate.	6 To monitor differences and detect trends. Any irregularities should be brought to the attention of the appropriate personnel.

NURSING CARE PLAN

Category	Frequency	Rationale
1 On admission	1 Once only, preferably when patient is settled in	1 To provide an accurate base-line.
2 Preoperative *or* pre-investigative	2 Once only	2 To provide an accurate base-line and to check that the patient's pulse is not irregular.

Category	Frequency	Rationale
3 Patients receiving blood transfusion	3 When unit is put up. Observe the patient at 5 minute intervals for the first 15-20 minutes and take again 1 hour later if condition warrants it. If pulse rate rises, record again and then as often as situation demands.	3 To record a base-line pulse and to detect any indication of reaction to the blood transfusion.
4 Postoperatively **a** Minor surgery **b** Major surgery	4 **a** On return from theatre only. **b** On return from theatre, then 4-6 hourly. Continue at discretion depending on nature of surgery.	4 To detect any cardiovascular changes and to monitor the patient's condition.
5 Patient with a central venous line	5 Four-hourly	5 To monitor the patient's cardiac function.
6 Patients with thyrotoxicosis, myxoedema	6 Four-hourly plus sleeping pulse	6 To monitor the patient's cardiac function.
7 Patients diagnosed as having cardiovascular problems	7 Depends on the condition	7 To monitor the patient's cardiac function.
8 Patients with signs or symptoms of local or systemic infection	8 Six-hourly until six normal recordings obtained	8 To monitor the development or course of the infection.

34

RESPIRATIONS

Definition

Respiration is the diffusion of gases between the air in the alveoli of the lungs and the blood in the alveolar capillaries.

Indications

The respiration rate is evaluated

1 To establish a base-line for respirations
2 To monitor fluctuations in respirations.

REFERENCE MATERIAL

The movements of respiration are essential in keeping the alveolar air constant and their observation is an important contribution to the general assessment of the patient.

Ventilation

Ventilation results from pressure changes transmitted from the thoracic cavity to the lungs. Inspiration is initiated by contraction of the diaphragm and external intercostal muscles so that the thoracic cavity expands both outwards and downwards (Figures 34.1 and 34.2).

The thoracic cavity and lungs are joined by a thin serous membrane, the pleura, which lines the ribs (parietal layer) and folds back on itself to cover the lungs (visceral layer) (Figure 34.3). As a result of this connection, the decreased intrathoracic pressure from the chest wall expansion is relayed to the intrapleural space and then to the lungs themselves. In response to a decrease in alveolar pressure, air rushes in. Expiration is a passive process by which stored energy is released and the lungs return to a resting state.

The degree to which the lungs stretch and fill during inspiration and return to their normal slight stretch during expiration is explained by the terms compliance and elastance.

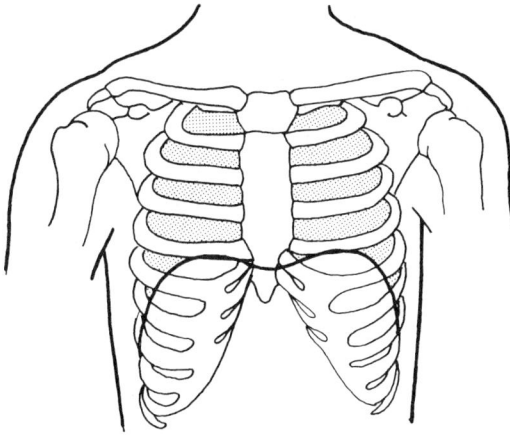

Figure 34.1 The lungs in the thorax. Note how high the diaphragm extends at the front of the chest

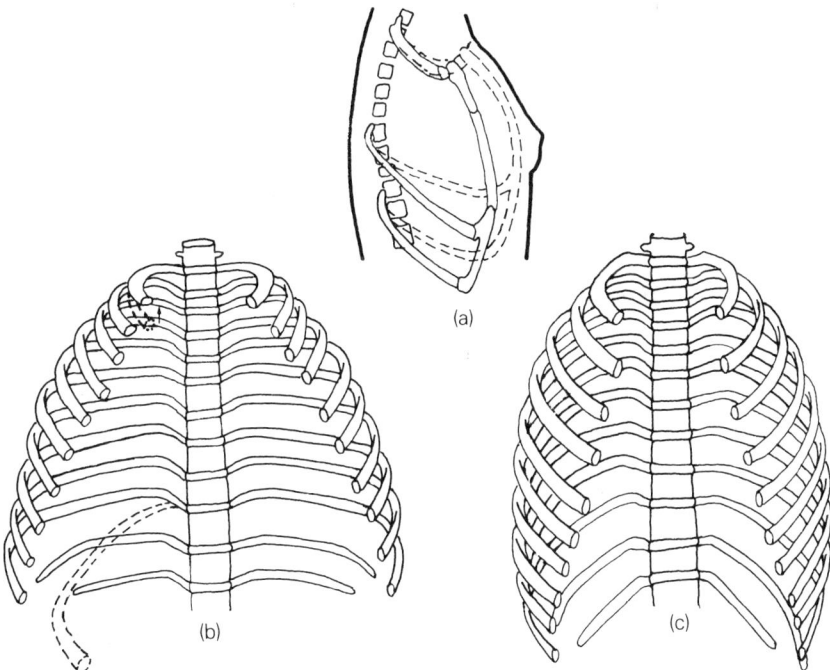

Figure 34.2 The movements of the rib cage in external respiration. **a** The solid outline shows the ribs in expiration, and interrupted outline the position of the same ribs in inspiration **b** The ribs seen from the front in inspiration, showing that the side diameter in the lower part of the chest is increased. **c** The ribs seen from the front in expiration

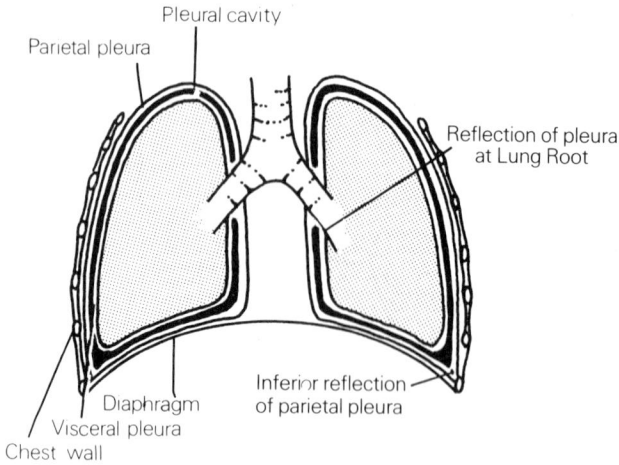

Figure 34.3   Diagram to show the relations of the pleura

Compliance is defined as the change in volume that occurs for a given change in pressure and varies according to lung size.

Elastance refers to the extent to which the lungs are able to return to their barely stretched position. Lung recoil is enhanced by the elastic properties of the lung tissue itself.

Resistance within the airways affects ventilation. Normally airway resistance is slight, so that minimal opposition to airflow occurs. To overcome the various resistances, the respiratory muscles must function.

Volume of Air Breathed (Figure 34.4)

Tidal Volume

The tidal volume is the volume of air inspired or expired in a single breath (about 500 ml).

Residual Volume

The residual volume is the volume of air in the lungs at the end of maximum expiration (about 1200 ml).

Expiratory Reserve Volume

The expiratory reserve volume is the maximum volume that can be expired from a resting expiratory level (about 1200 ml).

Total Lung Capacity

The total lung capacity is the volume of air in the lungs at the end of a maximum inspiration (about 6000 ml).

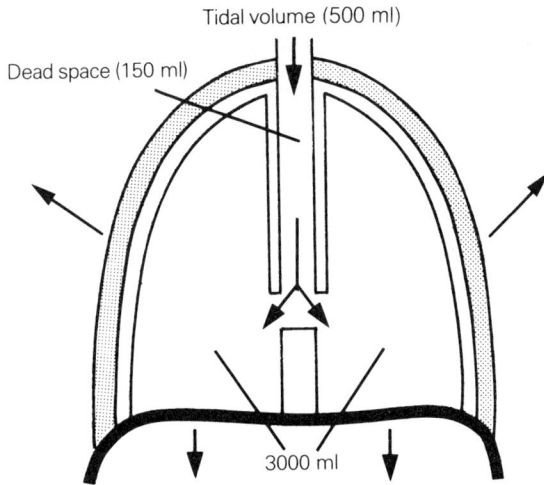

Figure 34.4 Inspiratory capacity

Vital Capacity

The vital capacity is the maximum volume of air that can be expired after a maximum inspiration (about 3800 ml).

Inspiratory Capacity

The inspiratory capacity is the maximum volume of air that can be inspired from a resting expiratory level (about 2500 ml).

Composition of Inspired and Expired Air

Inspired Air

Oxygen	20%
Carbon dioxide	0.04%
Nitrogen	80%

Expired Air

Oxygen	16%
Carbon dioxide	4%
Nitrogen	80%

Alveolar Air

Oxygen	14%
Carbon dioxide	5.5-6%
Nitrogen	80%

Exchange of Gases

The purpose of ventilation is to transport air to and from the alveoli (Figure 34.5). Adjacent to the alveoli is a dense vascular network.

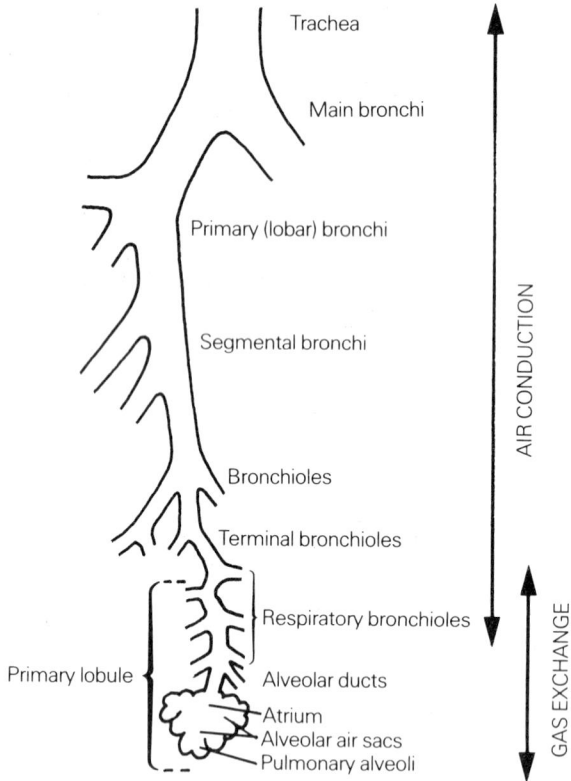

Figure 34.5 The air passages

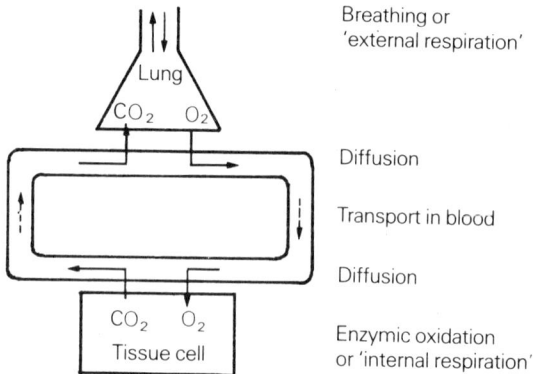

Figure 34.6 Respiratory processes

Movement of gas from alveolus to capillary and from capillary to alveolus occurs by simple diffusion. Oxygen moves into the alveolar capillaries and carbon dioxide moves out (Figure 34.6). Exchange of gases is measured by investigating the levels of the arterial blood gases.

Respiratory Centre

The respiratory centre in the brain comprises groups of nerve cells in the reticular formation of the medulla oblongata. Regular impulses are sent by these cells to the motor neurones in the anterior horn of the spinal cord which supply the intercostal muscles and the diaphragm. When the motor neurones are stimulated the muscles contract and inspiration occurs. When the neurones are inhibited, the muscles relax and expiration follows.

Respiratory centre activity is regulated in two ways, as described below (Figure 34.7).

Chemical Control

An increase in the amount of carbon dioxide in the blood supplying the respiratory centre stimulates the respiratory centre and breathing becomes faster and deeper.

During exercise, carbon dioxide is produced in the muscles by the oxidation of carbohydrate. The amount of carbon dioxide in the blood increases and this stimulates the respiratory centre, producing an increase in depth and rate of respiration. More oxygen is made available in the alveoli for the blood to transport to the muscles, at the same time eliminating more carbon dioxide.

As well as carbon dioxide, any substance that lowers the pH of the blood will stimulate the respiratory centre.

Nervous Control

Lung tissue is stretched on inspiration and this stimulates afferent fibres in the vagus nerve. These impulses cause inspiration to cease and expiration occurs. Emotion, pain and new sensations also cause an increased respiratory rate.

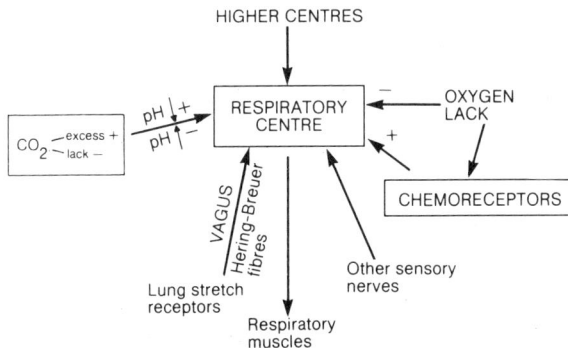

Figure 34.7 Factors controlling respiration

Lung Defence Mechanisms

The upper airway is designed to warm, humidify and filter inspired air. The nasal passages absorb noxious gases and trap inhaled particles. Smaller particles are removed by the cough reflex.

Observation of Respiration

Respirations should be observed for quality, rate, depth and pattern.

Quality

Normal relaxed breathing is effortless, automatic, regular and almost silent.

Rate

Rate and depth determine the type of respiration. The normal rate at rest is 12-18 breaths per minute in adults. It is faster in infants and children. The ratio of pulse rate to respiration rate is approximately 5 : 1.

Depth

The depth of respiration is the volume of air moving in and out with each respiration. This tidal volume is normally about 500 ml in an adult and should be constant with each breath. A spirometer is used to measure the precise amount.

Pattern

Changes in the pattern of respiratory rate may be defined as follows:

Tachypnoea   Tachypnoea is an increased respiratory rate, seen in fever, for example, as the body tries to rid itself of excess heat. Respirations increase by about 4 breaths a minute for every 1°F rise in temperature above normal (equivalent to about 7 breaths per minute for every 1°C). They also increase with pneumonia, other obstructive airway diseases, respiratory insufficiency, and lesions in the pons of the brainstem.

Bradypnoea   Bradypnoea is a decreased but regular respiratory rate, such as that caused by the depression of the respiratory centre in the medulla by opiate narcotics or a brain tumour.

Apnoea   Apnoea is the total absence of breathing; it may be periodic.

Hypernoea   Hypernoea is an increased rate of respiration.

Hypoventilation   Hypoventilation is an alteration in the pattern of respiration, which becomes irregular or slow, and the depth, which becomes shallow. This is caused by drugs, carbon dioxide narcosis and anaesthetics.

Hyperventilation   Hyperventilation is an increase in both the rate and depth of respiration. This follows extreme exertion, fear and anxiety, fever, hepatic coma, midbrain lesions of the brainstem, and acid-base imbalance such as diabetic ketoacidosis (Kussmaul's respiration) or salicylate overdose (in both these, compensation for the metabolic acidosis is attempted through respiratory alkalosis), as well as an alteration in blood gas concentration (either increased carbon dioxide or decreased oxygen). The breathing pattern is normally regular and consists of inspiration, pause, longer expiration, and another pause. But this may be altered by some defects and diseases. In adults, more than 20 breaths per minute is considered moderate, more than 30 severe.

Cheyne-Stokes Respiration This is a cycle in which respirations gradually increase in rate and depth and then decrease over a cycle of 30-45 seconds. Periods of apnoea (20 seconds) alternate with the cycles. Caused by increased intracranial pressure, severe congestive heart failure, renal failure, meningitis, and drug overdose. This type of breathing is also associated with the dying patient.

Biot's Respiration This is an interrupted breathing pattern, like Cheyne-Stokes respiration, except that each breath is of the same depth. It may be seen with spinal meningitis or other central nervous system conditions.

Kussmaul's Respiration This is a breathing pattern characterized by increased rate (more than 20 per minute) and increased depth, a panting, laboured kind of respiration seen in metabolic acidosis or renal failure.

Apnoeustic Respiration This is a pattern of prolonged, gasping inspiration, followed by extremely short, inefficient expiration, seen in lesions of the pons in the midbrain.

References

Bell G H et al. (1980) Textbook of Physiology, 10th edition, Churchill Livingstone, pp. 202-221.

Glennister T W A Ross R W (1974) Anatomy and Physiology for Nurses, 2nd edition, William Heinemann Medical Books, pp. 322-339.

Green J H (1973) Basic Clinical Physiology, 2nd edition, Oxford University Press, pp. 45-57.

Jarvis C M (1980) Vital signs: a preview of problems, in Assessing Vital Functions Accurately, Intermed Communications, pp. 25-28.

Roberts A (1980) Systems and signs. Respiration 1, 2, Nursing Times 76: Systems of life nos 71, 72, p. 8

Rokosky J S (1981) Assessment of the individual with altered respiratory function, Nursing Clinics of North America 16 (2): 195-199

GUIDELINES: RESPIRATIONS

Procedure

Action	Rationale
1 Do not explain the procedure to	1 Awareness on the patient's part of

Action	Rationale
the patient. Attempt to count the respirations when the patient is at rest. This may be done while you are still appearing to record the pulse.	the procedure often produces changes in the respiratory rate.
2 Ensure that the patient is in a comfortable, but also the required position.	2 To ensure that the patient is comfortable and relaxed. To ensure accurate observations.
3 Observe the movements of the chest wall.	3 To detect any respiratory obstruction. To assess excessive use of the intercostal and accessory muscles or respiration. To observe for dyspnoea.
4 Evaluate the sounds made when the patient breathes.	4 To detect respiratory obstruction and to assess whether suction or deep breathing exercises are required.
5 Count the chest movements for 60 seconds. One inhalation and one exhalation together count as one respiration.	5 To allow sufficient time to detect irregularities or other defects.
6 Record the number of respirations.	6 To monitor differences and to detect trends. Any irregularities should be brought to the attention of the appropriate personnel.

NURSING CARE PLAN

Category	Frequency	Rationale
1 On admission	1 Once only, preferably when patient settled in	1 To provide an accurate base-line.
2 Preoperative *or* pre-investigate	2 Once only	2 To provide an accurate base-line.
3 Patients diagnosed as suffering from diseases of the respiratory and cardiovascular system	3 Affected by the nature and course of the disease	3 To monitor the condition of the patient so that necessary action can be instigated.
4 Patients receiving blood transfusions	4 When the unit is put up observe the patient at 5 minute intervals for the first 15-20 minutes and again 1 hour later if the condition warrants it. If the patient shows	4 To record base-line respirations and to detect any indication of reaction to the blood transfusion.

Category	Frequency	Rationale
	signs of reaction to the transfusion, record again and then as often as the situation demands.	
5 Patients receiving oxygen inhalation therapy	5 Affected by the reasons for the therapy	5 To monitor the patient's reaction to the therapy.
6 **a** Postoperative (minor) **b** Postoperative (major)	6 **a** On return from theatre only **b** On return from theatre, then 4-6 hourly. Continue at discretion depending on the nature of the surgery.	6 To assess the return of normal respiratory function.
7 Patients with a central venous line	7 Four-hourly	7 To identify respiratory complications as a result of the catheterization.
8 Patients prescribed any drugs that may affect the respiratory system, e.g. opiates	8 Depends on the prescribed drug and its known side effects	8 To monitor the patient's respiratory function.
9 Patients receiving artificial ventilation; unconscius patients; patients suffering trauma to head and/ or the thoracic region	9 Depends on the condition of the patient	9 To monitor the patient's respiratory function.
10 Pyrexial patients	10 At least 6-hourly; more frequently if temperature grossly abnormal	10 To monitor the condition of the patient so that any necessary action can be instigated.
11 Asthmatic patients	11 Depends on the condition of the patient	11 To monitor the patient's respiratory function. Asthmatic patients experience difficulty in expiration due to the spasm of smooth msucle in the bronchi and bronchioles, which narrows the lumen of the air passages. Sitting the patient in an upright position with his/her limbs supported on a table will enable the

Category	Frequency	Rationale
		accessory muscles of expiration, i.e. the anterior abdominal wall and latissmus dorsi muscles, to function.
12 Patients suffering from chronic obstructive airways disease	12 Depends on the condition of the patient	12 To monitor the patient's respiratory function. Positioning of the patient as above will allow all the accessory muscles of respiration to function.

35

SCALP COOLING

REFERENCE MATERIAL

Doxorubicin (Adriamycin) is one of the most active cytotoxic agents currently used in cancer chemotherapy. It belongs to the anthracycline antibiotic group of drugs and has a wide spectrum of activity. Unfortunately administration of Adriamycin is associated with alopecia in approximately 90% of cases. This is often total. Hair loss is distressing for the patient and may lead to refusal to accept treatment.

Initial research into methods to prevent hair loss, using a scalp tourniquet or crushed ice, was carried out in America. Promising results led to follow up research at the Royal Marsden Hospital. The method developed differs on a number of points from previous work and the results achieved are considerably better. The success rate in the research project was 85% and this has been maintained in everyday practice. Two factors affect the amount of hair loss experienced by the patient:

1   Involvement of the liver with metastatic disease leads to elevated plasma levels of Adriamycin for a longer period. Extension of the cooling period does not seem to improve results.
2   Inadequate cooling because of exceptionally thick hair may lead to partial loss. It has been demonstrated that maximum cooling occurs 20 minutes after the cap has been placed in position. The weight of the cap, as well as the temperature, is a factor, as this ensures that the contact is maintained over the complete scalp. Success doesnot appear to be a dose dependent as first thought.

Scalp cooling, when Adriamycin is prescribed, is not performed routinely. The consultant's permission must be obtained as there is a risk of protecting scalp micrometasteses, especially where there is the possibility of circulating cells, e.g. in cases of leukaemias and lymphomas. The patient must consent when fully informed of the nature and length of the procedure. The patient may discontinue scalp cooling at any time if he/she finds it too traumatic, physically or psychologically, or if hair loss occurs.

Patients should be carefully selected for scalp cooling and should be well motiviated to undertake the procedure. Comments now show that cooling can be more distressing than originally thought, and patients have reported 'ice phobias' following treatment.

The effectiveness of scalp cooling has only been demonstrated satisfactorily with Adriamycin. However, patients receiving other cytotoxic drugs which may cause alopecia have undergone the procedure. Unfortunately the data collected is insufficient for evaluation at the time of writing.

References and Further Reading

Anderson J et al. (1981) Prevention of Doxorubicin-induced alopecia by scalp cooling in patients with advanced breast cancer, British Medical Journal 282: 423-424

Benjamin R S (1975) A practical approach to Adriamycin toxicology, Cancer Chemotherapy Reports 6: 319-327

Benjamin R S et al. (1974) Adriamycin chemotherapy — efficancy, safety and pharmacologic basis of an intermittent, single, high dosage schedule, Cancer 33: 19-27

Dean J C et al. (1979) Prevention of Doxorubicin-induced hair loss with scalp hypothermia, New England Journal of Medicine 301: 1427-1429

Edelstyn G A et al. (1977) Doxorubicin-induced hair loss and possible modification by scalp cooling, Lancet ii: 253-254

Hayward J L (1977) Assessment of response to therapy in advanced breast cancer, British Journal of Cancer 35: 292-298

Hunt J et al. (1982) Scalp hypothermia to prevent Adriamycin-induced hair loss, Cancer Nursing: 25-31

Middleton J et al. (1982) Prevention of Doxorubicin-induced alopecia by scalp hypothermia: relation to degree of cooling, British Medical Journal 284: 1674

Timothy A R et al. (1980) Influence of scalp hypothermia on doxorubucin-related alopecia, Lancet i: 663

Tormey D C (1975) Adriamycin in breast cancer. An overview of studies, Cancer Chemotherapy Reports 6: 319-327

GUIDELINES: SCALP COOLING

Equipment

1 A scalp cooling cap
   a Commercial make
   b Home made from eight hot/cold packs, as manufactured by 3M. These must be taped together with tape, such as 'sleek', and moulded around a wig stand. Whe bandaged in position the cap is placed in a deep freeze (temperature approximately −18 °C) for 24 hours.
2 Ear protection — gauze, cotton wool pads
3 Two crepe bandages — 10 cm or 15 cm wide
4 Two towels
5 Comfortable chair (recliner) or bed
6 Extra pillows and blankets as required

Procedure

Before commencing it is important to explain the procedure fully to the patient and obtain his/her consent. The patient should understand that he/she can discontinue the scalp cooling at any time and that this will not jeopardize chemotherapy. The patient may refuse the procedure.

Action	Rationale
1 Check that the cap has been in the deep freeze for 24 hours.	1 To ensure that the cap is cold enough to be effective.
2 Wet the patient's hair thoroughly.	2 To aid conduction of the cold.
3 Place the ear protection in position.	3 To prevent cold injury.
4 Soak one crepe bandage in cold water and use it to bandage the patient's head tightly. The bandage should be applied evenly and should provide a thin layer over the scalp.	4 To aid conduction of the cold. To compress the hair and prevent any trapping of air betwen the cap and scalp.
5 Place the cap on the patient's head, making sure it fits closely and covers the whole hairline.	5 To ensure cooling over the head, including all the hair roots.
6 Add supplementary packs if necessary.	
7 Bandage the cap in place.	7 To maintain even and close contact of the cap to the scalp and provide some insulation of the cold.
8 Add pillows, etc., as required.	8 To provide support for the head and neck, and reduce the weight of the cap, approximately 2-3 kg.
9 Place a dry towel around the patient's shoulders.	9 To catch any water if the cap defrosts.
10 Offer the patient the use of a blanket.	10 To prevent any chilling.
11 Leave the patient for at least 15 minutes prior to injection of the drug.	11 To obtain initial cooling of the scalp.
12 Administer Adriamycin by intravenous injection.	
13 Leave the patient for a further 45 minutes.	13 To maintain cooling until plasma levels of Adriamycin have dropped.
14 When sufficient time has elasped, remove the cap and bandages carefully.	14 To prevent damage to the scalp and hair.
15 Encourage the patient to rest, if desired.	15 To prevent faintness due to the weight being lifted off.
16 Towel the patient's hair dry and allow the patient to style it gently.	16 To prevent damage to the hair. To ensure that the patient is comfortable and has a chance to rearrange his/her hair before leaving the hospital.

NURSING CARE PLAN

Problem	Cause	Suggested Action
1 Inadequate cooling		1 Follow the procedure meticulously. Check that the cap is as cold as possible. If the patient has very thick hair, use the heaviest cap available.
2 Excess cooling	2 Thin hair	2 Use extra layers of bandage between the cap and the scalp. If it is still painful, discontinue the procedure.
3 Complaints of headache	3 Weight and coldness of the cap	3 Provide support and blankets as required.
4 Distressed patient	4 Claustrophobia	4 Support and reassure the patient. If necessary remove the cap.
5 Hair loss		5 Offer the patient the opportunity to discontinue the scalp cooling.
6 'Ice phobia'		6 Be aware of this possible problem; encourage the patient to discuss his/her feelings.

36

SPECIMEN COLLECTION

Definition

Specimen collection is the collection of a required amount of tissue or fluid with the aim of preserving any organism that may be present while at the same time preventing contamination from other organisms.

Indications

Specimen collection is required when microbiological investigation is indicated. Nursing staff should be able to identify the need for microbiological investigations and, if appropriate, initiate the taking of specimens. Specimen collection is often a first crucial step, in that microbiological investigations may define the nature of the disease and determine the mode of treatment and diagnosis.

REFERENCE MATERIAL

General Principles

Laboratory diagnosis of disease begins with proper collection of the right specimen at the appropriate time. Good liaison is essential between laboratory, medical and nursing staff if this is to be achieved. The nurse's role in this teamwork is to collect the desired material and to arrange for its transportation to the laboratory promptly.

The more material sent for laboratory examination, the greater the chance of isolating a causative organism. It is preferable to send a few millimetres of pus aspirated with a sterile syringe than to send a swab. A swab can only take up a small amount of material, dries quickly and traps in its fibres important cells and organisms that will fail to be transferred to smears of culture media.

Specimens are readily contaminated by poor techinique or by the use of unsuitable equipment. Specimens should be collected in sterile containers with close fitting lids unless instructions are given otherwise. Swabs should nevet be removed from their sterile tubes or specimen jars until everything has been prepared for taking the required samples.

Ideally samples should be collected before beginning any treatment, e.g.

antibiotics or antiseptics. If the patient is receiving such treatment at the same time the specimen is collected, the laboratory staff must be informed. Both antibiotics and antiseptics may destroy organisms that are, in fact, active in the patient and will affect the outcome of the laboratory tests.

Documentation

Requests for microbiological investigations must include the following information:

1 Patient's name, ward and/or department
2 Hospital number
3 Date collected
4 Time collected
5 Diagnosis
6 Relevant signs and symptoms
7 Relevant history, e.g. recent foreign travel
8 Any antimicrobial drug being taken by the patient
9 Type of specimen
10 Consultant's name
11 Name of doctor who ordered the investigation, as it may be necessary to telephone the result before the typed report is dispatched.

Transportation of Specimens

The sooner a specimen arrives in the laboratory, the greater is the chance of organisms present surviving and being identified. Delays will cause changes that may radically alter the result. The laboratory count of bacteria in a delayed specimen could be out of all proportion to that of the specimen when it was collected.

If specimens cannot be sent to a laboratory immediately, they should be stored as follows:

1 Blood culture samples in a 37°C incubator.
2 All other specimens in a specimen refrigerator at a temperature of 4°C.

Sterile transport media should also be available. The tip of a swab stick may be broken by snapping it against the inside neck of the specimen container, taking care not to contaminate this part of the swab shaft with the fingers, and inserting it into the container. This will then preserve the organism in the same condition and numbers. Some swabs are commercially produced in two sections; one being the actual swab, the other being a tube that contains a transport medium. When the swab has been taken, it is placed in the medium and dispatched, with the relevant documentation, to the laboratory.

Any specimen may contain pathogens. To avoid spreading organisms to other people or the environment, it is important not to contaminate the outside of any specimen container and to ensure that such containers are closed securely. Accidental spillage must be cleaned away immediately using the appropriate equipment and solutions. If a specimen container leaks, not only are the porter and laboratory staff at risk, but also contaminating bacteria may enter the container. Any tests carried out on such a specimen will be void. Ideally, all specimens should be placed in double self-sealing plastic bags, with one compartment containing the request form and the other the specimen in its container. Specimens should then be carried to the laboratory in a washable basket or tray.

Any specimen suspected of being highly infectious, such as hepatitits B positive specimens, must be identified clearly. Such specimens must be transported in the required container. When in doubt, the laboratory staff should be consulted. (For further information, see the procedure on hepatitis B, pages 184-188.)

Types of Investigations

Bacterial

There is a wide range of methods available for obtaining cultures and identifying organisms from a specimen or swab. To employ all these tests would be time consuming and costly. Testing, therefore, tends to be selective. It is at this stage that the laboratory request form plays a particularly important part. A faecal specimen, for example, from a patient with diarrhoea who also has a recent history of foreign travel, would be investigated for organisms not normally looked for in faecal specimens from patients without such a history.

The majority of specimens undergo microscopic investigation. This is valuable as an early indication of the causative organisms in an infection. The specimen is often cultured for 24-48 hours longer in the case of blood cultures. This is followed by antibiotic sensitivity testing on any pathogenic organisms that are isolated. Normally this takes a further 24 hours.

Viral

Three types of technique are available for the diagnosis of viral infections:

1 Electron microscopy
2 Culture
3 Serology.

For culture specimens the use of viral transport media and speed of delivery to the laboratory are important as viruses do not survive well outside the body. With good liaison, the nursing personnel should obtain the specimen when the laboratory staff have the transport ready to take it to the virus laboratories. If delays occur, the specimen should be refrigerated at a temperature of 4°C.

The time at which specimens are collected for viral investigations is important. Many viral illnesses have a prodromal phase during which the multiplication and shedding of the virus is at a peak and the patient is at his/her most infectious.

Serological for Detection of Antibodies

Ten millilitres of clotted blood are obtained at 10-14 day intervals to determine current or past infections. This is usually indicated by the presence or absence of a rising antibody titre.

Fungal

Infections by *Candida* species arise in the mouth and / or genital tract and may even invade the bloodstream, resulting in bacteraemia or septicaemias. Fungal investigations may also be carried out on parings and scrapings of skin, nails and hair.

Blood

For information on the collection of blood see the procedure on venepuncture (pages 464-467).

References and Further Reading

Ayton M (1982) Microbiological investigations, Nursing 2 (8): 226-229, 232
Hargiss C O Larson E (1981) How to collect specimens and evaluate results, American Journal of Nursing 81: 2166-2174
Parker M J (1982) Microbiology for Nurses, 6th edition, Ballière Tindall
Smith A L (1973) Principles of Microbiology, 7th edition, C V Mosby, pp. 114-125
Wilson M E Mizer H E (196) Microbiology in Nursing Practice, Macmillian, pp. 160-163

GUIDELINES: SPECIMEN COLLECTION

Procedure

Action	Rationale
1 Explain the procedure to the patient and ensure privacy while the procedure is being carried out.	1 To obtain the patient's consent and cooperation.
2 Wash your hands.	2 Hand washing greatly reduces the risk of infection transfer.
3 Place specimens and swabs in the appropriate, correctly labelled containers.	3 To ensure that only organisms for investigation are preserved.
4 Dispatch specimens to the laboratory with the completed request form promptly.	4 To ensure the best possible conditions for any laboratory examinations.

Eye Swab

1 Using either a plastic loop or a cotton wool-covered wooden stick, hold the swab parallel to the cornea and gently rub the conjunctiva in the lower eyelid.	1 To ensure that a swab of the correct site is taken. To avoid contamination by touching the eyelid.

Action	**Rationale**
2 If possible, smear the conjunctival swab on an agar plate at the bedside.	2 Eye swabs are often unsatisfactory because of the action of tears, which contain the enzyme lysozyme which acts as an antiseptic. Conjunctival scrapings are preferable. This procedure is usually performed by medical staff.

Nose Swab

1 Moisten the swab beforehand with sterile water.	1 To prevent discomfort to the patient. The healthy nose is virtually dry and a dry swab may cause discomfort.
2 Move the swab from the anterior nares and direct it upwards into the tip of the nose (Figure 36.1)	2 To swab the correct site and to obtain the required sample.
3 Gently rotate the swab.	

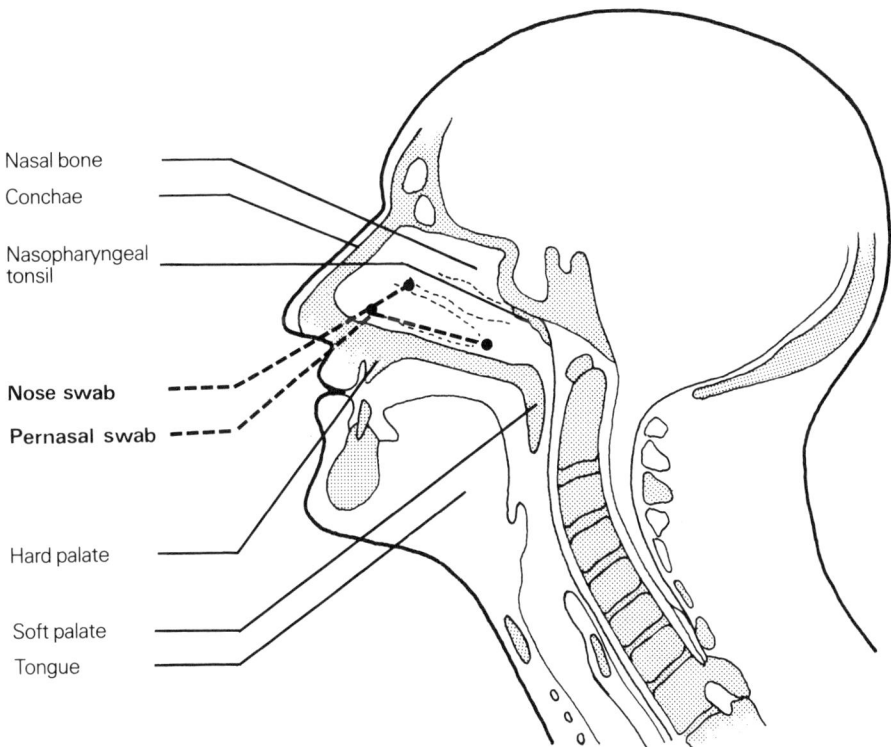

Figure 36.1 Area to be swabbed when sampling the nose

Action	**Rationale**

Pernasal Swab (for Whooping Cough)

1 Using a special soft wire mounted swab, pass it along the floor of the nasal cavity to the posterior wall of the nasopharynx (see Figure 36.1).	1 To minimize trauma to nasal tissue. To obtain a swab from the correct site.
2 Rotate the swab gently.	

Sputum

1 Use a specimen container that is free from organisms of respiratory origin. This need not, therefore, be a sterile container.	1 Sputum is never free from organisms since material originating in the bronchi and alveoli has to pass through the pharynx and mouth, areas that have a normal commensal population of bacteria.
2 Care should be taken to ensure that the material sent for investigation is sputum, not saliva.	
3 Encourage patients who have difficulty producing sputum to cough deeply first thing in the morning. Alternatively, a physiotherapist should be called to assist.	3 To facilitate expectoration.
4 Send any sputum specimen to the laboratory immediately.	4 The bacterial population alters rapidly and rapid dispatch should ensure accurate results.

Throat Swab

1 Ask the patient to sit in such a position that he/she is facing a strong light source. Depress the patient's tongue with a spatula.	1 To ensure maximum visibility of the area to be swabbed. The procedure is one that is likely to cause the patient to gag and the tongue will move to the roof of the mouth, contaminating the specimen.
2 Quickly, but gently, rub the swab over the prescribed area, usually the onsillar fossa or any area with a lesion or visible exudate (Figure 36.2).	2 To obtain the required sample.
3 Avoid touching any other area of the mouth or tongue with the swab.	3 To prevent contamination by other organisms.

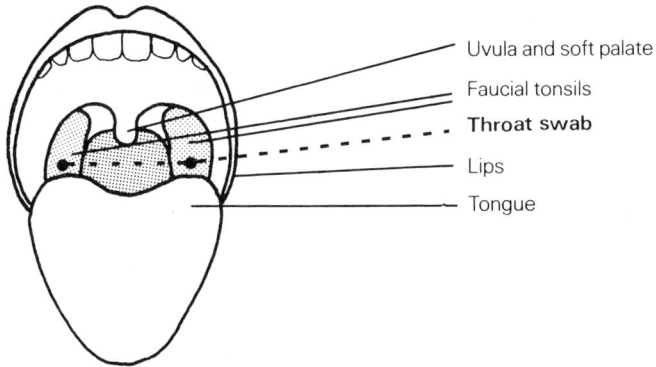

Figure 36.2 Area to be swabbed when sampling the throat

Action	Rationale

Ear Swab

1 No antibiotics or other chemotherapeutic agents should have been used in the aural region three hours before taking the swab.

2 Place the swab into the outer ear as shown in Figure 36.3. Rotate the swab gently.

1 To prevent contamination from other organisms. To prevent collection of traces of such therapeutic agents.

2 To avoid trauma to the ear. To collect any secretions.

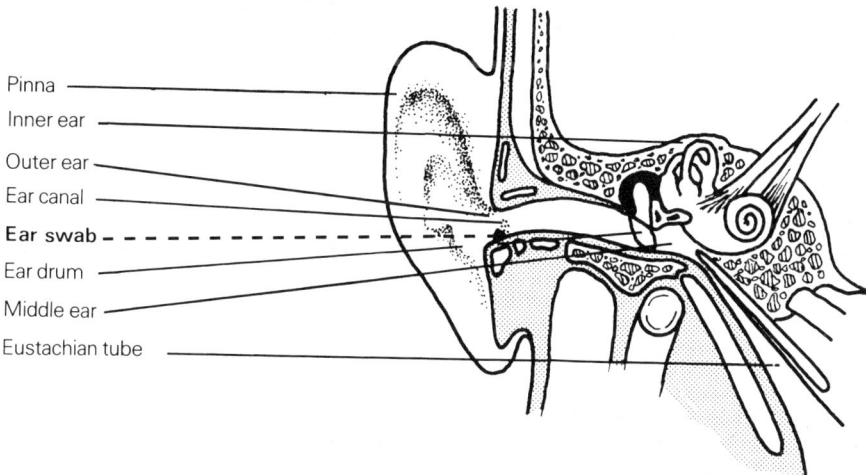

Figure 36.3 Area to be swabbed when sampling the outer ear

Action	**Rationale**

Wound Swab

1 Take any swabs required before dressing procedure begins.

1 To prevent collection of any therapeutic agents that may be employed in the dressing procedure.

2 Rotate the swab gently.

2 To collect samples. It is preferrable to send samples of purulent discharge to swabs.

Note: The use of disposable gloves is recommended in the following procedures in order to prevent cross-infection.

Vaginal Swab

1 Introduce a speculum into the vagina to separate the vaginal walls. Take the swab as high as possible in the vaginal vault.

1 To ensure maximum visibility of the area to be swabbed. To ensure that the swab is taken from the best site. If infection by *Trichomonas* species is suspected, a charcoal-impregnated swab is recommended as this organism survives longer in this medium.

Penile Swab

1 Retract prepuce.

1 To obtain maximum visibility of area to be swabbed.

2 Rotate swab gently in the urethal meatus.

2 To collect any secretions.

Rectal Swab

1 Pass the swab, with care, through the anus into the rectum.

1 To avoid trauma. To ensure a rectal not an anal sample.

2 Rotate gently.

3 In patients suspected of suffering from threadworms, take the swab from the perianal region.

3 Threadworms lay their ova on the perianal skin.

Faeces

1 Ask the patient to defaecate into a clinically clean bedpan.

1 To avoid unnecessary contamination from other organisms.

2 Scoop enough material to fill a third of the specimen container using a spatula or a spoon, often incorporated in the specimen container.

2 To obtain a useable amount of specimen.

To prevent contamination.

Action	**Rationale**
3 Examine the specimen for such features a colour, consitency and odour and record your observations.	3 To monitor any fluctuations and trends.
4 Segments of tapeworm are easily seen in faeces and any such segments should be sent to the laboratory for indentification.	4 Unless the head is dislodged, the tapeworm will continue to grow. Laboratory confirmation of the presence of the head is essential.
5 Patients suspected of suffering from ameobic dysentry should have any stool specimens dispatched to the laboratory immediately.	5 The parasite causing amoebic dysentry exists in a free-living ninmotile cysts. Both are characteristic in their fresh state but are difficult to identify when dead.

Urine

1 Specimens of urine should be collected as soon as possible after the patient wakens in the morning and at the same time each morning if more than one specimen is required.	1 The bladder will be full as urine has accumulated overnight. If specimens are taken at other times, the urine may be diluted. All specimens will be comparable if taken at the same time each morning.
2 Dispatch all specimens to the laboratory as soon after collection as possible.	2 Urine specimens should be examined within 2 hours of collection or 24 hours if kept refrigerated at a temperature of 4 °C. At room temperature overgrowth will occur and lead to misinterpretation. The cellular elements of urine break up quickly. Boric acid is sometimes used in specimen containers as a urine preservative.

Midstream Specimen of Urine: Male

1 Retract the prepuce and clean the skin surrounding the urethal meatus with soap and water, saline or a solution that does not contain a disinfectant.	1 To prevent other organisms contaminating the specimen. Disinfectants may irritate or be painful to the urethal mucous membrane.
2 Ask the patient to direct the first and last part of his stream into a urinal or toilet but to collect the middle part of his stream into a sterile container.	2 To avoid contamination of the specimen with organisms normally present on the skin.

Action	Rationale

Midstream Specimen of Urine: Female

1 Clean the urethal meatus with soap and water, saline or a solution that does not contain a disinfectant.	1 To prevent other organisms contaminating the specimen. Disinfectants may irritate or be painful to the urethal mucous membrane.
2 **a** Use a separate wool swab for each swab.	2 **a** To prevent cross-infection.
b Swab from the front to the back.	**b** To prevent perianal contamination.
3 Ask the patient to micturate into a bedpan or toilet. Place a sterile receiver or a wide-mouthed container under the stream and remove before the stream ceases.	3 To avoid contamination of the specimen with organisms normally present on the skin.
4 Transfer the specimen into a sterile container.	

Specimen of Urine from an Ileal Conduit

For further information see the relevant section in the procedure for stoma care (pages 395-396).

Catheter Specimen of Urine

For further information see the relevant section in the procedure for urinary catheterization (pages 454-455).

37

STOMA CARE

Definition

'Stoma' is a word of Greek origin meaning 'mouth' or 'opening'. A bowel or urinary stoma is usually created on the abdominal wall as a diversionary procedure because the urinary or colonic tract beyond the position of the stoma is no longer viable.

Indications

Stoma care is required for the following purposes:

1 To achieve and maintain patient comfort and security
2 To maintain good skin and stoma hygiene.

REFERENCE MATERIAL

Types of Stoma

Colostomy

In a colostomy the stoma may be formed from any section of the large bowel, e.g. 'end' or 'terminal' sigmoid colostomy (Figure 37.1).

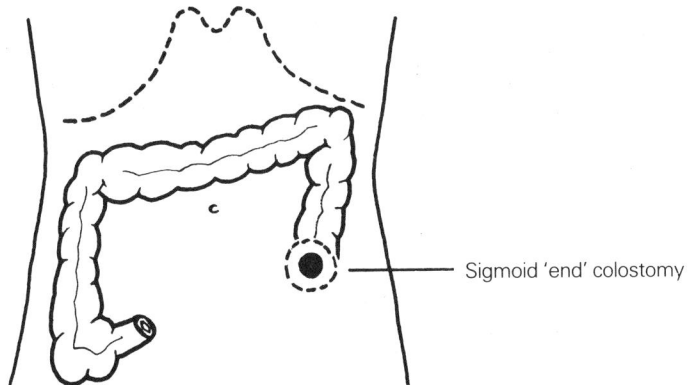

Figure 37.1 Sigmoid 'end' colostomy

A temporary colostomy may be raised to divert the faecal output, thus allowing healing of an anastomosis further along the colon. With a loop colostomy, a rod or bridge may be used to maintain a hold on the abdominal surface. Such a rod or bridge is removed 7-10 days after insertion (Figure 37.2).

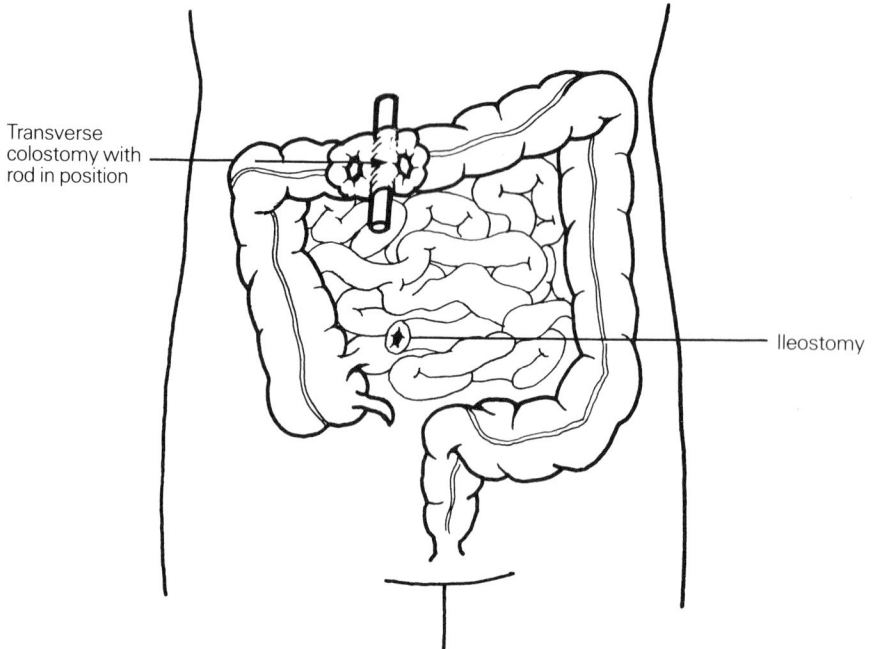

Figure 37.2 Ileostomy

Ileostomy

In an ileostomy the ileum is brought out on to the abdominal wall (Figure 37.2), as when, for example, the large colon is affected by inflammatory disease.

Ileal Loop, Ileal Conduit or Urostomy

The performance of such operations requires the ureters to be transplanted from the bladder into a length, approximately 15 cm, of ileum which has been isolated, along with its mesentery, from the remainder of the small bowel. One end of the ileum, with the resected ureters, remains inside the abdomen, while the other is brought out on to the abdominal wall and everted to form a slightly protruding stoma (Figure 37.3).

Other Types of Urinary Diversion

Other types of urinary diversions include ureterostomy, a procedure that brings the ureters out on to the abdominal wall together (one stoma) or separately (two stomas).

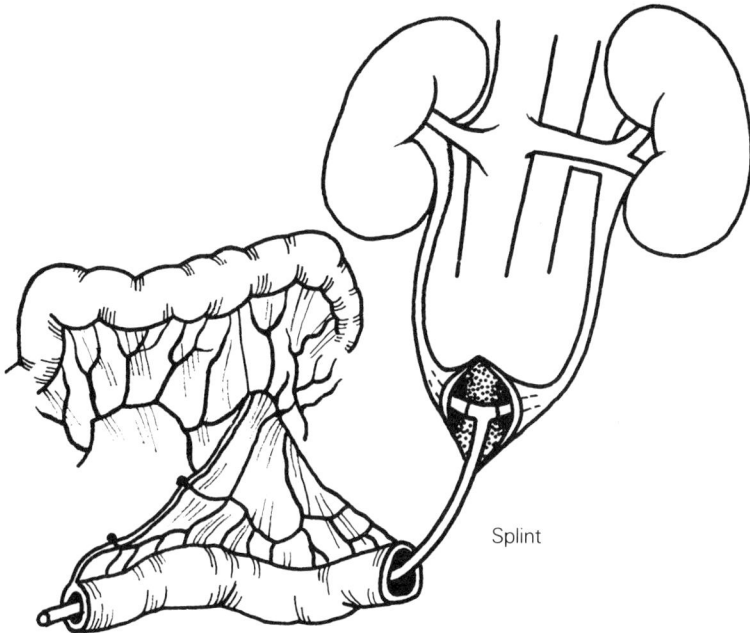

Figure 37.3 Urostomy

Indications for Surgery

1 Carcinoma of the bladder
2 Carcinoma of the bowel
3 Carcinoma of the pelvis
4 Trauma
5 Neurological damage
6 Congenital disorders
7 Ulcerative colitis
8 Diverticular disease
9 Familial polyposis
10 Intractable incontinence
11 Crohn's disease

Preoperative Preparation for Stoma Surgery

Physical preparation of the patient will vary according to the type of operation and the policies of individual surgeons and hospitals. This will involve the usual preparation for anaesthesia, preparation of the area of the body involved and of the bowel. Other specific procedures may also be included.

Psychological preparation of the individual facing stoma surgery should begin as soon as surgery has been considered. Boore (1978) and Hayward (1978) have illustrated the importance of preoperative information and explanation in reducing postoperative physical and psychological stress. The aims of presenting such information are as follows:

1   To help the individual with a stoma to return to his/her previous place in society whenever possible
2   To help in the process of adapting to a changed body image
3   To reduce anxiety. The individual's perception of life with a stoma may have a positive or detrimental influence on his/her rehabilitation. There may be myths and wrong information to dispel and his/her awareness of the experiences of another ostomist to discuss.
4   To explain that the presence of a stoma need not adversely affect any previous quality of life such as hobbies, work, social life or any other interests, although the underlying disease might
5   To prepare the individual for the appearance and likely behaviour pattern of the stoma
6   To reassure the individual that he/she will be able to manage an appliance whatever the environment
7   To assure the individual that he/she will be supported fully while in hospital and will not be discharged until he/she is confident about the stoma's care, and that continuing support will be available in the community.

Such preoperative education has been shown to increase cooperation and trust and to reduce anxiety, the length of time the individual remains in hospital and the amount of postoperative analgesia required. It should be borne in mind that any information given should be relevant to the patient's needs. Family and/or close friends may also be involved when appropriate.

Diet

Colostomy   It should be pointed out that certain foods may cause diarrhoea or excess flatus. It is suggested that rather than eliminate these items from the diet, the foods identified should be tried again in smaller portions. No food item affects everyone in the same way and it is best for the individual to experiment. He/she may may prefer to reduce the portion and prepare for the consequences. Beer may cause excess flatus. Other forms of alcohol will affect the ostomist as they do everyone else.

Ileostomy   Certain foods will cause excess flatus and pulses, cabbage, dried fruit, peanuts and coconut will be digested slowly. If eaten, therefore, they will need to be masticated well before swallowing.

Urostomy   There are no dietary restrictions. It must be stressed, however, that an adequate fluid intake must be maintained to minimize the risk of urinary infection. Approproximately 1.5 litres or 12 cups per day is recommended. The slow return of a normal appetite is a common feature following this operation and it gives cause for much anxiety. The individual should be warned of this and advised to take small, light meals supplemented by nutritious drinks. Normal appetite may not return for 2-3 months after the operation.

Fear of Malodour

This is a common fear often based on hearsay or experience with other ostomists in hospital or the community. Appliances are usually odour free when fitted correctly. Flatus may be released via charcoal filters and deodorizers are available. The individual must be reassured, however, that any problems that occur postoperatively will be investigated, with a good possibility of it being solved by such means as the use of alternative appliances or alteration of diet.

Sex and the Ostomist

The possibility of sexual impairment for both men and women after stoma surgery depends on the nature of the operation and ensuing damage to the nerves and tissues involved. Impairment may be permanent or temporary. In the latter case, resolution of the difficulty may take anything up to 2 years. Pre-and post-operative counselling may be required for both patient and partner. In cases of male impotence, surgical intervention, such as insertion of penile implants, may be offered if impairment becomes permanent. A useful survey of the psycho-social and sexual aspects will be found in Devlin and Plant (1979) and MacDonald (1982).

Acceptance of a change in the individual's body image may take months or years, as may as the loss of bladder or bowel control.

Personnel who may be Expected to Provide Information

1 Medical staff
2 Stoma care nurse
3 Nursing staff on the ward
4 Primary care team
5 Another suitable ostomist. 'Visitors' are trained by the voluntary associations and should be, ideally, of similar age, sex and background to the patient.

Useful Aids

1 Information booklets
2 Samples of the various appliances
3 Diagrams

These aids are valuable to reinforce and clarify the verbal information.

Preoperative Assessment

It is important to determine whether an individual will be able to manage a stoma by assessing the following:

1 Eyesight
2 Manual dexterity
3 The presence of other debilitating diseases, e.g. Parkinson's disease or arthritis
4 Mental confusion

5   Loss of limb
6   Skin conditions
7   Abdominal contours, e.g. the changes that occur with spina bifida.

Siting of the stoma is one of the most important preoperative tasks to be carried out by the doctor, stoma care nurse or experienced ward nurse (Figure 37.4). This minimizes future problems such as skin diseases or interference by the stoma with clothes. Among the priorities to be considered should be the following:

1   A flat area of the skin to facilitate safe adhesion of appliance
2   Avoidance of bony prominences such as hips or ribs
3   Avoidance of skin creases, especially in the region of the groin or the umbilicus
4   Avoidance of scars
5   Avoidance of waistline or belt areas
6   Maintenance of the stoma within the rectus sheath, as this reduces the risk of herniation later. The muscle may be identified by asking the patient to lie flat and then to raise his/her head. The muscle may also be palpated and is easily felt when the patient coughs.
7   The individual must be able to see the stoma site.

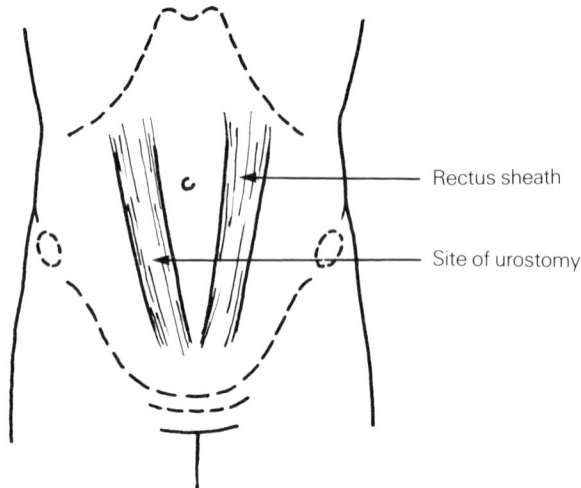

Figure 37.4   Site of urostomy

The individual must be observed lying, sitting in a comfortable chair, with the abdominal muscles relaxed, and standing. Consideration must be given to any bending or lifting involved with his/her work and any other activities in which he/she partakes. Account must also be taken of any weight gain or loss in the post-operative period.

Postoperative Period

Control of Stoma Action

Ileal Loop   Urine will dribble from the stoma every 20-30 seconds. The output may be slightly less after periods of reduced fluid intake, e.g. at night. An appliance has to be worn at all times.

Ileostomy   The ileostomy output, normally 500-800 ml every 24 hours, is of a porridge-like consistency and contain enzymes that will excoriate the skin if contact is allowed. While the effluent cannot be controlled, the ostomist may find that the stoma is more active after main meals.

Colostomy   The transverse colostomy output may benefit from 'bulking', using one of several agents. Individuals with a sigmoid colostomy may find that bran assists in producing a formed stool once or twice daily, as might synthetic agents such as Isogel and Celevac. Medications that reduce peristaltic action, e.g. codeine phosphate, may also be used to control diarrhoea. The only means of controlling a sigmoid colostomy, however, is by regular irrigation, if used. This method must be taught under supervision to suitable ostomists.

Postoperative Stages

Stage I   The patient is unable to perform his/her own stoma care but will observe those caring for him/her and may discuss it with them. Looking at the stoma may be very difficult for him/her and he/she may be over-aware of other people's reactions to it.

Stage II   As the individual's condition improves, he/she will be given a demonstration change of his/her appliance with full explanations of the principles of stoma care. This will be followed by further opportunities to discuss any problems or raise new queries. It is useful to involve the patient's partner or close friends or relatives at this stage. Their acceptance of the stoma may encourage the patient and help to restore his/her self-esteem. In the following days the patient will be encouraged to participate in and gradually assume responsibility for his/her own stoma care. He/she may now be ready to discuss appliances and choose the one that he/she wishes to use at home. Preparation for discharge will be discussed.

Stage III   The individual should now be independent, eating a normal diet, and ready for discharge. He/she should be confident in his/her stoma care.

The family should be closely involved during all three stages. They are also likely to require support and information so that they are in a position to help the ostomist.

Specific Discharge Plans

Follow-up Support   The patient is discharged with written reminders of how to care for his/her own stoma, how to obtain supplies of appliances, and any other information that may be required. The patient should have details of nonmedical stoma clinics, details about the relevant agencies and information about voluntary associations. Arrangements should also have been made for a home visit from the stoma care nurse and/or the community nurse.

Obtaining Supplies   All National Health Service patients with a permanent stoma are entitled to free prescriptions for their stoma care products, and should complete the relevant exemption from payment forms. Appliances can then be obtained from the local chemist or directly from the appropriate manufacturers.

Stoma Appliances and Accessories

Many of the appliances available today are very similar in style, colour and efficiency and often there is very little to choose between them when the time comes for the ostomist to decide what he/she would like to wear.

The aim of good stoma care is to return the individual to his/her place in society. One of the ways in which this can be achieved is to provide him/her with a safe, reliable appliance. This means that there must be no fear of leakage or odour and the appliance should be comfortable, unobtrusive and easy to handle. It is also necessary to ensure a problem-free skin and stoma.

Appliances

Choosing the Right Size of Appliance   Bags are labelled according to the size of the opening that fits around the stoma. To keep the skin unblemished, it must be protected from the stoma output. The size chosen, therefore, should be one that fits snugly around the stoma to within 0.5 cm of the stoma edge. This narrow edge of skin is left exposed to prevent any of the adhesives, some of which are more rigid than others, rubbing against the stoma. The appliances usually come with measuring guides to allow for correct choice of size. During the first weeks the oedematous stoma will reduce in size and the bags or flange of the two-piece type appliances will have to be changed accordingly.

Types of Appliance   Although some people whose stomas were created several years ago are wearing nondisposable rubber bags, most appliances used today are made of a specially designed laminate composed of three types of plastic. This should ensure that the appliances are

1   Leak proof
2   Odour proof
3   Unobtrusive
4   Noiseless
5   Disposable

The appliances differ slightly according to the stoma for which they are meant. All types, however, fall within one of two broad categories:

1   *One-piece*   This comprises a bag with an adhesive attached, e.g. Hollister or

Coloplast. When the bag is renewed, the adhesive is removed from the skin. Its advantage is that it is easy to handle, e.g. by an ostomist suffering from rheumatism.

2   *Two-piece*   This comprises a flange, for the skin, and a bag that clips on to the flange, e.g. System 2 or Eschmann 2 piece. Its advantages is that it can be used with ostomists who have a sore or sensitive skin as when bags are removed the skin is left undisturbed. Its disadvantage is that it is more difficult to handle as the bags must be clipped on securely and the flange hole needs to be cut out.

Drainable Bags

1   Bowel stoma bags
    Suitable for: Ileostomy, other large bowel stomas
    Stoma output: Fluid to semiformed (volume is too great for closed bags)
    Use: Emptied frequently, taking care to rinse outlet afterwards; may be left on for up to 3 days.
    Additional features: Flatus filters are absent in some as the fluid would obstruct the charcoal, rendering it useless, or will leak through the small opening; the outlet may have a separate clip or fixed 'roll up' closure
    Colour: Clear, white, pink/beige
2   Urinary stoma bags
    Suitable for: Urostomy
    Stoma output: Urine
    Use: Emptied frequently via a fixed tap; may be left on for up to 3 days
    Additional features: May be used with large collecting bag and tubing for night drainage
    Colour: Clear or white
3   Closed bags
    Suitable for: Sigmoid colostomy
    Stoma output: A normal stool
    Use: Changed once or twice a day
    Additional features: Some have incorporated flatus filters that allow the release of flatus through charcoal patches that absorb the odour
    Colour: Clear, white or pink/beige

Some of the bags may be fitted with protective adhesive especially for sensitive skin and all may be fitted with cotton covers.

Accessories

The specific products in this section have been mentioned as examples of what aids are available and reference to them is not necessarily intended as a recommendation.

Solutions for Skin and Stoma Cleaning   Soap and water, or water only, are sufficient. Detergents, disinfectants and antiseptics cause dryness and irritation and should not be used routinely. The stoma is not a wound or a lesion and should be regarded as a resited urethra or anus.

Skin Barriers

1   Creams
Unless made specifically for use on peristomal skin, these should not be used, as the residual surface film of grease prevents adherence of the appliance. Creams usually have a smoothing and moisturing effect.
Use: For sensitve skin, as a preventive measure.
Method: Use sparingly; massage gently into the skin until completely absorbed; excess grease may be wiped off with a tissue
Example: Chiron barrier cream (aluminium chlorohydrate 2% in an emulsified base)
Precaution: Not to be used in broken or sore skin

2   Skin gels/sealants
Use: Act as a film on the skin, firstly to prevent irritation, and secondly to give protection as it is removed with the adhesive of the bag, thus preventing removal of the stratum corneum of the skin.
Method: Use sparingly; pat on to the skin gently; dries quickly
Example: Skin Gel, Skin Prep
Precaution: Should not be used on broken skin as they contain alcohol and cause stinging

3   Lotions/Sprays
Use: As above
Method: Applied gently
Example: Skin Prep spray, OpSite spray, tincture of benzoin compound lotion
Precaution: As above. Tincture of benzoin is a mixture of 10% benzoin and 90% alcohol. Benzoin, a balsamic resin, is ground and combined with alcohol. Sensitivities to it are common. If applied to erythematous skin it causes pain, more irritation and weeping. When applied to good skin it acts as a protective and enhances adhesion of the appliance.

4   Protective wafers
Use: These are hypoallergenic and are designed to cover and protect skin, and allow healing if the skin is sore or broken. May be useful in cases of skin reaction or allergy to the adhesive of an appliance.
Method: The wafers may be cut to the required shape and fitted on to the skin. The appliances are then attached to the wafer. The rim of the wafer should not press against the stoma but should fit to 0.5 cm around it
Examples: Stomahesive, Comfeel and Seel a Peel. (Stomahesive is composed of gelatin, pectin, sodium carboxymethycellulose, and polyiso-butylene; it adheres painlessly to normal, erythematous, moist or broken skin; it is available in three sizes.)
Precautions: Allergy may occur, but rarely

5   Protective rings
Use: Protective rings are used to provide skin protection around the

stoma; they will protect a smaller area than the wafers mentioned above. They are also useful to fill in 'dips' or 'gulleys' in the skin.

Method: Like the wafers, they have an adhesive side and may be applied directly to the skin. They form an integral part of some of the appliances.

Example: Karaya rings, Seel a Peel rings and Cohesive washers (Karaya is a natural product developed from an Indian plant.)

Precautions: See section on protective wafers above.

6 Pastes

Use: Useful to fill in crevices and gulleys in the skin to provide a smooth surface for an appliance

Examples: Stomahesive paste, Colobase paste, Karaya gum paste and Orobase paste

Method: Stomahesive Either leave for 60 seconds after applying to the skin, when the surface will be dry, making the paste easier to mould into the skin contour, or apply with a spatula, or wet the finger first to prevent the paste sticking and mould the paste immediately. Will sting on raw areas as it contains alcohol. Apply a little Orahesive powder to these areas first.

Colobase paste: Use as above. Do not use on sore areas

Orobase paste: Similar to stomahesive in composition but with the addition of liquid paraffin. For protection of raw areas. Does not contain alcohol so will not cause local irritation

7 Powders

Use: For proctection of sore or raw areas without impeding adhesion of the appliance

Method: Sprinkle on affected areas

Examples: Karaya powder and Orahesive powder

Adhesive Preparation

1 Sprays

Use: Only required when appliance does not adhere well to the skin, e.g. due to leakage problems, difficult stoma site, or with abdominal fistulae

Method: Spray on appliance, not on the skin. Follow specific instructions on packaging. Removal should not be difficult.

Examples: Dow Corning Adhesive

Precaution: The individual products differ considerably in their method of application and it is recommended that the user consults the manufacturer's instructions

2 Lotions

Use: As above

Method: Pat gently on to skin. The individual products differ considerably in their method of application and it is recommended that the user consults the manufacturer's instructions

Examples: Saltair solution and tincture of benzoin compound

Deodorants

1 Aerosols
 Use: Absorb odour
 Method: One or two puffs into the air before emptying or removal of appliance
 Examples: Atmacol and ozone
2 Drops and powders
 Use: For deodorizing bag contents
 Method: One drop into appliance
 Examples: Dor (drops), Ostobon (powder), and Nilodor (drops)
 Precaution: Beware of overenthusiastic use which may result in a strong and distinctive odour that will become associated with stoma care
3 Other traditional methods
 Examples: Crushed aspirin, charcoal tablets and natural yoghurt
4 Flatus filters (charcoal filled)
 Use: To allow gradual release of flatus from the bag while allowing absorption of odour by the charcoal. The charcoal may only be effective for between 6 and 12 hours, depending on brand of filter. The filter will then require replacing with a fresh one
 Method: The individual products differ considerably in their method of application and it is recommended that the user consults the manufacturer's instructions
 Examples: Double sure, Filtrodor and Clinimed
 Precautions: Use of faltus filters is not advised when the stoma effluent is very fluid as the charcoal may become moist and the air outlet blocked. Many bags now have built-in filters

Useful Addresses

1 Association of Spina Bifida and Hydrocephalus, Tavistock House North, Tavistock Square, London SW1V 1PS (Tel: 01-388 1382/5)
2 Colostomy Welfare Group, 38/39 Eccleston Square, London SW1V 1PB (Tel: 01-828 5175)
3 Ileostomy Association of Great Britain, Amblehurst House, Chobham, Woking, Surrey GU24 9PZ (Tel: 09905-8277)
3 Urinary Conduit Association, Central Office, 36 York Road, Denton, Manchester M34 3HL (Tel: 061-226 8818)
4 Sexual and Personal Relationships of the Disabled, 286 Camden Road, London N7 0BJ (Tel: 01-607 8851/2)

References and Further Reading

Bailey A J (1977) Nursing the patient with a colostomy, Nursing Times 73: 382-385

Boore J R P (1978) A Prescription for Recovery: the Effects of Preoperative Preparation of Surgical Patients on Postoperative Stress, Recovery and Infection, Royal College of Nursing

Breckman B (1981) Stoma Care, Beaconsfield Publishers

Broadwell D C Jackson B J (1982) Princples of Ostomy Care, C V Mosby

Brooke B N et al. (1982) Stomas, W B Saunders

Cassel P (1980) Management of ulcerative colitis, Nursing 1st series no. 17: 727-729

Coloplast (undated) Back on Your Feet Again, Coloplast

Devlin H B Plant J (1979) Sexual function — an aspect of stoma care, British Journal of Sexual Medicine (1): 33-34, 37, (2): 6, 22, 26

Gray A (1980) A new lease of life, Nursing Times 76: 1616-1620

Hayward J (1978) Information — A Prescription Against Pain, Royal College of Nursing

MacDonald L (1982) Problems of the colostomy population, Stoma Care News 1: 45

Nursing Mirror (1983) Clinical Forum 8: Stoma Care. Nursing Mirror 157 (11): Supplement

Squibb Surgicare (undated) Understanding Urostomy, Squibb Surgicare

Squibb Surgicare (undated) Understanding Colostomy, Squibb Surgicare

Turner A G (1979) Urinary diversion, Journal of Community Nursing 2 (10): 20-21, 28

Whitethread M (1981) Ostomists: a world of difference, Journal of Community Nursing 5 (2): 4-5, 10

GUIDELINES: STOMA CARE

These procedural guidelines contain the basic information needed for changing a stoma appliance. Modifications may be made according to the following factors:

1 The place of change, i.e. bathroom, bedside, availability of sink, etc.
2 The person changing the appliance, i.e. nurse or patient
3 Type of appliance used, e.g. one- or two-piece, closed or drainable
4 Any accessories used, e.g. flatus filters, hypoallergenic tape, barrier creams, etc.

Equipment

1 Clean tray holding
   a Tissues
   b New appliances
   c Disposal bags for used appliances and tissues
   d Relevant accessories, e.g. flatus filters, tape, etc.
2 Bowl of warm water
3 Soap
4 Jug for contents of appliance

Procedure

Action	Rationale
1 Inform the patient of the proposed activity.	1 To obtain the patient's consent and cooperation.
2 Explain the procedure.	2 To familiarize the patient with the procedure.
3 Ensure that the patient is lying in a suitable and comfortable position where the patient will be able to watch the procedure, if he/she is well enough.	3 To allow good access to the stoma for cleaning and for secure application of the stoma bag. The patient will become familiar with the stoma and will also learn much about the care of the stoma by observation of the nurse.
4 Use a small protective pad to protect the patient's clothing from drips if the effluent is fluid.	4 Prevents the necessity of renewing clothing or bedclothes and demoralization of the patient due to any soiling.
5 If the bag is of the drainable type, empty the contents into a jug before removing the bag.	5 For ease of handling the appliance and prevention of spillage.
6 Remove the appliance. Peel the adhesive off the skin with one hand while exerting gentle pressure on the skin with the other.	6 To reduce trauma to the skin. Erythema as a result of removing the appliance is normal and quickly settles.
7 Remove excess faeces or mucus from the stoma with a dry tissue.	7 So that the stoma and surrounding skin are clearly visible.
8 Examine the skin and stoma for soreness, ulceration or other unusual phenomena. If the skin is unblemished and the stoma is a healthy red colour, proceed.	8 For the prevention of complications or the treatment of existing problems.
9 Wash the skin and stoma gently until they are clean.	9 To promote cleanliness and prevent skin excoriation.
10 Dry the skin and stoma gently but thoroughly.	10 The appliance will attach more securely to dry skin.
11 Apply a clean appliance.	
12 Dispose of soiled tissues and the used bag. Rinse the bag through in the sluice with water, wrap it in a disposable bag and place it in an appropriate plastic bin. At home the bag should be emptied into the toilet; a closed bag may be cut at the lower end, then rinsed using a jug or by holding it under the flushing water. Wrap the bag in newspaper, tie it in a plastic bag and dispose of it in a rubbish bag.	12 Faecal material in waste bags is a potential source of infection. Excreta should be disposed of down the sluice.

Action	Rationale
13 Wash your hands thoroughly.	13 To prevent spread of infection by contaminated hands.

GUIDELINES: COLLECTION OF A SPECIMEN OF URINE FROM AN ILEAL CONDUIT OR UROSTOMY

Equipment

1 Sterile dressing pack
2 Soft catheter — tracheal type, not larger than 12 or 14 gauge
3 Sterile gloves
4 Disposable plastic apron
5 Universal specimen container
6 Skin cleansing solution, e.g. Savlodil
7 Alcohol-based hand wash solution, e.g. Hibisol
8 Clean stoma appliance
9 Clean topical swabs

Procedure

Action	Rationale
1 Explain the procedure to the patient.	1 To gain the patient's consent and cooperation.
2 Ensure that the patient is in a comfortable position, e.g. sitting up, supported by pillows, and that the stoma is easily accessible.	
3 Screen the bed, then wash and dry your hands.	3 For the patient's privacy and to reduce the risk of cross-infection. Curtains are drawn at this stage so that dust and airborne organisms disturbed by the curtains do not settle on the sterile trolley.
4 Prepare the trolley and take it to the patient's bedside.	
5 Put on a disposable plastic apron.	5 To prevent cross-infection.
6 Remove the sterile dressing pack, catheter and receiver from their outer wrappings. Place them on the top shelf of the trolley.	
7 Remove the appliance from the stoma and cover the stoma with a clean topical swab.	To absorb spillage from the stoma.
8 Clean your hands with an alcohol-based hand wash solution, such as Hibisol, and put on sterile gloves	8 To reduce the risk of introducing infection into the stoma during the procedure.

Action	Rationale
before opening the sterile field on the trolley.	
9 Remove the gauze with forceps and discard it. Arrange a sterile towel to absorb spillage from the stoma.	9 To keep the areas as clean as possible and to protect the patient and the bedclothes from spilled urine.
10 Clean around the stoma with a skin cleansing solution, such as Savlodil, from the centre outwards. Dry the area.	10 Good cleansing of the area reduces the risk of introduction of surface pathogens into the ileal loop.
11 Insert the catheter tip gently to a depth of 2.5-5 cm only and wait for urine to drain through. Collect the sample in the specimen container. The recommended volume is 3-5 ml.	11 Gentle handling reduces the risk of ileal perforation and is more comfortable for the patient.
12 Remove the catheter and seal in the specimen container. Remove your gloves and attend to stoma care and apply a pouch as usual. Make the patient comfortable.	
13 Dispose of equipment.	
14 Wash and dry your hands.	14 To prevent cross-infection.
15 Check that the specimen is labelled correctly and dispatch it to the laboratory with the appropriate forms.	

NURSING CARE PLAN

Problem	Cause	Suggested Action
1 Leakage of urine or faeces	1 **a** Ill fitting appliance	1 **a** The opening of the appliance should fit snugly around the stoma.
	b Skin creases or 'gulleys' preventing correct application of adhesive	**b** Build up indented areas and fill in gulleys to create a smooth surface, e.g. using Stomahesive paste.
	c Infrequent emptying of drainable bag leading to stress on adhesion	**c** Drainable bags should be emptied frequently, e.g. 2-3 hourly if necesssary.
2 Sore skin	2 **a** Leakage	2 **a** As above.

Problem	Cause	Suggested Action
	b Skin reaction to adhesive	**b** Change the make of appliance or apply a protective square between skin and adhesive. Anti-inflammatory agents may be required for very severe reactions.
	c Poor hygiene	**c** Improve the technique of nurses or patients.
3 Odour	3 **a** Ill fitting appliance; lack of seal between skin and adhesive	3 **a** Fit the appliance with care. Consider a change of the type of appliance.
	b Poor hygiene	**b** Improve the technique of nurses or patient.
	c Poor technique, e.g. when emptying drainable bag	**c** Empty the bag, then rinse the end with water to ensure that it is clean before closing.
	d Ineffective flatus filters	**d** Use another type of filter or change the filter more frequently. (Filters should be peeled off and replaced as necessary.) Effectiveness lasts 6-12 hours.

Urostomy Specimen

1 Stoma specimen of urine contaminated	1 Contaminants introduced during specimen collection	1 Take a repeat specimen, observing aseptic procedure and cleaning the stoma well.
2 Ileum perforated during urine specimen collection	2 Catheter too hard or inserted too roughly	2 Report to a doctor immediately.
3 Difficulty passing catheter into conduit	2 **a** Small degree of retraction of ileum	2 **a** Apply gentle pressure to the area around the stoma to make it protrude.

Problem	Cause	Suggested Action
	b Unpredicable direction of ileum	**b** Insert your little finger gently into the stoma to determine the direction of the conduit. Insert the catheter tip along this line.

38

SURGICAL WOUNDS AND DRAINS

The following procedures offer a guide to the management of a selection of surgical wounds and drains.

SURGICAL WOUND MANAGEMENT

Definition

Surgical wounds are classified in various ways. A generally accepted model is to divide them into

1   *Simple wounds,* i.e. wounds where no tissue has been lost, as in a simple appendicectomy
2   *Complex wounds,* i.e. wounds where tissue has been lost and where skin grafting may be required.

REFERENCE MATERIAL

Types of Surgical Wounds

Cruse and Foord (1980), in a definitive study of the epidemiology of wound infection carried out over a 10 year period and embracing over 62 000 wounds, identified four types of surgical wounds:

Clean Wounds

In such wounds, no infection is encountered; there is no break in the aseptic technique; and no hollow muscular organ has been opened. Three operations, viz. cholecystectomy, appendicectomy in passing and hysterectomy are included in this category, provided that no acute inflammation is present.

Clean Contaminated Wounds

Here a hollow muscular organ is opened but minimal spillage of contents has occurred.

Table 38.1 Westaby's stages of wound repair

Stage	Phase	Time	Action
I	Traumatic inflammation	0 - 3 days	The wound is red, swollen and hot. Blood vessels bleed and platelets and fibrin cause clotting. Histamine is released, causing dilation of capillary blood vessels and thus allowing serum and white blood cells to enter the injured area, which results in oedema, increased colour and heat.
II	Destructive phase	1 - 6 days	Polymorphs and macrophages clear the wound of dead and inessential tissue. Wounds cannot heal in the absence of macrophages, which not only remove bacteria but are responsible for the formation and replication of fibroblasts, without which collagen cannot be produced.
III	Proliferative phase	3 - 4 days	Macrophages continue to clear the wound of debris. Fibroblasts continue to produce collagen, the main constituent of many body tissues. In the absence of lactate ions and vitamin C there will be a great reduction in the ability of fibroblasts to produce collagen. Adequate nutrition is, therefore, essential. The interaction of the various tissues during this period helps to produce granulation tissue. The amount of granulation tissue is dependent on the degree of inflammation. During Stage I, excessive inflammation may lead to over granulation with increased scar tissue (keloid and hypertrophic scars). In this phase the wound is very fragile and care must be exercised during dressings and mobilization.
IV	Maturation phase	24 days - 1 year	The scar changes colour from pink to white due to decrease in the activities of the healing process already mentioned. Collagen continues to be produced for some months to strengthen the wound. Thereafter production ceases and the wound gradually assumes the texture and pliancy of normal skin.

Contaminated Wounds

Here a hollow muscular organ is opened accompanied by gross spillage of contents or acute inflammation, without pus, is encountered. Also included in this category are fresh (within 4 hours) traumatic wounds, wounds that result from opening of the colon or wounds resulting from surgery where there has been a major break in aseptic technique.

Dirty Wounds

Such wounds include those where pus or a perforated viscus is encountered at surgery, and traumatic wounds of longer than 4 hours duration.

Wound Healing

To manage postoperative wounds appropriately, nurses must be skilled in the recognition of the normal mechanisms of healing, Westaby (1981) describes four stages of repair, which are given in Table 38.1.

Care of surgical wounds should be aimed at providing the ideal microenvironment in which wound healing can take place. Management must be relevant and the nurse should be able to support nursing interventions by written evidence or nursing research findings.

There are numerous wound agents and dressings available at present. New products constantly appear on the market with varying as claims to their efficacy. Nurses must not accept such claims at face value until they themselves have evaluated the product or dressing in the clinical situation. (For further information on a selection of such products, see the procedure on pressure sores, pages 341-350.)

SURGICAL WOUND DRAINS

Definition

A surgical wound drain is any piece of equipment used in surgery to drain off liquid or allow it to flow away slowly.

Indications

The use of surgical wound drains is indicated under the following conditions:

1   To drain intra-abdominal collections of pus, empyema or purulent pericarditis
2   Whenever collections of fluid are likely to occur postoperatively, when an

anastamosis or closure of a large organ produces a discharge or when haemostasis has not been achieved at surgery

3 To redirect body fluids to allow a new suture line time to heal.

REFERENCE MATERIAL

Types of Surgical Drains

There are several types of drain in general use:

1 *Redivac*   Plastic tube attached to a sterile vacuum drainage bottle
2 *Wick drain (Penrose)*   Soft latex tube with a gauze wick
3 *Paul's tubing*   Soft rubber tubing
4 *Corrugated drain*   Flat strips of corrugated rubber, plastic or latex
5 *Norton Morgan*   Paul's tubing with a corrugated drain inserted
6 *Suction drain and sump drain*   Rubber or latex catheter attached to a suction pump.

References and Further Reading

Bernhard L A (1982) Wound healing, Association of Operating Room Nurses Journal 35: 1067

Brubacher L L (1982) To heal a draining wound, Registered Nurse 45 (3): 30-35

Brunner L S Suddarth D K (1982) Lippincott Manual of Medical Surgical Nursing, Harper and Row, Volume 1, Chs 4-5

Cruse P J E Foord R (1980) The epideminology of wound infection, Surgical Clinics of North America 60 (1): 27-40

Knight B (1981) The history of wound treatment, Wound Care no. 2, Nursing Times 77: 5-8

Westaby S (1981) Healing — the wound mechanisim — 1, Wound Care No. 3, Nursing Times: 9-12

Westaby S (1982) Wound closure, Wound Care no. 6, Nursing Times 78: 21-24

GUIDELINES: CLEAN WOUND WITHOUT EXUDATE

Equipment

1 As for aseptic technique procedure (see page 10)
2 Sterile semiocclusive nonadherent dressing

Procedure

Action	Rationale
1 Explain the procedure to the patient.	1 To obtain the patient's consent and cooperation.
2 Perform dressing using an aseptic technique.	2 To prevent infection. (For further information on asepsis see the

Action	Rationale
	procedure on aseptic technique, pages 10-11.
3 Disturb the wound as little as possible.	3 To allow natural healing to occur.
4 When necessary cover the wound with a nonadherent dressing.	4 To provide the best possible environment for wound healing to take place. To reduce the risk of infection. To prevent a suture line rubbing against clothing.
5 Describe the wound carefully in the appropriate documentation.	5 For accurate evaluation of progress in wound healing.

GUIDELINES: CLEAN WOUND WITH EXUDATE

Equipment

1 As for aseptic technique procedure (see page 10)
2 Wound swab or sterile syringe

Procedure

Action	Rationale
1 Explain the procedure to the patient.	1 To obtain the patient's consent and cooperation.
2 Perform dressing using an aseptic technique.	2 To prevent infection. (For further information on asepsis, see the procedure on aseptic technique, pages 10-11.)
3 Moisten the dressing with an appropriate sterile solution, such as normal saline.	3 To facilitate removal of the dressing without destruction of granulation tissue.
4 Obtain a specimen of discharge with a wound swab or syringe.	4 To ascertain whether infection is present.
5 Clean the wound with an appropriate sterile solution, such as normal saline.	5 To prevent infection.
6 If exudate is excessive, cover the wound with a sterile dressing pad.	6 To prevent escape of and to absorb the exudate.
7 Assess the condition of the surrounding skin.	7 To preclude deterioration of skin leading to excoriation.
8 Describe the wound and the type of exudate in appropriate documentation and amend the care plan accordingly.	8 For accurate evaluation of progress in healing of the wound.

GUIDELINES: DEHISCENT WOUND WITH MINIMAL EXUDATE

Equipment

1 As for aseptic technique procedure (see page 10)
2 Wound swab
3 Sterile padded dressing
4 Sterile adhesive sutures, such as Steristrips

Procedure

Action	Procedure
1 Explain the procedure to the patient.	1 To obtain the patient's consent and cooperation.
2 Perform dressing using an aseptic technique.	2 To prevent infection (For further information on asepsis, see the procedure on aseptic technique, pages 10-11.)
3 Moisten the dressing with an appropriate sterile solution, such as normal saline.	3 To facilitate removal of the dressing without distruction of granulation tissue.
4 Clean the wound with an appropriate sterile solution, such as normal saline.	4 To prevent infection.
5 Obtain a specimen of the discharge with a wound swab or syringe.	5 To ascertain whether infection is present.
6 If possible, close the wound and apply adhesives sutures, such as Steristrips.	6 To maintain the apposition of wound edges and thus to promote healing.
7 Apply a nonadherent dressing.	7 To facilitate atraumatic dressing changes and minimize the risk of infection.
8 Assess the condition of surrounding skin.	8 To prelude deterioration of skin leading to excoriation.
9 Apply a sterile dressing pad.	9 To prevent escape of and to absorb the exudate.
10 Change the dressing only when necessary.	10 Frequent dressing changes reduce the skin surface temperature, delaying healing and allowing greater opportunity for infection to occur.
11 Describe the wound and type of exudate in appropriate documentation and amend the care plan accordingly.	11 For accurate evaluation of progress in healing of the wound.

GUIDELINES: DEHISCENT WOUND WITH COPIOUS EXUDATE

Equipment

1 As for aseptic technique procedure (see page 10)
2 Wound swab or sterile syringe
3 Sterile padded dressing
4 Sterile adhesive sutures, such as Steristrips
5 Wound irrigation device with stomahesive, such as Surgicare
6 Sterile irrigation syringe
7 Karaya paste

Procedure

Action	Rationale
1 Explain the procedure to the patient.	1 To obtain the patient's consent and cooperation.
2 Obtain a specimen of the discharge with a wound swab or syringe. Repeat after 7 days.	2 To ascertain whether infection is present.
3 Perform dressing using an aseptic technique.	3 To prevent infection. (For further information on asepsis, see the procedure on aseptic technique, pages 10-11).
4 Gently syringe the wound with an appropriate solution, such as normal saline.	4 To clean the wound and remove debris.
5 Assess the condition of the surrounding skin.	5 To preclude deterioration of skin leading to excoriation.
6 Where possible close the wound and apply adhesive sutures, such as Steristrips.	6 To maintain apposition of wound edges, thus promoting healing.
7 Make an opening in the stomahesive backing of the wound irrigation device, not larger than the wound defect.	7 A well fitted irrigation device prevents exudate from washing on to surrounding tissue, leading to excoriation.
8 Fill crevices and skin folds with karaya paste.	8 To ensure a smooth surface for the irrigation device and thus prevent leakage of exudate.
9 Remove the backing sheet from the stomahesive and place the device over the wound.	9 The irrigating device has a clear chamber through which the wound can be observed without removing the device.
10 Irrigate the wound as necessary.	10 To prevent excessive accumulation

Action	Rationale
	of exudate. Purulent and exudating wounds may be irrigated by connecting the inlet valve to sterile normal saline, or topical antibiotic, as prescribed, and the outlet valve to a drainage bag. This ensures a closed system of drainage.
11 Close the inlet and outlet valves of the irrigation chamber.	11 To prevent loss of exudate and minimize the risk of infection.
12 Leave the irrigating device untouched for as long as possible.	12 The wound should remain untouched as long as the device is patent and until exudate lessens to a sufficient degree to allow resuturing or healing by secondary intention.
13 Describe the wound and type of exudate in appropriate documentation.	13 For accurate evaluation of progress in healing of the wound.
14 Record the amount of irrigation.	14 To assess fluid loss due to exudate, and to ensure a balance between input and output of irrigating fluids.
15 Encourage the patient to take a nutritious diet, ensuring sufficient intake of Vitamin C and trace elements.	15 Where exudate output is excessive there may be severe protein depletion. Vitamin C and trace elements help promote healing

GUIDELINES: DRAIN DRESSING (REDIVAC AND CLOSED DRAINAGE SYSTEMS)

Equipment

1   As for aseptic technique procedure (page 10)
2   Keyhole dressing
3   Sterile padded dressing

Procedure

Action	Rationale
1 Explain the procedure to the patient.	1 To obtain the patient's consent and cooperation.
2 Perform dressing using an aseptic technique.	2 To prevent infection. (For further information on asepsis, see the procedure on aseptic technique, pages 10-11.)
3 Clean the surrounding skin with an appropriate sterile solution, such as normal saline.	3 To prevent infection.
4 Ensure that the skin suture holding the drain site in position is intact.	4 To prevent the drain from leaving the wound.
5 Cover the drain site with a keyhole	5 To protect the drain site and to

Action	Rationale
dressing and sterile padded dressing.	prevent infection entering the site.
6 Tape securely.	
7 Ensure that the drain is primed or that the suction pump is in working order.	7 To ensure continuity of drainage.

GUIDELINES: CHANGE OF VACUUM BOTTLE (REDIVAC AND CLOSED DRAINAGE SYSTEMS)

Equipment

1 Sterile topical swabs
2 Artery forceps — tip to be covered with rubber
3 Sterile drainage bottle

Procedure

Action	Rationale
1 Explain the procedure to the patient.	1 To obtain the patient's consent and cooperation.
2 Wash your hands.	2 To minimize the risk of infection.
3 Clean the nozzle of wall suction apparatus with an appropriate solution and prime a sterile vacuum bottle.	3 To ensure sterility and to prepare the bottle for attachment to the drainage tube.
4 Measure the contents of the bottle to be changed and record this in the appropriate documents.	4 To maintain an accurate record of drainage from the wound.
5 Clamp the tube with artery forceps and remove the bottle.	5 To prevent air and contamination entering the wound via the drain.
6 Clean the end of the tube and attach it to the sterile bottle.	6 To maintain sterility.
7 Remove the artery forceps.	7 To re-establish the drainage system.
8 Ensure that the bottle is primed.	8 To ensure that drainage continues.
9 If the vacuum is constantly lost, take down the dressing and examine the entry site of the drain.	9 To ensure that the drain has not become dislodged.
10 Re-dress as for a closed drainage system.	

GUIDELINES: REMOVAL OF DRAIN (REDIVAC AND CLOSED DRAINAGE SYSTEMS)

Equipment

1 As for aseptic technique procedure (page 10)
2 Sterile scissors or suture cutter

Procedure

Action	Rationale
1 Check the patient's operation notes.	1 To establish the number and site(s) of sutures.
2 Explain the procedure to the patient.	2 To obtain the patient's consent and cooperation.
3 Perform the procedure using an aseptic technique.	3 To prevent infection. (For further information on asepsis, see the procedure on aseptic technique, pages 10-11.)
4 Only clean the wound if necessary, using an appropriate sterile solution, such as normal saline.	4 To prevent microorganisms invading the suture pathway at removal.
5 Hold the knot of the suture with forceps and gently lift it upwards.	5 To allow space for the scissors or suture cutter to be placed underneath.
6 Cut the shortest end of the suture as close to the skin as possible.	6 To allow the suture to be liberated from the drain without any part of the exposed suture travelling through subcutaneous tissue.
7 Gently remove the drain.	
8 Cover the drain site with a sterile dressing and tape securely.	8 To prevent infection entering the drain site.
9 Measure and record the contents of the drainage bottle in the appropriate documents.	9 To maintain an accurate record of drainage from the wound.

GUIDELINES: DRAIN DRESSING (PENROSE, PAUL'S TUBING, CORRUGATED AND NORTON MORGAN DRAINAGE SYSTEMS)

Equipment

1   As for aseptic technique procedure (page 10)
2   Sterile padded dressings
3   Stomahesive wafers
4   Keyhole dressing
5   Drainable stoma bag

Procedure

Action	Rationale

Minimal Drainage

1 Explain the procedure to the patient.	1 To obtain the patient's consent and cooperation.
2 Perform the procedure using an	2 To prevent infection. (For further

Action	**Rationale**
aseptic technnique.	information on asepsis, see the procedure on aseptic technique, pages 10-11.)
3 Clean the surrounding skin with an appropriate sterile solution, such as normal saline.	3 To prevent infection.
4 Cut a hole slightly larger than the site in a stomahesive wafer and apply the wafer to the skin surrounding the drain.	4 To protect the skin from the drainage, which may cause excoriation. The wafer should fit as close to the drain as possible without interrupting the flow of effluent.
5 Leave the stomahesive wafer in position until the drain is removed.	5 To continue to protect vulnerable skin.
6 Cover the drain site and the stomahesive wafer with a keyhole dressing and sterile dressing pad. Tape securely.	6 To prevent spillage of drainage. To prevent infection.
7 Change the dressing whenever it becomes soiled.	7 To ensure patient comfort. To prevent infection. To maintain the integrity of the surrounding skin.
8 Describe the wound and type of drainage in appropriate documents and amend the care plan accordingly.	8 For accurate evaluation of progress of drainage.

Copious Drainage

1 Follow the procedure as above to the stage where stomahesive has been applied (i.e. items 1-5).	
2 Cover the drain with a drainable stoma bag.	2 To allow effluence to drain into the bag.
3 Ensure that the drain is enclosed by the aperture of the bag.	3 To prevent excoriation of the surrounding skin. To contain any odour.
4 Secure the bag with suitable tape if necessary.	4 To prevent the bag from becoming detached from the skin.
5 Empty the contents of the bag regularly and record the amount in appropriate documents.	5 To prevent accumulated fluid from detaching the bag from the skin due to its weight. To maintain an accurate record of drainage.

GUIDELINES: SHORTENING OF DRAIN (PENROSE, ETC., DRAINAGE SYSTEMS)

Equipment

1 As for aseptic technique procedure (see page 10)

2   Sterile scissors or suture cutter
3   Sterile safety pin
4   Drainable stoma bag

Procedure

Action	Rationale
1 Check the patient's operation notes.	1 To establish the length of drain to be shortened.
2 Explain the procedure to the patient.	2 To obtain the patient's consent and cooperation.
3 Remove the dressing or stoma bag and measure the contents.	3 To record accurately the amount of drainage.
4 Perform dressing using an aseptic technique.	4 To prevent infection. (For further information on asepsis, see the procedure on aseptic technique, pages 10-11.)
5 Only clean the wound if necessary, using an appropriate sterile solution, such as normal saline.	5 To prevent microorganisms invading the wound.
6 Hold the knot of the suture with forceps and gently lift upwards.	6 To allow space for the scissors or suture cutter to be placed underneath.
7 Cut the shortest end of the suture as close to the skin as possible.	7 To allow the suture to be liberated from the drain without any part of the exposed suture travelling through subcutaneous tissue.
8 Using forceps, gently ease the drain out of the wound to the length requested by the surgeon (usually 3-5 cm)	
9 Place a sterile safety pin through the drain as close to the skin as possible.	9 To prevent retraction into the wound.
10 Cut 3-5 cm from the distal end of the drain.	10 To ensure that there is not an unnecessary amount of drain in the drainage bag. To ensure patient comfort.
11 Place a clean, suitably sized drainage bag over the drain site.	11 To allow effluent to drain into the bag. To prevent excoriation of the surrounding skin. To contain any odour.
12 Secure the bag with a suitable tape if necessary	12 To prevent the bag from becoming detached from the skin.

GUIDELINES: REMOVAL OF DRAIN (PENROSE, ETC., DRAINAGE DRESSING)

Equipment

1 As for aseptic technique procedure (page 10)
2 Sterile scissors or suture cutter.

Procedure

Action	Rationale
1 Explain the procedure to the patient.	1 To obtain the patient's consent and cooperation.
2 Check the patient's operation notes.	2 To establish the number and site(s) of sutures.
3 Perform the procedure using an aseptic technique.	3 To prevent infection. (For further information on asepsis, see the procedure on aseptic technique, pages 10-11.)
4 Only clean the wound if necessary, using an appropriate sterile solution, such as normal saline.	4 To prevent microorganisms invading the suture pathway at removal.
5 Hold the knot of the suture with forceps and gently lift upwards.	5 To allow space for the scissors or suture cutter to be placed underneath.
6 Cut the shortest end of the suture as close to the skin as possible.	6 To allow the suture to be liberated from the drain without any part of the exposed suture travelling through subcutaneous tissue.
7 Using sterile forceps, gently remove the drain.	
8 Cover the drain with a sterile dressing and secure it with hypoallergenic tape.	8 To prevent infection entering the drain site.
9 Record removal of the drain in the appropriate documents and alter the nursing care plan.	9 To maintain an accurate record.

39

TEMPERATURE

Definition

Body temperature represents the balance between heat gain and heat loss as measured by a thermometer.

Indications

Measurement of body temperature is carried out for two reasons:

1 To establish a base-line temperature
2 To monitor fluctuations in temperature.

REFERENCE MATERIAL

The Temperature Recording Site

Oral

The pocket of tissue at the base of the tongue lies immediately above the sublingual artery. The proxmity of this artery to the external carotid artery means that changes in core temperature are quickly reflected here.

Oral temperatures are affected by the temperatures of ingested foods and fluids and by the muscular activity of chewing. Smoking will also affect the thermometer reading. It is recommended that the nurse waits 15 minutes following any of these activities before inserting the thermometer to allow the temperature to return to base-line level.

It is important that the thermometer is placed in the sublingual pocket and not in the area under the front of the tongue as there may be a temperature difference of up to 1.7 °C between these areas. The sublingual pockets are more protected from the air currents which cool the frontal areas and would result in a false low reading of a thermometer placed there.

Rectal

The rectal temperature is often higher than the oral temperature because this site is more sheltered from the external environment. However, this does not necessarily imply an increase in accuracy as the rectum is far from the central circulation and is inferior to the oral site in reflecting changes in temperature in the vital central organs. The presence of soft stool may separate the thermometer from the bowel wall and give a false reading, especially if the central temperature is changing rapidly. In infants this method is not recommended as it provides a risk of rectal ulceration or perforation.

A rectal thermometer should be inserted at least 4 cm in an adult to obtain the most accurate reading.

Axilla

The axilla is considered a less desirable site than the others since it is not close to major vessels and skin surface temperatures vary more with changes in temperature of the environment. It is a convenient site for patients who are unsuitable for or who cannot tolerate oral thermometers, e.g. after general anaesthetic.

To take an axillary temperature reading the thermometer should be placed in the centre of the armpit, with the patient's arm firmly against the side of the chest. The thermometer will take longer to register than when in the oral site.

Note: Whatever site is chosen for temperature measurement, it is important that this is then used consistently as switching between sites can produce a record that is misleading or difficult to interpret.

The Time for Recording Temperatures

The average person experiences circadian rhythms which make their highest body temperature occur in the late afternoon or early evening, i.e. between 4 p.m. and 8 p.m. The most sensitive time for detecting pyrexias appears to be between 7 p.m. and 8 p.m. (Angerami 1980). This should be considered when interpreting variations in 4-hourly or 6-hourly observations and when taking once-daily temperatures.

Instruments Used for Recording Temperatures

The most commonly used instruments are mercury in glass thermometers and electronic thermometers. A comparison of the use and effectiveness of these thermometers is made in Table 39.1.

References and Further Reading

Abbey J C et al. (1978) How long is that thermometer accurate? American Journal of Nursing 78: 1375-1376

Angerami E L S (1980) Epidemiological study of body temperature in patients in a teaching hospital, International Journal of Nursing Studies 17: 91-99

Blainey C G (1974) Site selection in taking body temperatures, American Journal of Nursing 74: 1859-1861

Litsky B Y (1976) A study of temperature taking systems, Supervisor Nurse 7: 48-53
Moorat D S (1976) The cost of taking temperatures, Nursing Times 72: 767-770
Stronge J L (1980) Electronic thermometers: a costly rise in efficiency? Nursing
    Mirror 151 (8): 29

Table 39.1   A comparison of mercury in glass and electronic thermometers

Mercury in glass thermometer	Electronic thermometer
Accuracy	
Accuracy of reading varies with the time the thermometer is left in the mouth. Premature removal, i.e. less than 2 minutes, may give a false, low result.	Audible tone and display light become apparent when the body temperature is reached — which reduces the risk of premature removal.
Reading on the scale must be interpreted by the nurse.	Digital readout minimizes the risk of interpretation error.
Instrument becomes increasingly likely to lose accuracy and be less reliable after use and/or storage (Abbey et al.1978).	Little research is available on long term accuracy, but a comparative accuracy study by Moorat (1976) showed that this type of thermometer demonstrated less fluctuation by comparison with mercury in glass or disposable types.
Hygiene	
Thermometers should be wiped clean after each use with a new swab saturated with isopropyl alcohol 70% and left dry. Wet or dirty thermometers support bacterial growth. Wool swabs in thermometer holders are not recommended for this reason.	Disposable cover slip over probe should be discarded after a single use. The nurse should keep the instrument around his/her neck and the patient must be discouraged from holding the end of the thermometer because of the risk of cross-infection.
Cost	
Materials are less expensive but temperature taking involves more time. The nursing time for trained staff increases the cost above that of electronic thermometers (Stronge 1980).	Materials are more expensive but the time factor is greatly reduced. Moorat (1976) suggested that a cost reduction of 300% could be achieved by utilizing this type of instrument.

GUIDELINES: TEMPERATURE

Equipment

1 Electronic thermometer and oral probe
2 Disposable probe covers.

The blue probe is for oral and axillar procedures; the red probe is for rectal procedures.

Procedure

Before use, remove the thermometer from its base unit; a neck strap is provided for convenience and its use is recommended.

Action	Rationale
1 Explain the procedure to the patient.	1 To obtain the patient's consent and cooperation.
2 Remove the probe from the stored position in the face of the thermometer and check that the reading is 34 °C.	2 If the readout does not register 34 °C the machine is faulty and should not be used.
3 Push the probe firmly into the probe cover.	3 The cover protects the tip of the probe and is necessary for correct functioning of the instrument.
4 Ask the patient to open his/her mouth and insert the probe under the tongue into the 'heat pocket' at the posterior base of the tongue.	4 The highest oral temperature reading is at the posterior base of tongue, which is least affected by environmental conditions.
5 Ask the patient to close his/her mouth.	5 To increase the patient's comfort and to minimize the risk of temperature lowering by the external environment.
6 Hold the thermometer in place until an audible tone is heard and the red light comes on.	6 Tissue contact must be maintained for an accurate reading to be obtained.
7 If figures on the display stop rising without an audible tone, tissue contact has been lost. Regain tissue contact and continue.	7 The probe must be supported outside the mouth as its top heavy shape tends to move the sensitive tip out of the heat pocket. The nurse should hold the probe in place as the patient may introduce cross-infection.
8 Remove the probe from the patient's mouth and note the temperature displayed.	8 An audible tone and a red light indicate that the patient's temperature is as displayed by the machine.

Action	Rationale
9 Discard the probe cover into a waste bag by pressing the probe top with your thumb.	9 Probe covers are for single use only. The discard mechanism prevents transfer of the patient's saliva to the nurse's hands.
10 Return the probe to its storage position in the face of the thermometer, cancelling the temperature reading.	10 The probe is best protected from damage in this storage position.
11 Return the thermometer to its base unit and ensure that the charge light is on.	11 The thermometer should be left charged and ready for its next use.

NURSING CARE PLAN

Category	Frequency	Rationale
1 On admission	1 Once only, preferably when the patient has settled in	1 To provide an accurate base-line.
2 Preoperative or pre-investigation	2 Once only	2 To provide an accurate base-line and to check that the patient is not pyrexial.
3 Pyrexial patients	3 At least 6-hourly; possibly hourly. Frequency is affected by direction of temperature movement, e.g. rising, falling or static.	3 To monitor the condition of the patient so that any necessary action can be instigated. *Note:* Patients receiving steroids may show only very slight rises in temperature even when suffering from severe infection.
4 Patients receiving blood transfusions	4 When the unit is put up, observe the patient at 5 minute intervals for the first 15-20 minutes and again 1 hour later if the patient's condition warrants it. If the patient's pulse rate rises or the patient shows other signs of reaction, record again, and then as often as the situation demands.	4 To record a base-line temperature and to monitor any reaction to the transfusion.
5 Postoperative (minor surgery)	5 On return from the theatre only	5 To detect postoperative hypothermia.

Category	Frequency	Rationale
6 Postoperative (major surgery)	6 On return from the theatre, then 4- to-6-hourly. Continue at your discretion, depending on the nature of the surgery.	6 To detect postoperative hypothermia and to monitor any pyrexia, e.g. due to infection.
7 Patient receiving steroids	7 Four-hourly	7 A very slight rise in temperature may be indicative of severe infection.
8 Patients receiving cytotoxic chemotherapy or antibiotics	8 Daily	8 To detect any development of infection or drug reaction.
9 Patients receiving radiotherapy	9 As necessary, depending on area and dose	9 To detect developing infections when defence mechanisms are lowered by the nature of the treatment.
10 Patients with radioactive caesium implants	10 Every 2 hours	10 Frequent monitoring is required to detect development of pelvic cellulitis due to a proflavin pack or postoperative complications, e.g. urinary tract infection or chest infection.
11 Patients with a central venous line	11 Every 4 hours	11 To identify any infection introduced by the central venous catheter as soon as possible.
12 Patients with a white blood cell count of less than 1000 cells/mm^3	12 Every 4-6 hours	12 To detect any developing infection as soon as possible so that appropriate therapy can be given.
13 Patients with a falling white blood cell count but having more than 1000 cells/mm^3	13 Daily	13 A falling white blood cell count increases the likelihood of infection.
14 Patients in close contact with a known source of infection	14 Daily	14 To check that infection has not been transmitted.
15 Patient with signs and/or symptoms of systemic or local infection	15 Every 6 hours until six normal recordings are obtained	15 To monitor the development or regression of infection.
16 Patient not feeling well or nurse concerned about patient	16 Once. However, if the temperature is elevated, check again 2-3 hours	16 To reassure the patient and the nurse. To check whether the

Category	Frequency	Rationale
	later and take appropriate action.	patient is pyrexial and if so ensure that appropriate action is taken.
17 Continuing care patients	17 Daily	17 Mainly because patients expect their temperatures to be taken. This is therefore omitted or increased at the nurse's discretion.

40

TRACHEOSTOMY CARE

The care of patients with a tracheostomy varies from hospital to hospital. The changing of a tracheostomy tube will usually be undertaken by a doctor or by a trained nurse who has been instructed in this procedure. It is important, however, that nurses are aware of the procedures and basic principles and know how to respond in an emergency situation.

Definition

A tracheostome is a surgical opening made from the skin into the trachea.

Indications

Tracheostomy may be carried out:

1 To provide and maintain a patent airway
2 To enable the removal of tracheobronchial secretions

A tracheostomy may be performed as a permanent, emergency or elective procedure.

REFERENCE MATERIAL

Types of Tracheostomy

Permanent

A permanent tracheostomy is the creation of a tracheostome following a total laryngectomy (see Figure 40.1a, b). The top three tracheal cartilages are brought to the surface of the skin and sutured to the skin in the form of a stoma. The 'end' tracheostome is permanent and the rigidity of the tracheal cartilage keeps the stoma open. The patient will breathe throught this stoma for the remainder of his/her life. As a result, there is no connection between the nasal passages and the trachea.

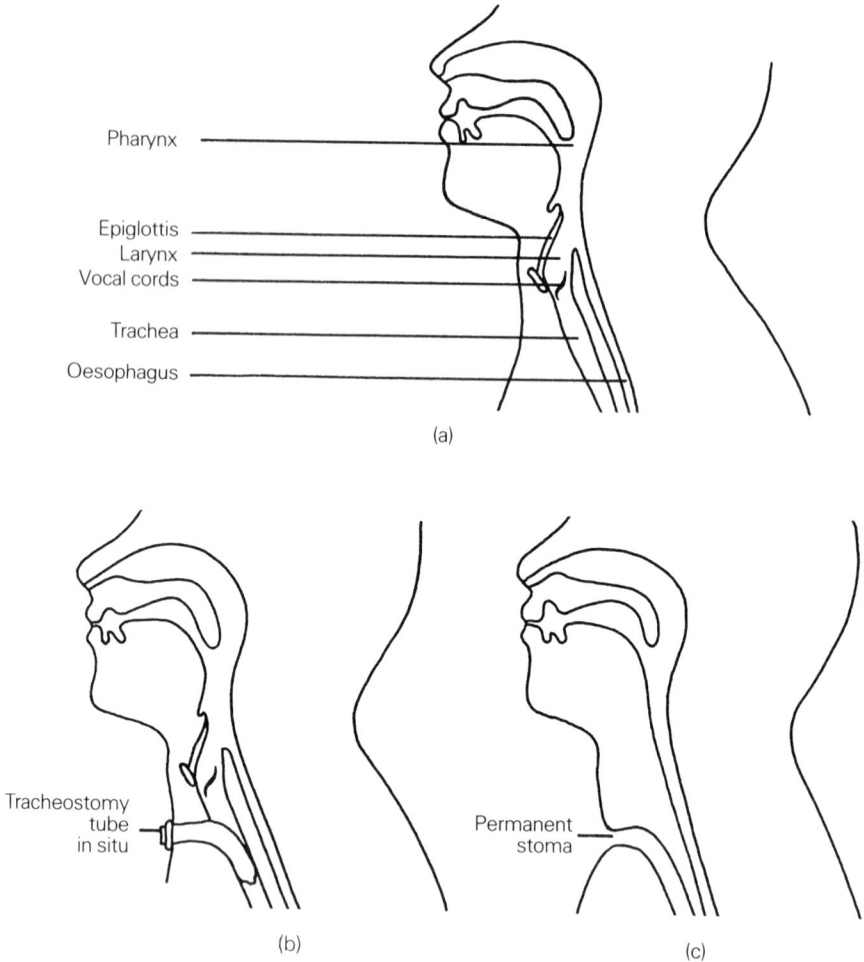

Pharynx
Epiglottis
Larynx
Vocal cords
Trachea
Oesophagus

(a)

Tracheostomy
tube
in situ

(b)

Permanent
stoma

(c)

Figure 40.1a   Anatomy of the head and neck. **b** Temporary tracheostomy. **c** Permanent tracheostomy (total laryngectomy)

Temporary

A temporary tracheostomy (see Figure 40.1c) is performed for patients as an elective procedure, e.g. at the time of major surgery.

Emergency

A tracheostomy may be performed as an emergency procedure when a patient is stridulous or when the airway is obstructed. Among the more common causes for such conditions are injury to the neck or the airways, poisoning, infection or neoplasms.

Types of Tubes

The choice of tracheostomy tube depends on the type of operation performed, the patient's ability to tolerate the tube and various external factors. A selection of tubes is listed below.

Temporary Tubes

Portex Cuffed Tracheostomy Tube A disposable plastic tracheostomy tube with introducer and inflatable cuff to give an airtight seal (Figure 40.2a). The cuff prevents blood reaching the lungs. The seal facilitates ventilation at the time of surgery.

Portex Uncuffed Tracheostomy Tube A disposable plastic tracheostomy tube with an introducer and inner tube (Figure 40.2b), used, for example, during radiotherapy, when a metal tube would cause tissue reactions.

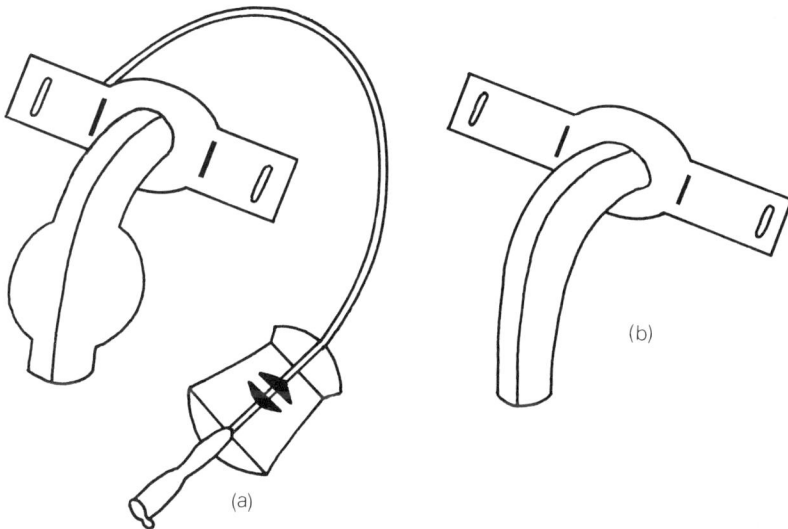

Figure 40.2 Tubes for temporary tracheostomies. **a** Portex cuffed tube. **b** Portex uncuffed tube

Jackson's Silver Tracheostomy Tube A silver tracheostomy tube with an introducer and inner tube (Figure 40.2c). The inner tube is locked in position by a small catch on the outer tube and may be removed and cleaned as necessary without disturbing the outer tube.

Negus's Silver Tracheostomy Tube A silver tracheostomy tube with an introducer and a choice of inner tubes, with and without speaking valves (Figure 40.2d). The outer tube does not have a safety catch, consequently the inner tube may inadvertently be coughed out.

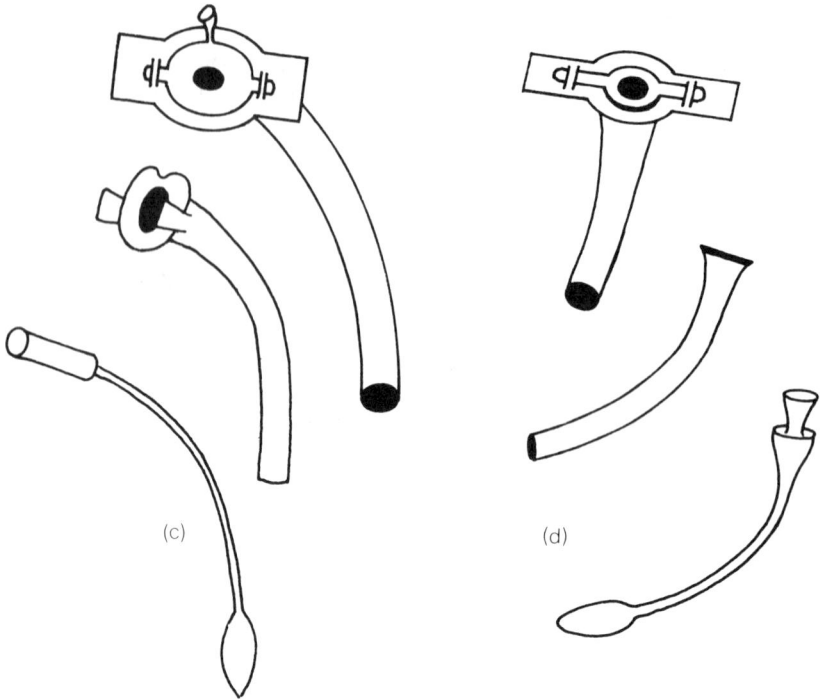

Figure 40.2c Jackson's silver tube. **d** Negus silver tube

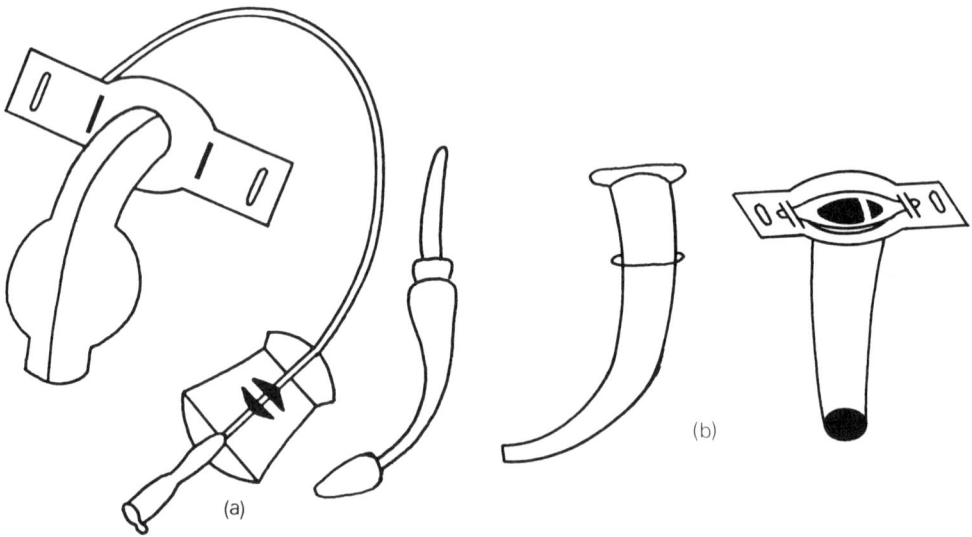

Figure 40.3 Tubes for permanent tracheostomies. **a** Portex cuffed tube. **b** Shaw's silver tube

Permanent Tubes

Portex Cuffed Tracheostomy Tube   A disposable plastic tracheostomy tube with an introducer and inflatable cuff to give an airtight seal (Figure 40.3a). The cuff prevents blood reaching the lungs. The seal facilitates ventilation at the time of surgery. This tube is used for laryngectomy patients for the first 48 hours post-operatively.

Shaw's Silver Laryngectomy Tube   A silver laryngectomy tube with an introducer and an inner tube beyond both lower and upper aspects of the outer tube (Figure 40.3b). Thus pressure dressings may be secured without occluding the stoma. The lower extension of the tube ensures that crusting does not occur when the tube is changed regularly. The silver catch on the outer tube keeps the inner tube in position.

Colledge Silver Laryngectomy Tube   A silver laryngectomy tube with an introducer (Figure 40.3c). This tube is usually fitted after drains have been removed postoperatively and bulky dressings are no longer necessary. The patient is discharged home with a set of such tubes.

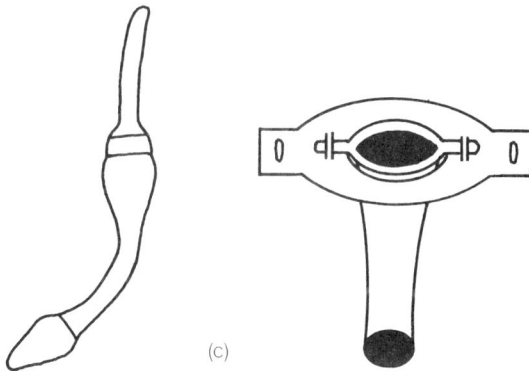

Figure 40.3c   Colledge silver tube

References and Further Reading

Davis J (1980) Surgical treatment — preparation of the patient, I — By the nurse, in Laryngectomy, Rehabilitation Seminars, Poole 1978, Abingdon 1980, National Society for Cancer Relief: pp. 67-72

McMinn R M H et al. (1981) A Colour Atlas of Head and Neck Anatomy, Wolfe Medical, pp. 102-103

Stell P M Maran A G D (1978) Head and Neck Surgery, William Heinemann Medical Books, pp. 36-48

Tiffany R (1979) Cancer Nursing: Surgical, Faber and Faber pp. 168-174

GUIDELINES: CHANGING A TRACHEOSTOMY DRESSING

Equipment

1 Sterile dressing pack
2 Tracheostomy dressing, such as Lyofoam, or a keyhole dressing
3 Tracheostomy tape
4 Cleaning solution, such as Hibisol
5 Alcohol-based hand wash solution, such as Hibisol

Procedure

Action	Rationale
1 Explain the procedure to the patient.	1 To obtain the patient's consent and cooperation.
2 Wash your hands and prepare the dressing tray or trolley.	
3 Screen the bed or cubicle.	3 To ensure the patient's privacy.
4 Perform the procedure using strict aseptic techique.	4 To prevent infection. For further information, see the procedure on aspetic technique (pages 10-11).
5 Remove the soiled dressing around the tube.	5 To avoid discomfort to the patient.
6 Replace with a tracheostomy dressing, such as Lyofoam, or a keyhole dressing.	6 To ensure the patient's comfort. To avoid pressure from the tube.

GUIDELINES: SUCTION AND TRACHEOSTOMY PATIENTS

The aim of suction is to maintain an airway and to prevent formation of crusts. The frequency of suction varies with individual patients according to their needs.

Equipment

1 Suction machine (wall source or portable)
2 Rubber connecting tube
3 Y connection
4 Sterile catheters (assorted sizes; see note below)
5 Disposable gloves
6 Jug of sodium bicarbonate solution
7 Spray, such as a Roger's spray, containing either sterile 1% sodium bicarbonate solution or normal saline
8 Disposable plastic apron
9 Alcohol-based hand wash solution, such as Hibisol

Note: It is advisable to use the right size catheter for the lumen of the tracheostomy tube: a 10FG catheter is appropriate for a 27-30FG tube, a 12FG catheter for a 33-36 FG tube; a 14FG catheter for a 39FG tube.

Procedure

Action	Rationale
1 Instruct the patient to use his/her spray, such as a Roger's spray, every 2 hours, i.e. two or three sprays directly into his/her tracheostomy. This will make him/her cough.	1 Suction will not be achieved if the secretions become too tenacious or dry. Spraying regularly minimizes this occurrence.
2 If the patient is able to perform his/her own suction, he/she should be taught this. Otherwise inform him/her precisely what is to be done.	2 To obtain the patient's cooperation. The procedure is unpleasant and can be frightening for the patient. Reassurance is vital. Self-control of the patient's suction is preferable if the patient is able to manage it.
3 Wash your hands with an alcohol-based hand wash solution, such as Hibisol, and put on a disposable plastic apron.	3 To reduce the risk of cross-infection. Most patients cough directly on to the nurse's clothes after spraying or suction.
4 Check that the Y connection is on the end of the suction tubing and set the suction machine to the appropriate level.	4 Sputum which is more tenacious requires more powerful suction.
5 Open the end of the suction catheter pack and use the pack to attach the catheter to the Y connection. Keep the rest of the catheter in the sterile packet.	5 To reduce the risk of transferring infection from your hands to the catheter and to keep the catheter as clean as possible.
6 Put on disposable gloves and withdraw the catheter from the sleeve.	6 Gloves minimize the risk of infection transfer to the catheter or from the sputum to the nurse's hands.
7 Introduce the catheter to about one-third of its length and apply suction by placing your thumb over the open limb of the Y connector.	7 Gentleness is essential; damage to the tracheal mucosa can lead to trauma and respiratory infection. The catheter should go no further than the carina to prevent trauma. The catheter is inserted with suction off so as not to irritate mucous membrane.
8 Withdraw the catheter gently with a rotating motion. Do not suction the patient for more than 15 seconds at a time.	8 To remove secretions from around the mucous membranes. Prolonged suction will result in infection.
9 Remove the catheter from the trachea having released your thumb from the Y connector.	9 To release suction and to prevent trauma to the tracheal mucosa. Catheters are used once only to

Action	Rationale
Remove gloves and discard them with the catheter.	reduce the risk of introducing infection.
10 Rinse the connection tube by dipping its end in the jug of sodium bicarbonate solution with the suction turned on.	10 To loosen secretions which have adhered to the inside of the tube.
11 If the patient requires further suction, repeat the above actions using new gloves and a new catheter.	
12 Repeat the suction until the airway is clear.	

GUIDELINES: CHANGING A TRACHEOSTOMY TUBE

Equipment

1   Sterile dressing pack
2   Tracheostomy dressing, such as Lyofoam, or a keyhole dressing
3   Tracheostomy tape
4   Cleaning solution, such as Normasol
5   Barrier cream
6   Lubricating cream
7   Sterile gloves
8   Disposable plastic apron
9   Alcohol-based hand wash solution, such as Hibisol

Procedure

Action	Rationale
1 Explain the procedure to the patient.	1 To obtain the patient's consent and cooperation.
2 Wash your hands and prepare a dressing trolley.	
3 Screen the patient's bed.	3 To ensure the patient's privacy.
4 Perform the procedure using strict aseptic technique.	4 For further information, see the procedure on aseptic technique (pages 10-11).
5 Assist the patient to sit in an upright position, supported by pillows with his/her neck extended.	5 To ensure the patient's comfort and to maintain a patent airway. If the neck is not extended, skin folds may occlude the tracheostomy when the tube is removed.
6 Remove the sterile dressing pack from its outer wrappings and open the tracheostomy dressing, such as Lyofoam.	6 Technique should be aseptic to reduce risk of cross-infection.

Action	Rationale
7 Put on a disposable plastic apron.	
8 Clean your hands with an alcohol-based hand wash solution, such as Hibisol.	
9 Put on disposable plastic gloves.	9 Gloves are necessary as the tube is difficult to manipulate with forceps.
10 Prepare the tracheostomy tube as follows:	10 So that the tube is ready for immediate insertion when required.
11 Thread one piece of tape through the slits in the flanges so that the tape passes behind the flange next to the stoma.	11 Tape is kept behind the flange to prevent it occluding the passage of air into the tracheostomy tube.
12 Put the tracheostomy dressing, such as Lyofoam, around the tube.	12 To prevent abrasion of the patient's skin by the tube.
13 Lubricate the tube sparingly with barrier cream. (If the patient is undergoing radiotherapy, a lubricating jelly, such as KY jelly, may be used instead.)	13 This acts as a barrier cream and cleansing agent. (Metallic elements of the cream may deflect ionizing rays from the desired target and increase the skin reaction.)
14 Remove the soiled tube from the patient's neck while asking the patient to breathe out.	14 Conscious expiration relaxes the patient and reduces the risk of coughing. Coughing can result in unwanted closure of the tracheostome.
15 Clean around the stoma with normal saline and dry gently. Apply barrier cream with topical swabs. (An aqueous cream may be used if the patient is having the site irradiated.)	15 To remove superficial organisms and crusts. Skin should not be left moist as this provides an ideal medium for the growth of micro-organisms.
16 Insert a clean tube with introducer in place, using an up and over action.	16 Introduction of the tube is less traumatic if directed along the contour of the trachea.
17 Remove the introducer immediately.	17 The patient cannot breathe while the introducer is in place.
18 Place the inner tube in position.	18 The inner tube may be changed several times when the outer tube is in position, thus minimizing the risk of trauma to trachea and stoma.
19 Tie the tape securely at the side of the neck.	19 To secure tube. Place the tie in an accessible place, at the same time ensuring that it will not cause discomfort to the patient.
20 Remove your gloves and ask the patient to breathe out on to the palm of your hand.	20 Flow of air will be felt if the tube is in the correct position.

21 Ensure that the patient is comfortable.

22 Clear away the trolley and equipment.

23 Scrub the soiled (silver) tube with a brush under cold running water. If the tube is very soiled, soak it in a solution of sodium bicarbonate for at least 15 minutes.	23 To remove debris that may occlude the tube and/or become a source of infection. The tube must be cleaned before boiling as heat coagulates any protein in the debris, which then becomes difficult to remove.

24 Sterilize the tube by boiling for at least 10 minutes.

Note: The quantity of secretions present will determine the frequency with which the inner tube is changed. The patient should be encouraged to perform his/her own tracheostomy care as soon as possible.

NURSING CARE PLAN

Problem	Cause	Suggested Action
1 Profuse tracheal secretions	1 Local reaction to tracheostomy tube	1 Suction frequently, e.g. every 1-2 hours.
2 Lumen of tracheostomy tube occluded	2 **a** Tenacious mucus in tube	2 **a** Spray frequently with sodium carbonate, e.g. every 1-3 hours, and suction. Change the inner tube regularly.
	b Dried blood and mucus in the tube, especially in the postoperative period	**b** Provide humidified air. (For further information, see the procedure on humidification, page 191)
3 Tracheostomy tube dislodged accidently	3 Tapes not adequately secured	3 Put in a spare tube. This should be clean and ready at the bedside. *Note:* Tracheal dilators must be kept at the bedside of patients with tracheostomies.
4 Unable to insert clean tracheostomy tube		4 Remain calm since an outward appearance of distress may cause the patient to panic and lose confidence.
	a Unpredicted shape or angle of stoma	**a** Lubricate the tube well and attempt to reinsert at various angles.

Problem	Cause	Suggested Action
	b Tracheal stenosis due to patient coughing, over-reacting or because the tube has been left out too long	**b** Insert a smaller size tracheostomy tube. If insertion still proves difficult, do not leave the patient but ask for a tube to be brought to the bed. Keep the tracheostomy patent with tracheal dilators if stenosis is pronounced until the tube is reinserted.
5 Tracheal bleeding following or during change of the tube	5 **a** Trauma due to suction or to the tube being changed **b** Presence of tumour.	5 Change the tube as planned if bleeding is minimal. For profuse bleeding, insert a cuffed tube, such as a Portex tube, and inflate. Inform the doctor. Suction the patient to remove the blood from the trachea.
6 Infected sputum	6 Nature of surgery and condition of patient often predispose to infection	6 Encourage the patient to cough up secretions and/or suction regularly. Change the tube and clean the stoma area frequently, e.g. 4-hourly. Protect permanent stomas with a bib or gauze.

41

TRACTION

Definition

Traction is a process whereby a force is exerted on a part or parts of the body. Countertraction is a process whereby a force is exerted that opposes the direct pull of the traction. The degree of countertraction depends on the amount of force necessary to counteract the pull of the traction.

Indications

Traction is indicated in the following circumstances:

1　To relieve pain and/or muscle spasm
2　To ensure rest for a limb or part of the skeletal system that may be diseased or broken until healing has occurred
3　To maintain correct anatomical alignment
4　To restore the length of a limb where, due to disease or trauma, shortening has occurred
5　To reduce dislocations of joints, as a preliminary measure, or in injury to the cervical vertebrae
6　To maintain the length of a limb where a fracture is unstable
7　As a preoperative measure prior to internal fixation.

REFERENCE MATERIAL

Types of Traction

Manual Traction

Manual traction is traction applied by the hands, as when a doctor reduces a fracture.

Fixed Traction

Fixed traction is traction between two fixed points. No weights or pulleys are used in this type of traction. The patient is attached to a device at one point and the affected part is pulled away from the point of fixation by extensions and cords which are tied to the device. The fixation point is the countertraction and the pulling extensions are the traction. This type of traction has the advantage of requiring a small degree of force only. It is frequently used to reduce or eliminate muscle spasm. An example of this type of traction would be the application of a Thomas' splint to a leg using skin extensions tied to the end of the splint.

Sliding or Balanced Traction

This is traction exerted against a weight. Extensions and cords are applied to the affected part or parts of a patient and fixed to the foot of the bed. When the foot of the bed is elevated, an inclined plane is formed down which the patient's body will slide, away from the point of fixation. The extensions serve as counter-traction; the sliding body forms the traction. An example of this type of traction would be Pugh's traction.

Weight and Pulley

A pulley is a wheel with a grooved edge suspended on an axle around which it rotates in a framework or block. A pulley block is a grouping of two or three pulleys on a single common axle in a frame. This type of traction may be a simple system using a single pulley to alter the direction of the force so that weights can be conveniently suspended, or a compound system using a number of pulleys in combination to increase the efficiency of the force applied as well as altering the direction. In all weighted traction, the weights must hang freely and not touch the side of the bed or the floor.

Single Fixed Pulley   This offers no mechanical advantage as the force (the weight) at one end of the cord is equal to the load. The advantage of this system is that traction cords can be passed in any convenient direction to reach a hanging weight, directing the force in a particular direction.

Paris of Pulley Blocks   Two pulley blocks are required at each point of suspension and are used to suspend plaster beds from overhead beams. The bed can be tilted in any direction by the patient or the nurse, thus increasing mobility and convenience.

Combination of Single Pulleys   In Hamilton-Russell traction the arrangement of a single pulley offers the advantage of suspending the patient's legs while allowing the direction of the traction force to be altered according to the principles of the parallelogram of forces.

Traction may be continuous, i.e. maintained without interruption, or intermittent, i.e. it may be discontinued for specified periods, such as mealtimes, or for toilet purposes.

Principal Sites Available for Traction

Skin Traction

Adhesive materials are applied to the skin and traction is achieved when a weight is added that pulls on tape, sponge rubber or plastic. The application of skin traction is contraindicated in the presence of an existing skin condition e.g. eczema or psoriasis, when the skin is thin and friable, where there are varicose veins, or where there is loss of normal skin sensation.

Skeletal Traction

Traction is applied to bone using wires, pins or tongs that are placed through bone. It affords a greater degree of comfort than skin traction and is the preferred method when traction is required over long periods.

Pulp Traction

A metal pin is passed through soft tissues and a stirrup is attached to the pin. Traction is applied via the stirrup.

Pelvic Traction

A canvas harness is fastened around the patient's pelvic region. The harness is attached to the foot of the bed by cords or straps. When the foot of the bed is elevated the patient's body slides down the inclined plane, forming the required traction.

Skull Traction

This may be applied by a harness, e.g. Glisson's sling, skull calipers or a half splint.

Application of Traction

Skin Traction

The application of skin traction may be painful. To minimize the patient's pain the following principles should be adhered to:

1   Skill and gentleness are required in handling the affected part.
2   Manual traction must be maintained.
3   The traction should be applied with speed and dexterity.
4   The length of any extension being applied is related to its purpose. If below-knee extensions (for knee tibial lesions) are applied to a hip or femoral lesion, the knee joint is strained by the traction being applied through the joint. If above-knee extensions (for femoral or hip lesions) are used, the knee joint must be supported.

Adhesive Types

Self adhesive   A self-adhesive medium is spread in a thin layer on a supporting material. The most commonly used medium is zinc oxide. The supporting material may be nonstretch perforated cloth in the form of zinc oxide plaster, or crosswise elastic fibre that may be perforated for ventilation. A disadvantage of zinc oxide preparations is that some patients develop a reaction to it in the form of contact dermatitis.

Diachylon adhesive   This is a lead-based adhesive material spread on various supporting materials. Such materials may be of ventilated elastic cloth or Holland cloth. This form of adhesive material can be reapplied after temporary removal and is less likely to cause contact dermatitis. A disadvantage is that the lead base may impede slightly the passage of the radiation if radiological investigations are required.

Unna's paste   This is a paste composed of 15% zinc oxide in gelatin, glycerin and water stored in airtight jars. Heat reduces the paste to a fluid state; it is then painted on to prepared calico extensions before application to the affected part. Setting takes 2 hours or more.

Nonadhesive Types

Latex Foam Pads or Bandages   These may be improvised extensions or, more commonly, commercially supplied extension kits. They have a disadvantage in that to serve as extensions they must be firmly bandaged to the skin, with the resulting danger of constricting the part bandaged.

Gamgee Tissue Under a Clove Hitch   An anklet of gamgee padding with a calico bandage arranged as a clove hitch attaching the affected part to the foot of an elevated bed may serve as a temporary extension while permanent extensions are being replaced or Unna's paste extensions are setting.

Skeletal   Strong pins, wires or tongs are passed through the bone, often under anaesthesia, by a surgeon using full aseptic technique. Commonly used are Steinmann's pins, Kirschner wires, Denham pins and Crutchfield tongs.

Specific Types of Traction

Illustrated descriptions of the types of traction currently in use can be found in Hilt and Cogburn (1980) and Roaf and Hodkinson (1980).

General Principles for the Care of Patients on Traction

Position

Patients may be required to adopt uncomfortable or unnatural positions for long periods. This may make the management of everyday functions such as eating, drinking, personal hygiene and toileting difficult. Help and sympathy from nursing personnel will be required until the pattient has adopted new ways of dealing with this situation.

Stasis

Prolonged immobilization produces many adverse reactions.

Pressure sores Skin and underlying tissues in direct contact with the bed may break down, become infected or even become necrotic. Frequent and consistent attention to the care of pressure areas is essential.

Kidneys Stasis of urine in the kidneys due to immobilization and position may result in renal complications. A high fluid intake is recommended to counteract any such complications.

Bowels Patients on traction for extended periods may become constipated. A high fibre diet should be introduced if permissable, to prevent such a complication developing.

Chest Stasis may lead to oedema of the lungs and respiratory distress. Physiotherapy, breathing exercises and suitable medication may be required to overcome such complications.

Psychological effects

Little knowledge is available on the psychological effect of prolonged traction on patients and/or nurses. Howard amd Corbo-Pelaia (1982) offer an assessment of a patient who received halo traction.

References and Further Reading

Brunner L S Suddarth D S (1982) The Lippincott Manual of Nursing Practice, 3rd edition, J B Lippincott, pp. 763-766

Cohen S (1979) Nursing care of a patient in traction, American Journal of Nursing 79: 1771-1798

Hilt N E Cogburn S B (1980) Manual of Orthopaedics, C V Mosby, pp. 517-552

Howard M Corbo-Pelaia S A (1982) Psychological after effects of halo traction, American Journal of Nursing 82: 1839-1843

Powell M (1982) Orthopaedic Nursing and Rehabilitation, 8th edition, Churchill Livingstone, pp. 24-27

Roaf R Hodkinson L J (1980) Textbook of Orthopaedic Nursing 3rd edition, Blackwell Scientific Publications, pp. 459-497

GUIDELINES: SKIN TRACTION

Equipment

Commercially prepared packs are now generally available. If this is not the case, then the items contained in the section on the application of skin traction in the reference materials section should be consulted (see page 432).

Procedure

Action	Rationale
Adhesive	
1 Explain the procedure to the patient.	1 To obtain the patient's consent and cooperation.
2 Ensure privacy for the patient while carrying out the procedure.	
3 Ensure that the affected part is clean	3 To prevent infection from developing
4 Shave any limb covered by thick tough hairs.	4 To ensure that adhesive sticks to the skin and not to the hairs. The part affected will be sore if the traction is applied to the hair follicles only.
5 If possible, leave the ankle joint free.	5 To allow full plantarflexion and dorsiflexion in the foot.
6 If the lower limb is for traction, apply pieces of felt or latex foam to the malleoli and other bony prominences.	6 To protect them from friction. To prevent the development of pressure sores.
7 Leave the patellae exposed and the knee 10-15° off full flexion.	7 To prevent limb deformity and joint stiffness.
8 Paint the limb with tincture of benzoin compound	8 To reduce moisture through perspiration. To increase the adhesive quality of the material used. To harden the skin. To act as a barrier to the adhesive in the event of the patient developing contact dermatitis.
9 Apply the extension strapping without folds or creases	9 To prevent discomfort. To prevent skin deterioration under the strapping.
10 Ensure that the part affected is in the correct anatomical position, e.g. feet and patellae pointing upwards when patient is in the supine position.	10 To prevent limb deformity.
11 Check the temperature and colour of the part affected as required	11 To ensure that the tension of strapping is correct.

Nonadhesive

As above, but omit the shaving and tincture of benzoin compound actions.

Skeletal

Action	Rationale
1 Use strict aseptic technique when	1 To prevent local and/or systemic

Action	Rationale
attending to the sites of entry of pins, wires and tongs	infection
2 Record vital signs as necessary	2 To monitor development of any infection.

NURSING CARE PLAN

Problem	Cause	Suggested Action

Skin

1 Patient is irritable, complains of pain, itching; elevated temperature; drainage through supporting material; foul odour	1 Skin breakdown is occurring or has occurred	1 Inform appropriate personnel. Remove supporting material if applicable.
2 Patient complains of paraesthesia, joint pain and/or coldness of part affected	2 Supporting material bound too tightly	2 Rebandage.
3 Increase in the distance between the sole of the foot, for example, and the spreader (a piece of wood, plastic or metal that serves to maintain the pull of the extensions along parallel lines as they are attached to the traction cord)	3 Skin extension material slipping	3 Reapply.
4 Localized sores	4 Bandage or extension material causing pressure	4 Reapply.
5 Drop foot	5 Pressure on the lateral politeal nerve	5 Realign the limb in the correct anatomical position. Ensure correct degree of knee flexion.
6 Joint irritation or displacement of bone at fracture site	6 Insufficient traction	6 Ensure sufficient traction.
7 Low grade osteo-myelitis	7 Infection at site of entry of pin, wires or tongs	7 Inform appropriate personnel. Ensure strict aseptic technique when attending to lesion.
8 Delayed union or nonunion of fracture	8 Over-distraction at fracture site	8 Realign.

Problem	Cause	Suggested Action
9 Necrosis of the bone adjacent to the pin, wires or tongs	9 Impaired blood supply	9 Inform appropriate personnel.
10 Pin slipping from one side to the other, carrying an area of nonsterile pin into the bone, or rotatory slipping	10 Pin is loose in the bone. May be an area of necrotic or osteo-porotic bone around the pin	10 Report to the medical staff.
11 Swelling, oedema, pain, discoloration below site of insertion of pin	11 May be indicative of venous thrombosis	11 Report to the medical staff.

42

THE UNCONSCIOUS PATIENT

Definition

Plum and Posner (1978) define unconsciousness as an unrousable, unresponsive state characterized by the absence of any psychologically understandable response to external stimulus or inner need. Spielman (1981) adds that such a definition is more accurate if based on a continuum from normal consciousness to deep coma with various stages of impaired consciousnes in between, e.g. confusion, lethargy and stupor. Jennett and Teasdale (1984) initiated the Glasgow Coma Scale as a means of assessing the integrity of the central nervous system on the basis of three behavioural responses that denote the patient's motor activity, verbal performance and eye opening ability. Myco and McGilloway (1980), in the introduction to their article, have a brief survey of the ways in which 'unconsciousness' has been defined. The authors conclude that 'consciousness' and 'unconsciousness' cannot be defined simply in physiological or sociological terms, but should be approached as containing, or lacking, elements of both.

Indications

The normal reflexes that protect the conscious patient have been lost and their protective function must be taken over by the nurse until the patient can function fully in his/her environment. In order to do this it will necessary

1 To establish and maintain a clear airway
2 To assess the level of consciousness
   a Evaluate verbal responses
   b Evaluate motor responses
3 To evaluate the vital signs
4 To maintain fluid and electrolyte balance
5 To carry out direct nursing care appropriate to the patient's condition.

REFERENCE MATERIAL

Causes of Unconsciousness

Poisons and Drugs

1 Alcohol
2 General anaesthetics
3 Overdose of drugs
4 Gases
5 Heavy metals.

Vascular Causes

1 Ischaemia
2 Hypertensive encephalopathy
3 Haemorrhage - subarachnoid, cerebral haemorrhage.

Infections

1 Septicaemia
2 Encephalitis
3 Meningitis
4 Protozoon (e.g. malaria)
5 Matazoon (e.g. cysticercus)
6 Fungal (e.g. torulosis).

Endocrine Causes

1 Myxoedema
2 Addison's disease.

Metabolic Causes

1 Diabetes
2 Uraemia
3 Hepatic coma
4 Tetany.

Seizures

1 Epilepsy
2 Eclampsia.

Other Causes

1 Neoplastic causes
2 Trauma, hypothermia, hyperthermia, dehydration.

Recording level of consciousness

There is no universally accepted method of assessing and recording a patient's level of consciousness. One of the more commonly used ones is the Glasgow coma scale. Useful descriptions of this scale may be found in Albeson (1982) and Jones (1979).

Attitudes of Nurses

Leon and Smyder (1980) came to the conclusion that, in general, nurses felt acceptance for the comatose patient and were challenged by such an assignment. Calmness pervaded the respondents' attitudes when providing care for these patients. These authors also felt, however, that further research was needed to gain insight into how nurses can effectively cope with their feelings of hopelessness and despair and with the questions surrounding whether or not to prolong life.

References and Further Reading

Albeson N M (1982) Observations of the neurosurgical patient, Curationis 5 (3): 32-37
Jennett B Teasdale G (1974) Assessment of coma and impaired consciousness. A practical scale, Lancet ii: 81-83
Jones C (1979) Glasgow coma scale, American Journal of Nursing 79 (9):1551-1553
Leon M Smyder M (1980) Care of the long-term comatose patient: a pilot study, Journal of Neurosurgery Nursing 12 (3): 134-137
Mason A Pratt J (1980) Touch, Nursing Times 76: 999-1001
Mountjoy P Wrythe B (1970) Nursing Care of the Unconscious Patient, Baillière Tindall and Cassell, p. 7
Myco F McGilloway F A (1980) Care of the unconscious patient: a complementary perspective. Journal of Advanced Nursing 5 (3): 273-283
Pulm F Posner J (1978) Diagnosis of Stupor and Coma, 2nd edition, F A Davis
Ricci M M (1979) Neurological assessment: keeping it ongoing, in Coping with Neurological Problems Proficiently, Intermed Communications, p. 33 ff.
Roberts A (1982) Systems and signs. Nervous System. Coma, Nursing Times 78 Systems of Life 6 October
Spielman G (1981) Coma: a clinical review, Heart and Lung 10 (4): 700-707

GUIDELINES: THE UNCONSCIOUS PATIENT

Equipment

1   Airway
2   Ambu bag with valve and mask
3   Suction equipment
4   Oxygen equipment
5   Neurological tray, thermometer, sphygmomanometer
6   Intravenous infusion equipment
7   Personal hygiene equipment
8   Eye toilet set
9   Oral toilet set

10 Catheter care set
11 Nasogastric tube feeding equipment
12 Well lit room (observation of patient's colour important)
13 Cot sides for the bed (patient may be restless)
14 Nursing observation charts (neurological, intravenous, turning, nasogastric)
15 Intubation and tracheostomy equipment for possible emergency use.

Procedure

Action	Rationale
1 The room should be well lit with an even temperature and good ventilation.	1 The observation of the patient's colour is important as an indication of the patient's wellbeing and minimal changes will not be noticed in a dim light, e.g. early signs of skin deterioration. An even temperature aids prevention of cross-infection and assists in the management of patients with hypothermia.
2 Nurse the patient in a bed with a firm, non-metallic base with a detachable head, and with padded cot sides.	2 To facilitate cardiac massage, if required. To prevent self-injury to a restless patient.
3 Insert a bed-cradle.	3 To allow for unhampered movement of limbs.
4 Place the patient in the left-lateral or semiprone position.	4 To prevent the tongue falling back against the pharyngeal wall, thus occluding the airway. To prevent respiratory complications by encouraging drainage of respiratory secretions and promoting oxygen and carbon dioxide exchange. To prevent contractures. Unequal strength in opposing sets of muscles fosters contractures.
5 Place the limbs as follows (Figure 42.1).	5 To promote comfort and maintain proper alignment of the body.

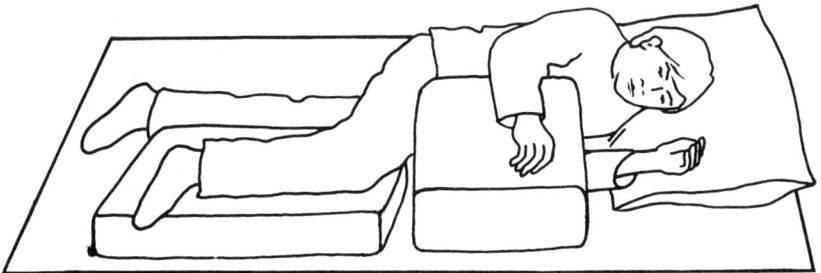

Figure 42.1 Positioning the unconscious patient

Action	Rationale
a *Head:* Put the patient's head on a pillow.	
b *Trunk:* Keep the spine straight and place pillows at the patient's back for support.	
c *Upper Limbs:* Bring the uppermost arm forward in front of the patient. Bend the elbow slightly but keep the wrist extended. Support the arm on a pillow and bring the bottom arm up alongside the face with the palm facing upwards.	To prevent oedema by inappropriate pressue on venous flow. To prevent internal rotation of the hip.
d *Lower Limbs:* Flex the uppermost leg and bring it forward. Support it on pillows. Keep the lower leg extended straight and in line with the spin. Make sure the patient's uppermost leg does not rest on his lower leg.	To avoid pressure sores.
Maintain the patient's feet at an angle of 90°. Use a footboard or special boots to achieve this position.	To prevent foot-drop.
6 Remove all dental prostheses.	6 ⎫
7 Use suction to remove excess secretions and/or vomitus.	7 ⎬ To obtain and maintain a clear, open airway.
8 Clean the patient's nostrils.	8
9 Insert an airway.	9 ⎭

Note: For methods of assessing and evaluating the following, see the procedure on neurological observations (pages 301-305)

10 Evaluate the patient's verbal responses, if any.	10 To assess the patient's level of consciousness.
11 Evaluate the patient's motor responses.	11 As the patient's condition deteriorates, he may no longer localize pain and respond to it in a purposeful way. General restlessness may be observed.
12 Assess the patient's pupillary activity.	12 Any pupillary changes may indicate involvement of cranial nerve III and possible brainstem damage.

Action	**Rationale**
13 Assess the patient's motor function by evaluating: **a** Muscle strength **b** Muscle tone **c** Posture **d** Coordination **f** Abnormal movements.	13 Damage to any part of the patient's nervous system can affect the ability to move.
14 Assess the patient's sensory function.	14 When disease or injury damages the sensory pathways, the sensory responses are always affected.
15 Assess the patient's vital signs: **a** Respirations **b** Temperature **c** Blood pressure and pulse	15 **a** Respirations are controlled by different areas of the brain. Any injury or disease in these areas will cause respiratory changes. **b** Damage to the hypothalamus, the temperature regulating centre, may result in grossly abnormal body temperatures. **c** Particularly important in unconscious patients as indicators of intracranial pressure.
16 Administer intravenous fluids as prescribed and record.	16 To maintain the patient's fluid and electrolyte balance.
17 Asepsis must be maintained throughout for any procedure involving the puncture site of a cannula.	17 To prevent local and/or systemic infection.
18 Maintain the nasogastric feeding. (See the procedure on nasogastric feeding, pages 287-293).	18 Feeding through a nasogastric tube ensures better nutrition than does intravenous feeding. Paralytic ileus is frequent in the unconscious patient and a nasogastric tube assists in gastric decompression.
19 Speak softly and use the patient's personal name. NEVER talk about the patient when in his hearing. Explain each procedure before carrying it out.	19 The sense of hearing frequently remains intact in the unconscious patient.
20 Touch the patient gently.	20 Through touch individuals establish themselves and their relationships with their environment. Being denied opportunities to touch can impair physiological, psychological and social development.

Action	**Rationale**
21 Give the patient a daily blanket bath.	21 To ensure that the patient's skin is kept clean, dry and supple.
22 Carry out eye toilet. (See the procedure on eye care, pages 169-175.)	22 The blink reflex is absent during unconsciousness. This may lead to corneal drying, irritation and ulceration.
23 Carry out oral toilet. (See the procedure on mouth care, pages 278-280.)	23 To maintain a clean, moist mouth. To prevent the accumulation of oral secretions. To prevent the development of mouth infection.
24 Observe the patient for signs of bladder distention. (See the procedure on urinary catheterization, pages 449-453.)	24 To prevent urinary complications. In males, an external sheath catheter may be used initially. Continuous bladder drainage may be necessary later. Catheterization may be immediately necessary for females. Regular catheter toilet will be necessary should this be the case.
25 Carry out bowel care. (See the procedure on bowel care, pages 49-71.)	25 To prevent constipation or diarrhoea. (For further information, see the procedure on bowel care, pages 62-70.)
26 Put the patient throught passive limb movements.	26 To prevent contractures. To aid circulation.
27 Change the patient's position regularly, e.g. every 2 hours, and record.	27 To relieve pressure areas. To prevent respiratory complications by allowing for postural drainage and for each side of the chest to receive a period when, free of compression by body weight, it can expand fully.

NURSING CARE PLAN

Problem	**Cause**	**Suggested Action**
1 Restlessness and/or confusion	1 **a** A degree of restlessness may be favourable since it may indicate that the patient is regaining consciousness. When a patient is regaining consciousness there is usually a period of clouding of consciousness, with confusion and disorientation. This may present itself in the form of aggression or uncooperative behaviour.	1 **a** Be assertive. Convey confident firmness implying an expectation that the patient will follow your suggestions and requests. **b** Ascertain that restlessness is not the result of some physical discomfort, e.g. constipation, patient too hot or cold. Carry out appropriate procedure.

Problem	Cause	Suggested Action
	Restlessness may be a manifestation of brain injury, however. It is common in cerebral anoxia, when there is a partially obstructed airway, distended bladder, bleeding or fracture.	c Summon help if the patient becomes aggressive or violent. d Ensure that the patient does not harm himself, e.g. place cot-sides in position.
2 Seizures	2 An unconscious patient is a potential candidate for seizures	2 a Maintain a clear, airway. b Protect the patient from self-injury. c Observe the patient during the seizure and record observations on a seizure chart. d Administer prescribed drugs.
3 Cerebrospinal fluid leakage through the nose and/or ears	3 May be indicative of a basilar skull fracture	3 Place a sterile topical swab against the nose and/or ears to collect drainage. Inform the medical staff.
4 Vomiting	4 May indicate that medulla oblongata is compromised	4 Maintain a clear airway. Inform the medical staff immediately.
5 Distended bladder	5 See the procedure on urinary catheterization (pages 449-453 for problems associated with catheterization.	
6 Inability to maintain own nutritional intake	6 See the procedure on nasogastric feeding (pages 287-292) for problems associated with this type of nutrition.	

URINARY CATHETERIZATION

Definition

Urinary catheterization is the insertion of a special tube into the bladder, using aseptic technique, for the purpose of evacuating or instilling fluids.

Indications

Male

In the male, urinary catheterization may be carried out for the following reasons:

1 To empty the contents of the bladder, e.g. prior to or after abdominal, pelvic or rectal surgery and prior to certain investigations
2 To determine residual urine
3 To allow irrigation of the bladder
4 To bypass an obstruction
5 To relieve retention of urine
6 To introduce cytotoxic drugs in the treatment of papillary bladder carcinomas
7 To enable bladder function tests to be performed
8 To measure urinary output accurately, e.g. when a patient is in shock, undergoing bone marrow transplantation or receiving high dose chemotherapy
9 To relieve incontinence when no other means is practicable.

Female

In the female, urinary catheterization may be carried out for the nine reasons listed above and for two further reasons:

10 To empty the bladder prior to childbirth, if thought necessary
11 To avoid complications during intracavity insertion of radioactive caesium.

REFERENCE MATERIAL

Common Sites of Cross-infection

The common sites of cross-infection of a catheterized patient are illustrated in Figure 43.1.

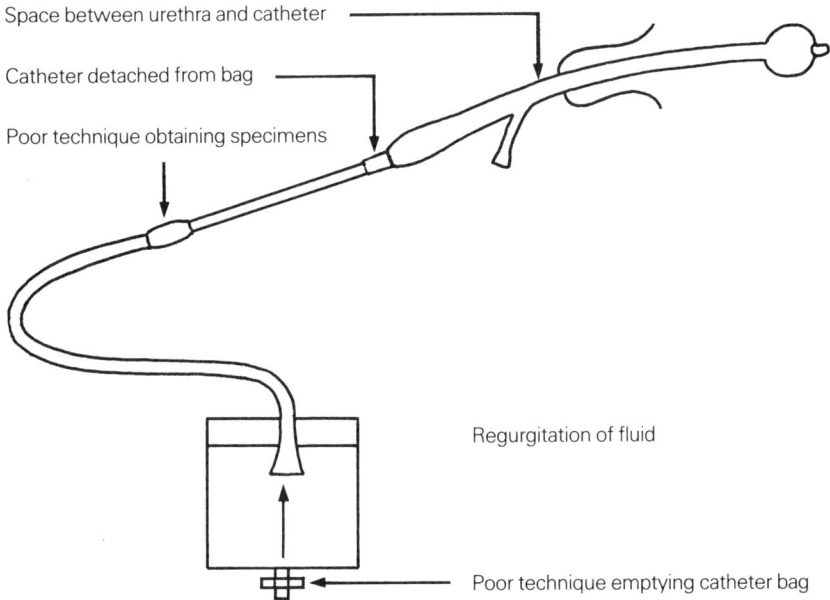

Space between urethra and catheter

Catheter detached from bag

Poor technique obtaining specimens

Regurgitation of fluid

Poor technique emptying catheter bag

Figure 43.1 Common sites of cross infection in a catheterized patient

Type of Material

Catheters are commercially available in a variety of materials.

Latex

Latex is a purified form of rubber and is the softest material from which catheters are made. It can provoke urethral reaction.

Teflon-coated Latex

Teflon-coated latex was produced to reduce urethral reaction. It is appropriate for short or medium term catheterization.

Silicone-coated or All Silicone

Silicone is a very soft, inert material ideal for long term drainage. This type of catheter is more expensive than those mentioned above and must be reserved for patients who require catheterization for two or more weeks.

Catheter Selection

Selection of catheter type and size is important if catheterization is to be effective. This also ensures that equipment is used efficiently and economically.

Types of catheters

Types of catheters are listed in Table 43.1, together with their applications.

Table 43.1 Types of catheters

Catheter type	Material	Uses
Foley two-way	Latex	The usual choice when short term indwelling catheterization is indicated. It may remain in position for up to 1 month.
Foley three-way	Latex	For those procedures where there is a need to irrigate the bladder or instill solutions into it. Potential infection is avoided by decreasing the need to break the closed system of drainage.
Red rubber	Rubber	Nondrainage procedures, e.g. residual urine or obtaining sterile specimen form an ileal conduit. Rubber is extremely irritating to urethral mucosa.
Silastic	Silicone	Long term indwelling catheterization with an approximate life span of 3 months.

Catheter Size

Catheter size is measured in French gauge. 1 FG indicates an external tube diameter of the catheter of $\frac{2}{3}$ mm.

Leg Drainage Bag

If an active patient has a permanent urinary catheter in position, he/she should be instructed in the use of a leg drainage bag as this will allow the resumption of a full range of normal activities. Such patient education should begin several days before his/her discharge so that any problems may be identified while the patient is still in hospital. If the patient has any physical or mental disabilities, a responsible relative or close friend should be taught the required catheter care before the patient is discharged. Catheter bags capable of holding larger volumes of urine than leg catheter bags are available for use at night.

References and Further Reading

Blannin J P Hobden J (1980) The catheter of choice, Nursing Times, 76: 2092-2093
Brunner L S Sudarth D S (1978) The Lippincott Manual of Nursing Practice, 2nd edition, J B Lippincott, pp 594-600
Chilman A M Thomas M (1978) Understanding Nursing Care, Churchill Livingstone, p. 307
Shafer K N et al. (1979) Medical-Surgical Nursing, 6th edition, C V Mosby, pp. 455-462

GUIDELINES: URINARY CATHETERIZATION

Equipment

1 Sterile catheterization pack containing gallipots, receiver, wool balls, topical swabs, disposable towels, disposable dissecting forceps
2 Disposable pad
3 Sterile gloves
4 Selection of appropriate catheters
5 Sterile anaesthetic lubricating jelly, such as Xylocaine gel
6 Universal specimen container
7 Antiseptic solution such as Savlodil
8 Alcohol-based hand wash solution, such as Hibisol
9 Gate clip
10 Hypoallergenic tape
11 Scissors
12 Sterile water or saline
13 Syringe and needle
14 Disposable plastic apron
15 Drainage bag and stand or holder

Procedure

Action	Rationale
Male	
1 Explain the procedure to the	1 To obtain the patient's consent and

Action	Rationale
patient.	cooperation.
2 **a** Screen the bed.	2 **a** To ensure the patient's privacy.
b Assist the patient to get into the supine position with his legs extended.	**b** To allow dust and airborne organisms to settle before the sterile field is exposed.
c Do not expose the patient at this stage of the procedure.	
3 Wash your hands.	
4 Put on a disposable plastic apron.	
5 Prepare the trolley, placing all equipment required on the bottom shelf.	
6 Take the trolley to the patient's bedside, disturbing screens as little as possible.	6 To minimize airborne contamination.
7 Remove cover that is maintaining the patient's privacy and position a disposable pad under his buttocks and thighs.	
8 Open the outer cover of the catheterization pack and slide the pack on to the top shelf of the trolley.	
9 Using an aseptic technique, open the supplementary packs.	9 The bladder is a sterile organ.
10 Clean your hands with an alcohol-based hand wash solution, such as Hibisol.	10 Your hands may have become contaminated by handling the outer packs.
11 Put on sterile gloves.	
12 Place sterile towels across the patient's thighs.	
13 Apply the nozzle to the tube of anaesthetic lubricating jelly.	
14 Wrap a sterile topical swab around the penis. Retract the foreskin, if necessary, and clean the glans penis with an antiseptic solution, such as Savlodil. Use forceps to manipulate the swabs.	
15 Insert the nozzle of the lubricating jelly into the urethra. Squeeze the gel into the urethra, remove the nozzle and discard the tube. Massage the gel along the urethra.	15 Adequate lubrication helps to prevent urethral trauma. Use of a local anaesthetic minimizes the discomfort experienced by the patient.
16 Grasp the shaft of the penis, raising it until it is almost totally extended. Maintain your grasp of the penis until the procedure is finished.	16 This manoeuvre straightens the penile urethra and facilitates catheterization. Maintaining a grasp of the penis prevents contamination

Action	**Rationale**
	and retraction of the penis.
17 Place the receiver containing the catheter between the patient's legs. Insert the catheter for 15-25cms until urine flows.	17 The male urethra is approximately 18 cm long.
18 If resistance is felt at the external sphincter, increase the traction on the penis slightly and apply steady, gentle pressure on the catheter. Ask the patient to strain gently, as if passing urine.	18 Some resistance may be due to spasm of the external sphincter. To help relax the sphincter.
19 Either remove the catheter gently when urinary flow ceases, or	
a When urine begins to flow, advance the catheter almost to its bifurcation.	**a** Advancing the catheter ensures that it is correctly positioned in the bladder.
b Inflate the balloon according to the manufacturer's directions, having ensured that the cateter is draining properly beforehand.	**b** Inadvertent inflation of the balloon in the urethra causes pain and urethral trauma.
c Withdraw the catheter slightly and attach it to the drainage system.	
d Tape the catheter laterally to the thigh or on the abdomen.	**d** This smooths out the urethral curve and eliminates pressure on the penoscrotal junction which can lead to the formation of a fistula.
e Ensure that the catheter is not taut on the skin.	**e** This allows room for movement should spontaneous erection occur.
20 Reduce or reposition the foreskin.	20 Retraction and constriction of the foreskin behind the glans penis (paraphimosis) may occur if this is not done.
21 Make the patient comfortable. Ensure that the area is dry.	22 If the area is left wet or moist, secondary infection and skin irritation may occur.
22 Measure the amount of urine.	
23 Take a urine specimen for laboratory examination, if required.	23 For further information, see the procedure on the collection of a catheter specimen of urine (pages 454-455).
24 Dispose of equipment in a disposable plastic bag and seal the bag before moving the trolley.	24 To prevent environmental contamination.
25 Draw back the curtains.	
26 Record information in any relevant documents.	

Action	**Rationale**

Female

1 Explain the procedure to the patient.	1 To obtain the patient's consent and cooperation.
2 **a** Screen the bed. **b** Assist the patient to get into the supine position with knees bent, hips flexed and feet resting about 60 cm apart. **c** Do not expose the patient at this stage of the procedure.	2 **a** To ensure the patient's privacy. **b** To allow dust and airborne organisms to settle before the sterile field is exposed.
3 Ensure that a good light source is available.	3 To enable the genital area to be seen clearly.
4 Wash your hands.	
5 Put on a disposable plastic apron.	
6 Prepare the trolley, placing all equipment required on the bottom shelf.	
7 Take the trolley to the patient's bedside, disturbing screens as little as possible.	7 To minimize airborne contamination.
8 Remove cover that is maintaining the patient's privacy and position a disposable pad under the patient's buttocks.	
9 Open the outer cover of the catheterization pack and slide the pack on to the top shelf of the trolley.	
10 Using an aseptic technique, open supplementary packs.	10 Catheterization requires the same aseptic precautions as a surgical procedure.
11 Clean your hands with an alcohol-based hand wash solution, such as Hibisol.	11 Your hands may have become contaminated by handling of outer packs, etc.
12 Put on sterile gloves.	
13 Place sterile towels across the patient's thighs.	
14 Separate the labia minora so that the urethral meatus is seen. Using sterile topical swabs, one hand should be used to maintain labial separation until catheterization is completed.	14 This manouevre helps to prevent labial contamination of the catheter and provides better access to the urethral orifice.
15 Clean around the urethral orifice with an antiseptic solution, such as Savlodil, using single downward strokes. Forceps should be used to	15 Inadequate preparation of the urethral orifice is a major cause of infection following catheterization.

Action	**Rationale**
handle the cleaning swabs.	
16 Dry the area well before proceeding.	
17 Lubricate the catheter with sterile anaesthetic lubricating jelly, such as xylocaine gel.	17 Lubricating the catheter reduces friction and trauma to the urethral mucosa. Use of a local anaesthetic minimizes the patient's discomfort.
18 Place the catheter, in the receiver, between the patient's legs.	
19 Introduce the tip of the catheter into the urtehral orifice in an upward and backward direction. Advance the catheter until 5-6 cm have been inserted.	19 The direction of insertion and the length of catheter inserted should bear relation to the anatomical structure of the area.
20 *Either* remove the catheter gently when urinary flow ceases, *or* **a** Advance the catheter 6-8 cm	**a** This prevents the balloon from becoming trapped in the urethra.
b Inflate the balloon according to the manufacturer's directions, having ensured that the catheter is draining adequately.	**b** Inadvertent inflation of the balloon within the urethra is painful and causes urethral trauma.
c Withdraw the catheter slightly and connect it to the drainage system.	
d Tape the catheter and drainage system to the thigh.	**d** This prevents traction and tension on the bladder and friction in the urethra.
21 Make the patient comfortable and ensure that the area is dry.	21 If the area is left wet or moist, secondary infection and skin irritation may occur.
22 Measure the amount of urine.	
23 Take a urine specimen for laboratory examination, if required.	23 For further information, see the procedure on the collection of a catheter specimen of urine (pages 454-455).
24 Dispose of equipment in a disposable plastic bag and seal the bag before moving the trolley.	24 To prevent environmental contamination.
25 Draw back the curtains.	
26 Record information in any relevant documents.	

Note: When the bladder is very distended a gate clip should be applied to the drainage bag or catheter tubing to regulate the flow rate after 500 ml of urine has been drained. This prevents shock due to sudden reduction in intra-abdominal pressure.

GUIDELINES: COLLECTION OF A CATHETER SPECIMEN OF URINE

Equipment

1 Swab saturated with isopropyl alcohol 70% such as Medi Swab
2 Gate clip
3 Sterile syringe and needle
4 Universal specimen container

Procedure

Action	Rationale
1 Explain the procedure to the patient.	1 To obtain the patient's consent and cooperation.
2 Screen the bed.	2 To ensure the patient's privacy.
3 If there is no urine in the tubing, clamp the tubing below the rubber cuff until sufficient urine collects.	3 To obtain an adequate urine sample.
4 Wash and dry your hands.	
5 Clean the rubber cuff with a swab saturated with isopropyl alcohol 70%.	5 To prevent cross-infection.
6 Using a sterile syringe and needle, aspirate the required amount of urine from the rubber cuff (Figure 43.2).	6 The rubber cuff is specially designed to occlude the puncture hole when the needle is withdrawn. If the catheter bag or tubing is

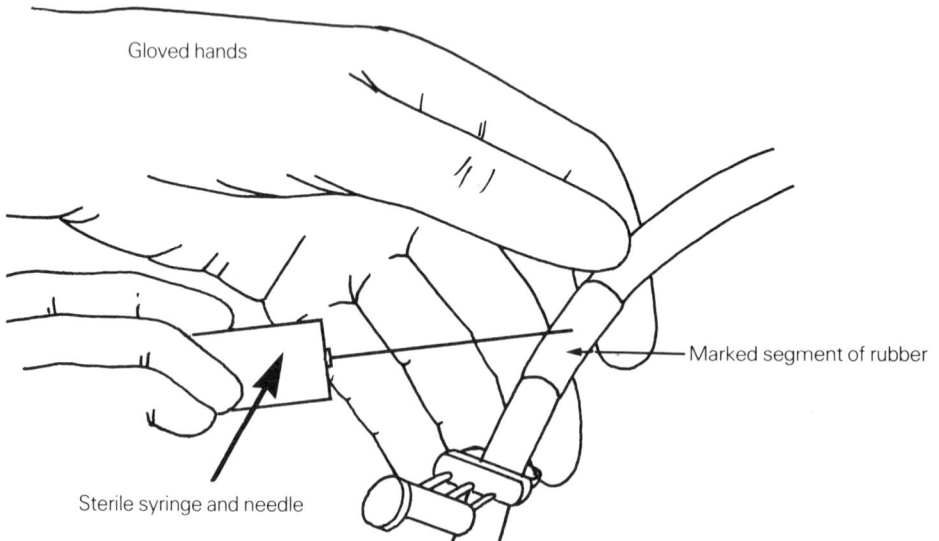

Gloved hands

Marked segment of rubber

Sterile syringe and needle

Figure 43.2 Taking a specimen

Action	Rationale
	punctured it causes leakage of urine and aspiration of air inwards, carrying organisms with it. Specimens collected from the catheter bag may give false results due to organisms proliferating there.
7 Place the specimen in a sterile container.	
8 Wash and dry your hands.	
9 Unclamp if necessary.	9 To allow drainage to continue.
10 Make the patient comfortable.	
11 Label the container and dispatch it to the laboratory with the completed request form.	

GUIDELINES: EMPTYING A CATHETER BAG

Equipment

1 Swabs saturated with isopropyl alcohol 70%, such as Medi Swab
2 Heat-disinfected jug or sterile jug
3 Disposable gloves

Procedure

Action	Rationale
1 Explain the procedure to the patient.	1 To obtain the patient's consent and cooperation.
2 Wash your hands and put on disposable gloves.	2 To prevent cross-infection.
3 Clean the outlet valve with a swab saturated with isopropyl alcohol 70%.	
4 Allow the urine to drain into the appropriate jug.	
5 Close the outlet valve and clean it again with a new alcohol-saturated swab.	5 To prevent cross-infection.
6 Cover the jug and dispose of the contents in the sluice, having noted the amount of urine if this is required for fluid balance records.	6 To prevent environmental contamination.
7 Heat-disinfect the jug after each use or return the jug for sterilization.	7 To prevent cross-infection.
8 Wash your hands.	

NURSING CARE PLAN

Problem	Cause	Suggested Action
With Catheter in Place		
1 Urinary tract infection introduced during catheterization	1 **a** Faulty aseptic technique **b** Inadequate urethral cleansing **c** Contamination of catheter tip	1 **a** Inform a doctor **b** Obtain a catheter specimen of urine.
2 Urinary tract infection introduced via the drainage system	2 **a** Faulty handling of equipment **b** Breaking the closed system **c** Raising the drainage bag above bladder level	2 **a** Inform a doctor. **b** Obtain a catheter specimen of urine.
3 No drainage of urine	3 **a** Incorrect identification of external urinary meatus (female patients) **b** Blockage of catheter	3 **a** Check that catheter has been correctly sited. **b** In the female, leave the catheter in position to act as a guide, re-identify the urethra and recatheterize the patient. Remove the inappropriately sited catheter.
4 Urethral mucosal trauma	4 **a** Incorrect size of catheter **b** Procedure not carried out correctly or skilfully **c** Movement of the catheter in the urethra **d** Creation of false passage as a result of too rapid insertion of catheter	4 **a** Recatheterize the patient using the correct size of catheter. **c** Check the strapping and reapply as necessary. **d** You may need to remove the catheter and wait for the urethral mucosa to heal.
5 Inability to tolerate indwelling catheter	5 **a** Urethral mucosal irritation **b** Psychological trauma	5 **a** You may need to remove the catheter and seek an alternative means of urine drainage. **b** Explain the need for and functioning of the catheter.

Problem	Cause	Suggested Action
6 Inadequate drainage of urine	6 **a** Incorrect placement of catheter	6 **a** Resite the catheter.
	b Kinked drainage tubing	**b** Inspect the system and straighten any kinks.
	c Blocked tubing, e.g. pus, urates, phosphates, blood clots	**c** If a three-way catheter, such as Foley's, is in place, irrigate it. If an ordinary catheter is in use, milk the tubing in an attempt to dislodge the debris; then replace it with a three-way catheter.
7 Fistula formation	7 Pressure on the peno-scrotal angle	7 Ensure that correct strapping is used.
8 Penile pain on erection	8 Not allowing enough length of catheter to accommodate penile erection	8 Ensure that an adequate length is available to accommodate penile erection.
9 Paraphimosis	9 Failure to retract foreskin after catheterization or catheter toilet	9 Always retract the foreskin.
10 Formation of crusts around urethral meatus	10 Infection involving urea-splitting organisms that cause deposits of salts to form around the catheter	10 Correct catheter toilet.
11 Leakage of urine around catheter	11 Incorrect size of catheter	11 Replace with the correct size of catheter.

After Removal of Catheter

1 Dysuria	1 Inflammation of the urethral mucosa	1 Ensure a fluid intake of 2-3 litres per day. Advise the patient that dysuria is common but will usually be resolved once micturation has occurred at least three times. Inform medical staff if the problem persists.
2 Retention of urine	2 May be psychological	2 Encourage the patient to increase his/her fluid intake. Offer the patient a warm bath. Inform medical staff if the problem persists.

Problem	**Cause**	**Suggested Action**
3 Urinary tract infection.		3 Encourage a fluid intake of 2-3 litres a day. Collect a specimen of urine. Inform medical staff if the problem persists. Administer prescribed antibiotics.

44

VENEPUNCTURE

Definition
Venepuncture is the term used for the procedure of entering a vein with a needle.

Indications
Venepuncture is carried out for two reasons:

1 To obtain a blood sample for diagnostic purposes
2 To monitor levels of blood components.

REFERENCE MATERIAL
Venepuncture is a routine procedure that is increasingly being performed by nursing staff. In order to do this safely the nurse must have a basic knowledge of the following:

1 The relevant anatomy and physiology
2 The criteria for choosing both the vein and device to use
3 The potential problems which he/she may encounter.

Certain principles, such as adherence to an aseptic technique, must be applied throughout. The circulation is a closed sterile system and a venepuncture, however quickly completed, is a breach of this system providing a method of entry for bacteria.

The nurse must be aware of the physical and psychological comfort of the patient. He/she must appreciate the value of adequate explanation and simple measures to prevent haematoma formation, a complication of venepuncture, not a natural consequence of it.

Anatomy and Physiology
The superficial veins of the upper limb are most commonly chosen for venepuncture. These veins are numerous and accessible, ensuring that the procedure can be performed safely and without discomfort. Occasionally the

veins of a lower limb may be utilized if this is unavoidable, as blood flow in this region is diminished and the risk of ensuing complications higher.

Criteria for Choosing a Site for Venepuncture

The Condition and Accessibility of the Peripheral Veins

Veins may be tortuous, sclerosed, fibrosed or thrombosed, inflamed or fragile and unable to accommodate the device to be used. If the patient complains of pain or soreness over a particular site, this should be avoided, as should areas that are bruised. Veins adjacent to foci of infection must not be considered.

Preference is given to a vessel which is unused, easily detected by inspection and/or palpation, patent and healthy. These veins feel soft, bouncy and will refill when depressed.

Anatomical Considerations

The venous anatomy of each individual differs, but care must always be taken to avoid adjacent structures, e.g. arteries and nerves. Accidental puncture of an artery may cause painful spasm and could result in prolonged bleeding. If a nerve is touched, this can result in severe pain and the attempted venepuncture should be stopped.

Palpation is of value in distinguishing structures clinically, e.g. arteries and tendons, due to the presence of a pulse or resistance, and detecting deeper veins.

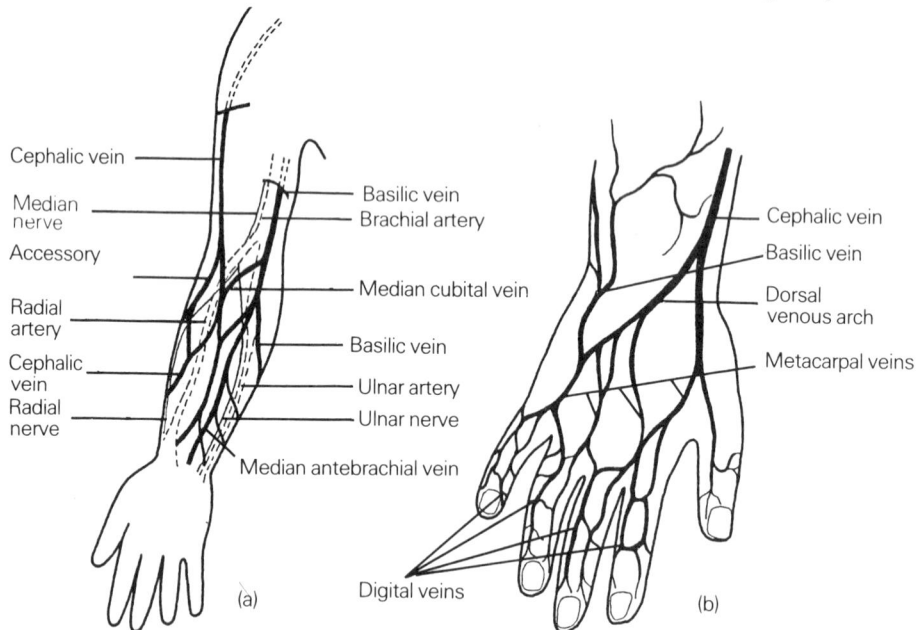

Figure 44.1a   Superficial veins of the forearm. **b** Superficial veins of the dorsal aspect of the hand

Use of veins which cross joints or bony prominences and those with little skin or subcutaneous cover, e.g. the inner aspect of the wrist, will subject the patient to more discomfort.

The sites of choice (Figure 44.1) are branches of

1 The basilic vein
2 The cephalic vein
3 The median cubital vein in the antecubital fossa.

These are sizeable veins capable of providing copious and repeated blood specimens. The brachial artery and median nerve are in close proximity and must not be damaged.

The choice of vein, however, must be that which is best for the individual patient. When using other sites it is advisable to avoid junctions within the venous network. Another feature in veins is the presence of valves. These are folds of the endothelium present in larger vessels to prevent a backflow of blood to the extremity. If detected, a puncture should be performed above the valve in order to facilitate collection of the sample .

The Clinical Status of the Patient

Injury or disease may prevent the use of a limb for venepunture. Amputation, fracture or cerebrovascular accident are good examples of conditions that affect venous access. Use of a limb may be contraindicated because of an operation on one side of the body, e.g. mastectomy. Impairment of lymphatic drainage can influence venous flow regardless of whether there is obvious lymphoedema. An oedematous limb should be avoided as there is danger of stastis predisposing to such complications as phlebitis and cellulitis. Positioning of the patient may dictate the site of venepuncture.

Physiological Factors

The tunica media, the middle layer of the vein wall, is composed of muscle fibres capable of constricting or dilating in response to stimuli from the vasomotor centre in the medulla via the sympathetic nerves. The nurse must be aware of the factors which can influence venous dilation. These are

1 Anxiety
2 Temperature
3 Mechanical or chemical irritation
4 The clinical state of the patient, e.g. hypovolaemia due to dehydration.

Anxiety may be reduced by presenting a confident manner together with an adequate explanation of the procedure. Careful preparation and an unhurried approach will help to relax the patient and his/her veins.

The temperature of the environment will influence venous dilation. If the patient is cold no veins may be evident on first inspection. Application of heat, e.g. in the form of a hot compress, will increase the size and visibility of the veins, thus increasing likelihood of a successful first attempt.

Venepuncture may cause the vein to collapse or go into a spasm. This will produce discomfort and a reduction in blood flow. Good technique will reduce the likelihood of this and stroking the vein or applying heat will help resolve it.

Good technical skill also prevents trauma to the tunica intima, the lining of the vein. Roughening of the smooth endothelium encourages the process of thrombus formation.

Choice of Device

The intravenous devices commonly used to perform a venepuncture for blood sampling are a straight steel needle and a steel winged infusion device. The optimum gauge to use is 21g (standard wire gauge). This enables blood to be withdrawn at a reasonable speed without undue discomfort to the patient or possible damage to the blood cells.

The nurse must choose the device dependent on the condition and accessibility of the individual patient's veins (see Table 44.1).

Skin Preparation

Asepsis is vital when performing a venepuncture as the skin is breached and an alien device introduced into a sterile circulatory system. The two major sources of microbial contamination are

1　The hands of the practitioner
2　The skin of the patient.

Good hand washing and drying techniques are essential on the part of the nurse. If handwashing facilities are unavailable, an alcohol-based hand wash solution is an acceptable substitute.

To remove the risk presented by the patient's skin flora, firm and prolonged rubbing with an alcohol-based solution, such as chlorhexidine 70% in spirit, is advised. This cleaning should continue for at least 30 seconds, although some authors state a minimum of 1 minute or longer. The area that has been cleaned should then be allowed to dry to facilitate coagulation of the organisms, thus ensuring disinfection. The skin must not be touched or the vein repalpated prior to puncture.

Skin cleansing is a controversial subject and it is acknowledged that a cursory wipe with an alcohol swab does more harm than no cleaning at all as it disturbs the skin flora. Good cleaning techniques in a hospital environment, where transient pathogens abound, are of value in controlling infection.

Summary

In order to perform a safe and successful venepuncture it is important that the nurse considers carefully the choice of vein and device and applies the principles of asepsis. Supervision by an experienced member of staff is desirable when the nurse begins to practice.

Table 44.1 The choice of intravenous device

Device	Gauge	Advantages	Disadvantages	Use
Needle	21	Cheap. Easy to use with large veins.	Rigid. Difficult to manipulate with smaller veins in less conventional sites. May cause more discomfort.	Large, accessible veins in the antecubital fossa. When small quantities of blood are to be drawn.
Winged infusion device	21	Flexible due to small needle shaft. Easy to manipulate and insert at any site. Causes less discomfort.	More expensive than steel needles.	Veins in sites other than the antecubital fossa. When quantities of blood greater than 20 ml are required from any site.
	23	As above.	As above, plus there can be damage to cells which can cause inaccurate measurements.	Small veins in more painful sites, e.g. inner aspect of the wrist, especially if measurements are related to plasma and not cellular components.

References and Further Reading

Plumer A L (1982) Principles and Practice of Intravenous Therapy, 3rd edition, Little, Brown

Sager D Bomar S (1980) Intravenous Medications, J B Lippincott

White J et al. (1970) Skin disinfection, John Hopkins Medical Journal 126: 169-170

GUIDELINES: VENEPUNCTURE

Equipment

1   Clinically clean tray or receiver
2   Tourniquet or sphygmomanometer and cuff
3   Syringe(s) of appropriate size
4   21g needle or 21g winged infusion device
5   Swab saturated with isopropyl alcohol 70%
6   Sterile cotton wool balls
7   Sterile adhesive plaster or hypoallergenic tape
8   Labelled blood specimen bottle(s)
9   Specimen requisition forms

Alternatively, there are a number of vacuum systems available that can be used for taking blood samples. These are simple to use and cost effective. The manufacturer's instructions should be followed carefully if one of these systems is to be used and the following items will replace syringes, needles and specimen bottles:

1   21g multiple sample needle *or* 21g winged infusion device and multiple sample luer adapter
2   Plastic shell to hold specimen tubes
3   Appropriate vacuumed specimen tubes, labelled.

Procedure

Action	Rationale
1 Approach the patient in a confident manner and explain the procedure to the patient.	2 To obtain the patient's consent and cooperation. To reduce anxiety.
2 Allow the patient time to ask questions and discuss any problems which have arisen previously.	2 A relaxed patient will have relaxed veins.
3 Assemble the equipment necessary for venepuncture.	3 To ensure that time is not wasted and that the procedure goes smoothly without unnecessary interruptions.
4 Carefully wash and dry your hands prior to commencement.	4 To minimize the risk of infection.
5 Check all packaging before opening	5 To maintain asepsis throughout

Action	**Rationale**
and preparing the equipment on the chosen clinically clean receptacle.	and to check than no equipment is damaged.
6 Take all the requirements to the patient, exhibiting a competent manner.	6 To put the patient at his/her ease.
7 In both an inpatient and an out-patient situation, lighting, ventilation, privacy and positioning must be checked.	7 To ensure that both patient and operator are comfortable and that adequate light is available to illuminate this procedure.
8 Consult the patient as to any preferences and problems he/she may have identified at previous venepunctures.	8 **a** To involve the patient in his/her treatment. **b** To acquaint the nurse fully with the patient's previous venous history. **c** To identify any changes in clinical status which may influence vein choice, e.g. mastectomy.
9 Support the chosen limb.	9 To ensure the patient's comfort.
10 **a** Apply a tourniquet to the upper arm on the chosen side, making sure it does not obstruct arterial flow. The position of the tourniquet may be varied, e.g. if a vein in the hand is to be used it may be placed on the forearm. A sphygomano-meter cuff may be used as an alternative.	10 **a** To dilate the veins by obstructing the venous return.
b The arm may be placed in a dependent position. The patient may assist by clenching and unclenching his/her fist.	**b** To increase the prominence of the veins.
c The veins may be tapped lightly. **d** If all these measures are un-successful, remove the tourniquet and apply moist heat, e.g. a hot compress, to the chosen limb.	**d** To promote blood flow and therefore distend the veins.
11 Select the vein using the aforementioned criteria.	
12 Select the device, based on vein size, site, etc.	
13 Wash your hands with soap and water or clean your hands using a suitable alcohol-based solution.	13 To maintain asepsis.
14 Clean the patient's skin carefully for at least 30 seconds using an appropriate preparation and allow	14 To maintain asepsis.

Action	Rationale
to dry. Do not repalpate the vein or touch the skin.	
15 Inspect the device carefully.	15 To detect faulty equipment, e.g. bent or barbed needles. If these are present, discard them.
16 Anchor the vein by applying manual traction on the skin a few centimetres below the proposed insertion site.	16 **a** To immobilize the vein. **b** To provide countertension, which will facilitate a smoother needle entry.
17 Insert the needle smoothly at an angle of approximately 30°. The shaft of a straight needle may be bent slightly at the hub to enable the entry to be as flush with the skin as possible.	17 To ensure a successful, pain-free venepuncture.
18 Level off the needle as soon a flashback of blood is seen in the tubing of a winged infusion device or when puncture of the vein wall is felt. If you are using a needle and syringe, pull the plunger back slightly prior to venepuncture and a flashback of blood will be seen in the barrel on vein entry.	
19 Advance the needle approximately 1 mm into the vein, if possible.	19 To stabilize the device within the vein and prevent it becoming dislodged during venepuncture.
20 Do not exert any pressure on the needle.	20 To prevent a through puncture occurring.
21 Withdraw the required amount of blood.	
22 Release the tourniquet. In some instances this may be requested at the beginning of sampling as inaccurate measurements may be caused by haemostatis, e.g. blood calcium levels.	22 To decrease the pressure within the vein.
23 Withdraw a small amount of blood into the syringe.	23 To reduce the amount of static blood in the vein and therefore the likelihood of leakage.
24 Pick up a sterile wool ball and place it over the puncture point.	
25 Remove the needle.	
26 Apply digital pressure directly over the puncture point.	26 To stop leakage and haematoma formation.
27 Do not apply pressure until the needle has been fully removed.	27 To prevent pain on removal.

Action	**Rationale**
28 Pressure should be applied until the bleeding has ceased, approximately 1 minute. Longer may be required if current disease or treatment interferes with clotting mechanisms.	28 To prevent leakage and haematoma formation.
29 The patient may apply pressure with his/her finger but should be discouraged from bending his/her arm if a vein in the antecubital fossa is used.	29 To prevent leakage and haematoma formation.
30 Transfer the blood to appropriate specimen bottles as soon as possible, making sure that the correct quantity is placed in each container.	30 **a** To prevent clotting in the syringe. **b** To ensure that an adequate amount is available for each test.
31 Mix well if the bottle contains a chemical to prevent clotting or aid accurate measurements.	31 To ensure that the blood is correctly presented to the laboratory and that the patient does not have to have a repeat specimen taken.
32 Label the bottles with the relevant details.	32 To ensure that the specimens from the right patient are delivered to the laboratory, the requested tests are performed and the results returned to the correct patient's records.
33 Inspect the puncture point before applying a dressing.	33 To check that the puncture point has healed.
34 Ascertain whether the patient is allergic to adhesive plaster.	34 To prevent an allergic skin reaction.
35 Apply an adhesive plaster or alternative dressing.	35 To cover the puncture and prevent leakage or introduction of bacteria until healing is complete.
36 Ensure that the patient is comfortable.	36 To ascertain whether he/she wishes to rest before leaving (if an outpatient) or whether any other measures need to be taken.
37 Discard waste, making sure it is placed it in the correct containers, e.g. 'sharps' into a designed receptacle.	37 To ensure safe disposal and avoid laceration or other injury of staff. To prevent reuse of equipment.
38 Follow hospital procedure for collection and transportation of specimens to the laboratory.	38 To make sure that specimens reach their intended destination.

NURSING CARE PLAN

Problem	Possible Cause	Suggested Action
1 Excessive pain	1 **a** Anxiety, fear, low pain, tolerance	1 **a** Confident, unhurried approach. Use all methods, including heat, to dilate veins. Avoid hesitancy and skin 'tickling'. Consider use of winged infusion device.
	b Frequently used vein	**b** Avoid this site, if possible, otherwise proceed as above.
	c Nerve touched	**c** Remove the needle immediately and proceed to a different site.
2 Very anxious patient	2 **a** Previous trauma **b** Needle phobia	2 Confident unhurried approach. Make sure the patient is comfortable, perhaps reclining/lying down. Use all methods, including heat, to dilate veins. Consider use of winged infusion device.
3 Limited venous access	3 **a** Repeated use, e.g. prolonged cytotoxic therapy	3 **a** Confident, unhurried approach. Use all methods including heat to dilate veins.
	b Phlebitis	**b** Use a winged infusion device of 21g or 23g. Only proceed if you are sure of a successful first attempt. Consider referral to a more experienced colleague.
	c Bruising due to (1) Fragile veins in the elderly (2) Anticoagulant therapy or low platelet levels	**c** As above plus apply tourniquet gently or do not use. Ensure adequate pressure to puncture site to prevent further damage.
	d Peripheral shutdown	**d** Use all methods to dilate veins as listed. A

Problem	Possible Cause	Suggested Action
		sphygomomanometer and cuff may enable more effective restriction of the venous return. Work quickly if the patient is in a collapsed state. Pull blood back into the veins by massaging above the venepuncture site.
4 Infection	4 Poor aseptic technique	4 Practice good hand washing and skin cleansing and take particular care with immune compromised patients.

Practical Problems

Problem	Possible Cause	Suggested Action
1 Missed vein	1 **a** Inadequate anchoring **b** Wrong positioning **c** Poor lighting **d** Less than 100% concentration.	1 Withdraw the needle almost to the bevel and manoeuvre gently to realign needle and vein. Readvance, but if it becomes painful, remove. Better preparation next time.
2 Spurt of blood on entry	2 Bevel tip of needle entering vein before entire bevel is under the skin, due to vein being very superficial	2 Ignore. Reassure the patient if a small blood blister develops.
3 Blood flow stops	3 **a** Overshooting vein or advancing needle while withdrawing blood **b** Vein collapse due to contact with valve or vein wall **c** Poor blood flow	3 **a** Gently ease needle back and continue. **b** Manoeuvre gently. Release and retighten tourniquet and continue. **c** As above and massage above the needle tip to pull blood into vein.
4 Haematoma	4 **a** Perforation of opposite wall of vein	4 **a** Insert needle at correct angle and stop when a flashback is

Problem	Possible Cause	Suggested Action
		seen in syringe or tubing of winged fashion infusion device. Do not advance needle during taking of sample.
	b Forgetting to remove tourniquet before removing needle	**b** Remember next time.
	c Inadequate pressure on puncture site	**c** Press. Supervise the patient doing the same.
5 Hardening of the veins due to scarring and thrombosis	5 Prolonged use of one site	5 Alternate venepuncture sites to prevent this. Do not use hard veins as this is often not successful and will cause the patient pain.
6 Mechanical problems	6 Faulty equipment, e.g. bent needle tips, cracked syringes	6 Check carefully before use and discard.
7 Transmittable diseases	7 Viruses pose the major risk, causing hepititis B, cytomegalovirus, acquired immune deficiency syndrome	7 **a** All blood should be handled with care and caution used when handling specimens of patients suspected of infection, e.g. Australia antigen positive persons. **b** Gloves should be worn when taking blood and handling samples. Hospital policy should be strictly observed.
8 Needle inoculation	8 **a** Lack of caution **b** Overfilling of 'sharps' containers	8 Dispose of equipment safely to prevent inoculation. If it does occur, follow accident procedure and report the incident immediately. An injection of hepatitis B immunoglobulin may be required.

45

VIOLENCE AND ITS MANAGEMENT

Definition
Violence is the exercise of physical force in such a way as to cause injury or damage to oneself, others or property. Aggression is the threat of violence.

Indications
Management of violence is necessary

1 When a patient makes an attack on another person
2 When a patient becomes disturbed to the extent that he/she is considered a danger to him/herself or others.

REFERENCE MATERIAL

Principles
Four principles underlie the management of violent patients:

1 The risk of physical injury should be minimized. (Any restraint employed must be of a degree appropriate to the actual danger or resistance shown by the patient.)
2 The agreed procedures for the nursing care of violent patients should be adhered to.
3 As far as possible, the therapeutic regime should be maintained.
4 All hospital personnel should see it as their obligation to render assistance if a violent incident occurs.

Violence and its Causes
Violence is one expression of aggression. Freud (1955) and Lorenz (1966) viewed violence as an inherent part of human nature. Bandura and Walters (1963) see violence as a learned response. Berkowitz (1962) and Dollard and Miller (1961) regard violence as a response to frustration. According to personality, environment or social culture, so this agression may be expressed in various ways.

Personality

Eysenck (1979) has shown that different individuals when provoked similarly react differently. Yet numerous studies of adopted children have shown that violent behaviour is more closely related to the pattern in the natural rather than in the adoptive parents even though the adoptive parents provide the child's entire social environment.

Environmental and Social Influences

Wertham (1968) has shown that 50% of all violent crimes are connected with alcohol. Failure of communication, at all levels, is also an important factor. Where communication ends, violence begins. There also exists in contemporary society an apparent commercial disrespect for life. Television companies screen programmes littered with scenes of violence, often at peak viewing times. Toys of violence abound. Poor housing, racial prejudice, unemployment, inadequate social services and drug abuse are other areas that have been identified as fertile soil for the growth of violence. On the more personal level, violent behaviour is rooted in negative emotions — jealously, greed, the distortion and frustration of sexual development, revenge, humiliations, irritations and rivalries. One group that may be identified as contributing to or even initiating violence at this level are the relatives and friends of patients.

Predispositions to Violent Behaviour

It is difficult to place violent behaviour in diagnostic categories. The major psychoses, alcoholism and drugs may all predispose to violent behaviour. Organic confusional states, hypoxia and toxic states may also produce such behaviour.

The Care of Violent Patients

Among the guidelines recommended by the Royal College of Nursing and the National Council for Nurses of the United Kingdom (1972) for the care of violent patients, were the following:

1   All staff within the vicinity of the violent incident must accept responsibility to intervene or give assistance.
2   Staff should receive instructions and guidance in the management of violence.
3   The violent patient is a sick person, regardless of behaviour, class, creed or colour.
4   Staff must control their own emotions. Prevention is the goal.
5   The attitude of staff should be calm, noncritical and nondomineering.
6   Physical confrontations should avoided.

There will be occasions when, for a variety of reasons, a patient will become violent. In these situations it is essential for the nurse to apply confidently the appropriate skills in order to manage the incident. Leiba (1980) isolates four aspects that need to be considered in the management of violence in the hospital setting:

1 Organization of the ward, department, etc.
2 Prevention
3 Management
4 Follow-up.

Organization of the Ward, Department, etc.

The way in which staff are deployed influences the likelihood and outcome of any violent incident. There must be adequate staffing levels to deal with the violence. There must be a hospital policy for the management of violence . All hospital personnel should then know what to do and how to do it. Teaching sessions on the management of violence should be held on a regular basis so that staff benefit from controlled practice of the required techniques for avoiding or containing violence. It is helpful if there is a team in the hospital that can be called on if such an emergency occurs. Teamwork is essential and the leader must be seen to be confident in making the necessary decisions.

Prevention

Potentially violent situations may be prevented from developing into frank violence by the skills of the staff present at the time. Knowledge of the propensities of individual patients will enable a nurse to recognize many of the signs of impending violence, thus allowing steps be taken to help patients find alternative outlets for their aggressive feelings.

Management

Once violence has occurred, the following may be regarded as among the important management decisions that need to be implemented:

1 All medical and nursing personnel must be involved immediately, the former as medication may be required as part of the management of the situation.
2 Some nurses must be delegated to attend to the needs of the remaining patients, to telephone for help, and to prepare any required medication.
3 If immobilization is needed, the agreed policy for restricting a patient must be implemented.

Follow-up

The incident should be regarded by staff as one from which something can be learned. Staff should be given the opportunity to discuss freely their feelings about the patient, other members of staff and the way the incident was handled as soon as possible after the incident has been resolved. Staff injured as a result of their involvement in the incident may be entitled to industrial injuries benefits or a payment under the criminal injuries compensation scheme and will need to be informed of their rights. All documentation required by law or hospital policy should be completed and forwarded to the appropriate departments.

In Conclusion

It is important to remember finally that many violent incidents arise from the patient feeling vulnerable. Attack may become the preferred means of defence. The manner in which such a patient is approached may be crucial in determining whether the patient will feel secure enough to cease his behaviour or continue to feel threatened, thus spurring him/her on to new acts of violence. The need to control a patient physically should not be seen as a failure of the use of other methods but as the application of the appropriate technique in that situation. Protection against any administrative or legal problems lies in following the appropriate guidelines and applying them in good faith and with due restraint.

References and Further Reading

Bandura A Walters R (1963) Social Learning and Personality Development, Holt, Reinhardt and Winston

Berkowitz L (1962) Aggression: A Social Psychological Analysis, McGraw-Hill

Bethlem Royal and Maudsley Hospitals (1976) Guidelines for the Nursing Management of Violence, Bethlem Royal and Maudsley Hospitals

DHSS (1975) Management of Violent and Potentially Violent Patients in Mental Illness and Subnormality Hospitals, HMSO

Dollard J Miller N E (1961) Frustration and Aggression, Yale University Press

Eysenck H J (1979) The Origins of Violence, Journal of Medical Ethics 5 (3): 105-107

Frued S (1955) The Complete Psychological Works of Sigmund Freud, Volume 18, Hogarth Press

Leiba P A (1980) Management of Violent Patients, Nursing Times Occasional Papers 76 (23): 101-104

Lorenze K (1966) On Aggression, Harcourt, Brace and World

Royal College of Nursing (1979) Seclusion and Restraint in Hospitals and Units for the Mentally Disordered, Royal College of Nursing

Royal College of Nursing and the National Council for Nurses of the United Kingdom (1972) The Care of the Violent Patient: Report of the Liaison Committee, Royal College of Nursing

Russell C Russell W M S (1979) The Natural History of Violence, Journal of Medical Ethics 5 (3): 108-117

Shaw S H (1982) Violence: a personal profile, The Practitioner 226: 281-283

South East Thames Regional Health Authority (1976) Managing the violent patient, Discussion and teaching document, South East Thames Regional Health Authority

Wertham F (1968) A Sign for Cain, Hale

West D J (1979) The response to violence, Journal of Medical Ethics 5 (3): 128-131

Video Material

Nursing Management of Violence, produced by the South East Thames Regional Health Authority, 1977

GUIDELINES: VIOLENCE AND ITS MANAGEMENT

Procedure

Action	Rationale

General Principles

1 Call for assistance by shouting or using any signalling system.

2 Ask another patient to summon help when appropriate.

3 Continue to hold on to the patient once he/she is immobilized.

4 Consider carefully the accessories you wear. Be aware of the length of your fingernails and the way long hair is dressed. Pens, badges and other items must be removed beforehand preferably.

1 It is easier to manage the situation with two or more people.

3 To contain the violence.

4 To minimize the risk of physical injury to patients and staff.

Personal Attack

1 Shout to the patient to stop.

2 Call for assistance.
3 Sound any signalling system.

If these fail, *either*

4 **a** Stay close to the patient.
b Grasp the patient's arm at elbow level and pull towards you.
c Change your grip quickly and encircle patient with your arms.
d Continue pulling the patient towards you.
e Quickly get behind the patient.
f Push the patient towards the nearest wall.
g Retain your grip and lean against the patient, pressing patient to the wall (Figure 45.1).

or

5 **a** Move to one side.
b Place your nearest leg behind the patient.

1 **a** A sharp command may bring the patient back to the reality of the situation.

4 To immobilize the patient by pressing his/her body forward against a wall.

5 To immobilize the patient by holding the patient face downwards on the floor.

Action

Rationale

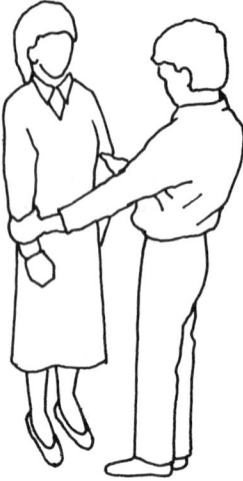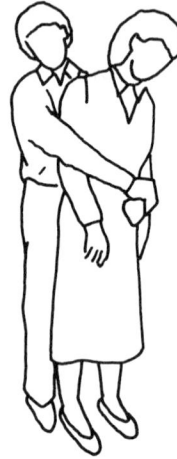

Figure 45.1   Managing the violent patient

c   Keep your foot firmly on the ground.

d   Push the patient over your leg (Figure 45.2).

e   Lower the patient and yourself to the floor, turning the patient at the same time so that the patient's face is towards the floor.

f   Lie across the patient's trunk.

g   If possible, wrap the patient in a blanket (Figure 45.3).

g   To restrict use of limbs even further and to minimize the risk of physical injury to patient and staff.

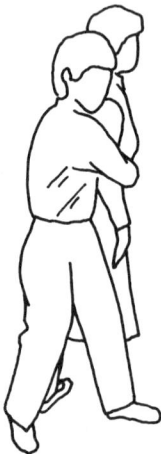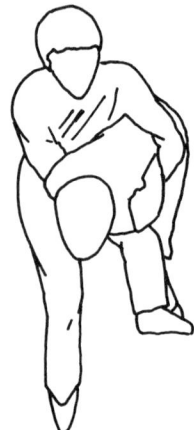

Figure 45.2   Managing the violent patient — a personal attack from behind

Action	**Rationale**
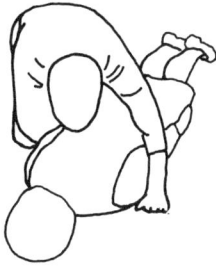	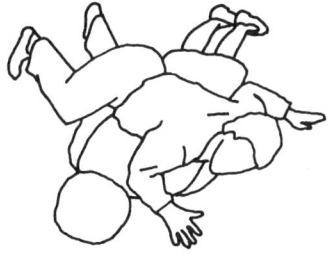

Figure 45.3 Managing the violent patient — a personal attack from behind

Attempted Choking

1 *With the patient in front of you:*

a Bend sharply forward from the waist (Figure 45.4).

b Cross your wrist in front of you and carry out the procedures for personal attack outlined above.

a To break the patient's grip.

b In case the patient brings his/her knee up.

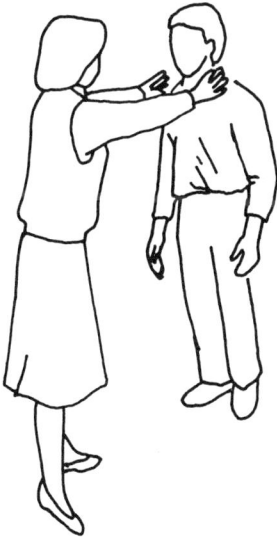	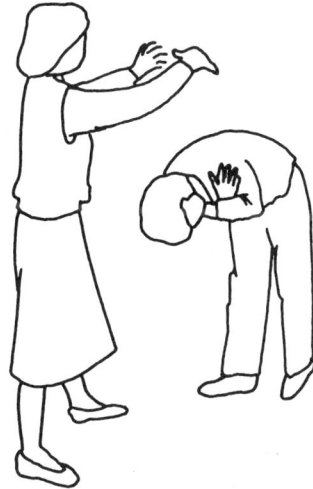

Figure 45.4 Managing the violent patient — attempted choking by a patient in front

2 *With patient behind you:* .

a Grasp a single finger of each of the patient's hands (Figure 45.5).

b Wrench outwards to the full extent of your reach.

a To break the patient's grip

Action	**Rationale**
c Prise the patient's fingers apart.	
d Pull the patient's arms forward, holding the patient close to your back.	**d** To immobilize the patient.
e Maintain this position.	
f Call for help.	

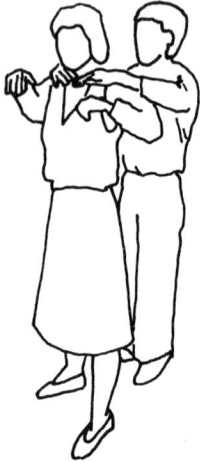

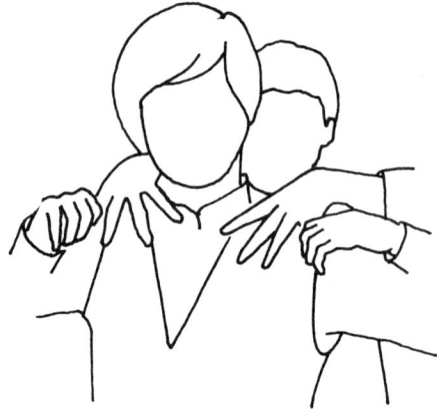

Figure 45.5 Managing the violent patient — attempted choking by a patient from behind

Hair and Tie Pulling

1 Grasp the patient's wrist, pulling his/her hands towards you.	1 To release the pressure on the hair or item of clothing being pulled.
2 Maintain this position (Figure 45.6).	
3 Call for help.	

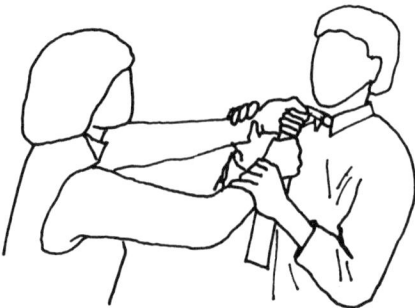

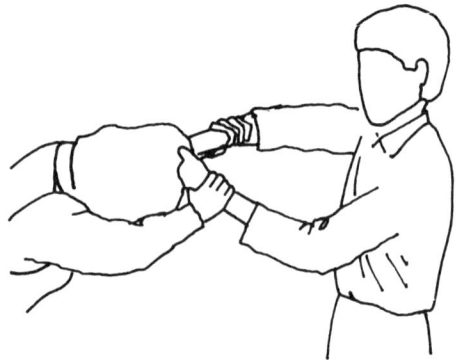

Figure 45.6 Countering hair and tie pulling

Action	**Rationale**

Attack with Objects

1 Back away from the situation.
2 Keep the patient in front of you.
3 Call for help.
4 If trapped, call for help and sound any signalling system.
5 Use a chair or similar object as a shield.
6 Keep to the middle of the room.
7 Defend yourself if attacked (Figure 45.7).

1 ⎫
2 ⎬ To minimize the risk of physical injury.
3 ⎭
4 ⎫

5 ⎬ To protect oneself.
6
7 ⎭

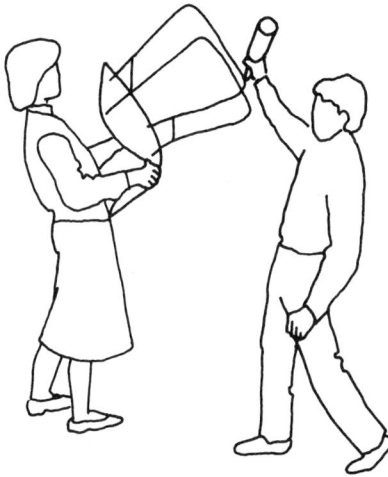

Figure 45.7 Countering an attack with a blunt object

8 *Blunt object:*
   a Close in quickly.
   b Grasp object.
   c Hold on tightly.
   d Call for help.
9 *Sharp object:*
   a Pick up any piece of clothing or material, the larger and thicker the better.
   b Use the material to absorb the impact of any blow.
   c Smother the weapon if possible with the material (Figure 45.8).
   d Call for help.

Action	Rationale

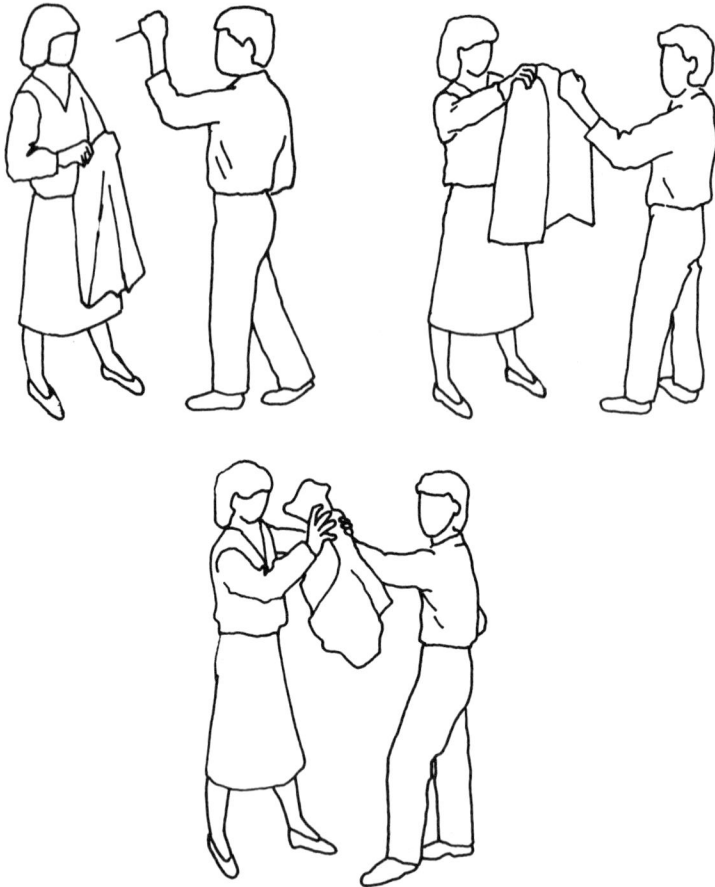

Figure 45.8 Countering an attack with a sharp object

Threat with Firearms

1 Do as the patient demands.	1 A life-threatening situation.

Management of Personnel Involved

1 Senior nurse or team leader should assess the situation and allocate roles. This should include allocating some nurses to care for the remaining patients and to contain violence in the area if possible.	1 Violent incidents are distressing and may trigger off more violence.
2 The first team member should help the nurse who is immobilizing the	2 To achieve full immobilization of the patient.

Action	**Rationale**
patient. He/she may need to disarm the patient and to get the patient to the floor as quickly as possible in the face downwards position of this has not already been achieved. This member should lie across the patient's trunk.	
3 The second member should assist the first two nurses, and should restrain the patient's legs.	
4 The third member should restrain the patient's head and shoulders and turn the patient's head to one side.	4 To maintain a clear airway.
5 The fourth member should help to restrain the patient's legs.	
6 One member, preferably someone who has a particularly good relationship with the patient, should continue talking to the patient.	6 To inform the patient what is happening and the reasons for it.
7 A doctor, preferably the patient's own, should be called and must come immediately.	7 Medication may be required in the management of the violent incident.
8 Attend to any patients and/or staff injured during the violent incident. Inform such people of their legal rights.	8 To comply with legal obligations and hospital policy.
9 Record details of any violent incidents in the appropriate documents.	9 To comply with legal obligations and hospital policy.
10 The entire team involved should discuss the incident.	10 To ventilate feelings. Violent incidents are to be regarded as learning situations.

INDEX

abdominal
  aorta, 2
  cavity, 2
  fluid, relief of the pressure of, 1
  paracentesis, 1-5
    equipment for, 2,3
    indications for, 1
  viscera & abdominal paracentesis, 1
acid base balance & treatment of cardiac arrest, 84, 90
acidosis, metabolic, 363
acquired immune deficiency syndrome, 470
adhesive preparations for stoma patients, 391
adhesives in traction, 432, 433, 435
adrenaline
  in cardiac arrest treatment, 84
  solution, prone to deterioration, 138
adriamycin, 367
aggression vs violence, 471
air
  composition of inspired & expired, 359
  embolism, a hazard of catheter insertion, 94,
    103, 104, 108, 228
airborne contamination, minimizing, 8, 8, 10
albumen, 259, 267
allergy, 226, 228
alopecia
  & administration of adriamycin, 367
  & scalp cooling, 367-370
  & systemic effects of handling cytotoxic drugs, 112
aluminium antacids & constipation, 51
alveoli, 306, 356, 361, 362
Ambu bag, 87, 88, 89, 90, 91, 238, 311
Ambulift, 255
aminoacid preparations administered
  intravenously, 209
  aminoacids & the liver, 259
aminophylline
  in treatment of cardiac arrest, 84
  suppositories, prone to deterioration, 138
amphetamines, 129
amyloidosis, liver biopsy indicated for, 257
anaemia, 44
anal fissures, rectal lavage contraindicated, 59
anal pruritis, suppositories & treatment of, 56
analgesic agent, Entonox as an, 156, 158
analgesics & constipation, 52
anaphylactic
  reaction, 211
  shock & death with green soap enema, 56
anastamosis, 402
anorexia nervosa & constipation, 51
anoxia, 83, 312
  cerebral, postoperative, 336
  & tissue death in pressure sores, 339
anthracycline antibiotic group of drugs, 367
anthrax & formaldehyde for terminal disinfection of, 15
antibacterial agents, effectiveness of, 26
antibiotic therapy & central venous catheterization, 92
antibiotics
  administered intravenously, 208
  barrier nursing of patients resistant to, 12
  conditions for the storage of, 136
  lumbar puncture & introduction of, 264, 267
  serological detection of, 374
anticholinergics & constipation, 51
anti-emetics, prophylactic, 234

antifungal agents, effectiveness of, 26
antihistamines, 167, 169
anti-inflammatory eye-drops,167
antiseptic skin cleansers, 91
anitviral oral hygiene agents, 276
apical drain & removal of air from intrapleural space,
  193
apical heart beat, 353
apneoa, 300, 362
apnoeustic respiration, lesions suggested by, 300
apomorphine, 177
appendicectomy, 399
aqueous humour, 164
Argyle 'double seal' system, 195
arterial pressure, consequences of changes in, 35
artery
  hepatic, catheterization of, 141
  superior gluteal & intramuscular injection, 138
ascitic fluid
  cessation of drainage, 4, 5
  clotting of, procedure in event of, 4
  composition of, 1, 4
  drainage of, 3, 4, 5
asepsis, principles of, 6, 7, 8, 9
aseptic technique, 6-11, 28 29
  aim of, 6, 7
  importance of, 6, 47, 90
  procedure, 10, 11, 104
aspirin
  time remaining in small intestine, 177
  tablets, prone to deterioration, 138
asthma, 306
ataxic breathing, lesions suggested by, 300
atropine
  sulphate in treatment of cardiac arrest, 84
auscultatory gap, 43

Babinski response, 304
bacteria, removal of in handwashing, 7
bacterial
  infections in neutropenia, 21
  investigations of specimens, 373
  vaccines, storage conditions for, 136
  bacteriological surveillance of staff, 14
balanced traction, 431
barium enema, 59
barrier nursing, 12-24
  attending to the patient, 18, 19, 20
  bathing & changing in, 15
  general procedures of, 14, 15, 16
  procedures on discharge of patient, 20, 21
  & source isolation, 13
basal
  blood pressure, 36, 37, 42
  drain, 193
basilic vein as catheterization site, 92, 93
bed type & relief of pressure, 342, 343
bedding as a source of infection, 13, 23
bedpan vs commode in evacuation of the bowels, 52
bends, patients with the, Entonox contraindicated for,
  157
Betadine, 9, 101, 102, 105
bigeminal pulse, 353
bile duct, puncturing of, 260, 263
biomechanics of lifting, 251
Biot's respiration, 363

bladder, 2, 3
    erosion & haematuria following chlorhexidine
        gluconate, 26
    function & abdominal paracentesis, 1
    irrigation, 25, 26, 28-34,
        care of patient during, 31, 32
        recording chart for, 32, 33
    lavage, 25-28
        indications for, 25, 127
        & irrigation, solutions used for, 25, 26
blapharoconjunctivitis, 168
Bleomycin, 1, 116, 117
blink reflex, 166, 168, 298, 303
blistering associated with mustine, 112
blood
    administered intravenously, 209
    — brain barrier, 133, 137, 267
    clots, removal of a bladder lavage, 25, 127
    count, 124
    pressure, 35-43
        diastolic, 36, 38, 39, 41
        factors affecting, 37
        falls in & shock, myocardial
        function & haemorrhage, 36
        methods of recording, 37
        prevention of fall in, 4
        & pulse, 36, 229
        rises in, factors affecting, 36
    product therapy in neutropenia, 22
    urea, 286
    viscosity, 37
    volume & central venous pressure, 96
        & blood pressure, 37
blower humidifier, 189, 191
Bocasan as an oral hygiene agent, 275, 281
bolus injection, dangers of in continous infusion, 210,
    214
bone marrow
    aspiration, 44-48
        anaesthetics for, 45, 47
        complications in, 46
        red, sites in adults, 44
        yellow & fatty, 44
boracic acid, 275
boracic lotion 166
bowel
    care, 49-71
    disease, inflammatory, 54, 59
    functioning, normal factors affecting, 52
    fungal infection of, in neutropenia, 22
    mucosa, enema used to soothe & treat irritated, 54
    surgery, 59
brachial
    plexus injury as hazard of catheter insertion, 94
    pulse site, 351, 352
    vein as site for catheterization, 92, 93
brachytherapy, 72, 73, 74
bradycardia, 299, 305
bradypnoea, 362
brain damage, 83
brainstem
    herniation & lumbar puncture, 264, 266
    damage, 297
bran vs other laxatives, 54
breast lesions, 239, 241
breast neoplasm causing malignant pleural effusion, 115
Breckenridge report & intravenous drug administration,
    205
Buddhists, religious requirements on death, 249
bulk, lack of & constipation, 51
bulk & laxatives, 53, 54

burns, redressing & Entonox, 157
Buchanan bib, laryngectomy & humidification, 190, 191

cachexia, 6
caesium, [137]
    applicators in gynaecology, 74, 75, 76
    implants & applicators, 72-82
    implant needles, insertion & removal of, 73, 74
    vs iridium [192], 72
calcium chloride in treatment of cardiac arrest, 84
canal of schlemm, 162, 167
canalicular fibrosis, 169
Candida albicans, in oral cavity, 21, 276, 280
capillary damage, 339
caps, masks & footwear in barrier nursing, 14
carbohydrates, oxidation of & carbon dioxide, 361
carbon dioxide narcosis, 307
    & hypoventilation, 362
carbon monoxide poisoning, 306, 312
carcinogenesis & mutagenesis, 113
carcinogenic effects of cytotoxic drugs at therapeutic
    levels, 112
carcinoma
    of the bladder, 383
    of the bowel, 383
    of the cervix & caesium [137], vs radium, 72
    of corpus of the cervix:
        Curietron afterloading applicator, 76
        & Fletcher applicator, 74, 75
        & Heyman's capsules, 76
        & Stockholm applicators, 74
    of the liver, primary & secondary, 257
    of the mouth & hypopharynx, 283
    of the pelvis, 383
    & pleural effusions, 115
    of the thyroid, treatment programme for, 229, 230
cardiac
    arrest
        causes of, 83, 84
        in asystole fibrillation, 83
        indicators of, 83
        in iodine [131], patient, emergency procedures for, 238
        resuscitation team, 86
        schematic of necessary procedures, 85
        treatment of, 84
        in ventricular fibrillation, 83
    arrythmias & green soap enema, 56
    competence & central venous pressure, 96
    failure, congestive, rectal lavage contraindicated for,
        59
    irritability & catheter insertion, 108
    myopathy, 84
    output & factors affecting blood pressure, 37
    problems, sodium containing laxatives contraindicated
        for patients with, 54
    rupture & catheter insertion, 108
    tamponade, 203
        & sternal puncture, 46
cardiopulmonary resuscitation 83-91
    criteria for suitability of patient for, 86, 87
    equipment for, 87, 88
    procedures for, 88, 89, 90
care, pre & postoperative, 329-338
carotid pulse site, 351, 352
carotid sinuses, 35
catalase, 274, 279
cataracts, posterior subcapsular, 169
catheter
    bag, guidelines for emptying, 455
    care
        principles of asepsis, 94, 95

principles of & maintenance of
closed system, 94, 95
central venous removal of non-skin tunnelled, 105-108
cleaning an obstructed & bladder lavage, 25
dangers of using acetone of silicone, 101
discharging patients with a central venous
in position, 97
embolism as hazard of insertion of, 94
for bladder lavage & irrigation, 26, 27
Hickman wide bore, 93, 95, 100, 102, 103, 104, 105
insertion of, 92-94
hazards of, 94
procedure for, 93
removal of skin tunnelled, 95, 110
selection, 447, 448
silicon for skin tunnelling, 93
catheterization
& Entonox, 157
female urinary, guidelines for, 452, 453
indications for, 446
male urinary, guidelines for, 449, 450, 451
indications for, 446
for peritoneal dialysis, 320, 321
urinary, 124, 446-458
cauda equina, 226
cellulitis due to sepsis, 226
central nervous system, lesions to & cardiac arrest, 84
central venous catheter: changing the dressing of, 100,
101, 102, 103
guidelines for taking blood samples from, 103, 104,
105
central venous catheterization: 92, 111
reasons for, 92
central venous pressure: 92, 95
blood volume & cardiac competence, 95, 96
reading, 95
cephalic vein at axilla, catheterization of, 92, 93
cerebral
abscess & cerebrospinal fluid, 267
circulation, 83
oedema, enema used to decrease, 55
cerebrospinal fluid 264, 265, 266, 267, 268, 269, 270,
271, 272
functions of, 265
pressure, 266, 269, 270, 271
cervix, carcinoma of the, 74, 75, 76
Chaga's disease & constipation, 51
chemical stimulants as laxatives, 53, 54
chemotherapeutic agents for cancer, hazards of
handling, 112
chemotherapy, systemic, 115
chest drains, 193, 194
chest infection: 82
& post-operative care, 338
chest wall, 358
Cheyne-Stokes respiration, 300, 363
childbirth
enema used to clean lower bowel prior to, 54
& Entonox, 157
Chloramphenicol, 168, 169
chlorexidine
alcoholic solution of:
& catheter sterilization, 97
effectiveness of, 7
detergent wash, effectiveness of, 7
gluconate as a bladder wash-out, 26
as an oral hygiene agent, 275, 276, 280
in spirit spray, 9
cholecystectomy, 399
choline theophyllinate tablets, 138
choroid, 162, 163

plexus, 265
ciliary body, 162, 163, 167
circadian rhythms & temperature, 413
circulatory overload 227, 322
dangers of tap-water enema, 55, 56
cirrhosis, liver biopsy indicated for, 257
cisternal puncture, 265
clavicles, 44
cleaning
hands & aseptic technique, 7
instruments & clothes, 7, 8
clinified tubes, 285, 287, 289, 291
clothes, cleaning & aseptic technique, 78
clothing & gowns in barrier nursing, 14
clotting time, prolonged & liver biopsy contraindicated,
257
cluster breathing, lesions suggested by, 300
coagulation defects, 44, 257
codeine & constipation, 51
codeine phosphate, 76
colon, 3, 49, 381,382
damage to motility of from chemical laxatives, 54
distal, 50
functions of, 49
sigmoid, 50
colonic
lavage vs suppositories, 57
obstruction, suppositories contraindicated, 57
stasis, water, absorption & constipation, 50
colostomy 9, 381, 387
& diet, 384
sigmoid, 381
temporary, 382
coma & levels of consciousness, 297
communicable diseases & barrier nursing, 12
confusion, delirium & levels of consciousness, 297
congenital disorders & stoma, 383
coning & lumbar puncture, 264, 266, 270, 271, 272
conjunctiva, 162, 163, 165
conjunctival hyperaemia, 168
consciousness, full, 296
constipation 49, 50, 51, 52
individual differences & definition of, 52
management of, 50, 51, 52
manual evacuation of bowels & Entonox, 157
reasons for, 51
constrictor pupillae, 168
contamination
airborne & aseptic technique, 8, 9
of bare hands with iodine [131],
emergency procedures for, 237
of staff clothing, 23
controlled drugs 128-130, 144
cornea, 162, 163, 164, 165
corneal
deposits, 169
permeability, 166
steeping, 169
ulcers, 166
coronary occlusion & cardiac arrest, 84
corpus, carcinoma of, 74, 75, 76
corrugated drainage system, 408, 409, 410, 411
corticosteroids, 169
preparations, conditions for storage, 136
costal cartilage, 8th, 259
costodiaphragmatic recess, 258
cough reflex, 190, 191, 275
coughing & systemic effects of handling cytotoxic drugs,
112
cranial nerve
third & control of pupillary activity, 297

fifth & seventh & blink reflex, 298
ninth & tenth, gag & swallow reflex, 298
Crohn's disease & stoma, 383
cross-infection
  common sites of, 446, 447
  of wounds, 9
Curietron afterloading applicator & treatment of
  carcinmoa of corpus or cervix, 76
cyanide poisoning, acute,& hyperbaric oxygen therapy,
  312
cyanosis, 203, 228, 290, 306
  & catheter insertion, 108
cyclophosphamide, 116
cycloplegia, 169
cycloplegics, 166, 167
cytology & cerebrospinal fluid, 267
cytomegalovirus, 470
cytotoxic
  agents given intravesically, 26
  chemotherapy
    & hair-loss, 367, 368
  neutropenia, 21
cytotoxic drugs
  handling & administration 112-127
    protection of environment when, 119
    protection of staff when, 116, 117, 118, 119
  insertion of, 1
  intramuscular & subcutaneous injection of, 122
  intravenous administration of, 120, 121
  intravesical administration of, 123, 124, 125, 126, 127
  introduction of & lumbar puncture, 264
  oral administration of, 121, 122
  proven local effects of direct contact, 112
cytotoxic therapy & central venous catheterization, 92

death
  documentation in event of, 245, 246, 247
  following an operation, procedures for, 247
  in caesium ⁻¹³⁷ patients, procedures for, 247
  in iodine ⁻¹³¹ patients, emergency procedures for, 247
  in iridium ⁻¹⁹² patients, procedures for, 247

  medical certificate of the cause of, 245
    & occurence of bacterial fermentation, 246
    relatives, dealing with in the event of, 248
    & religious requirements of:
      Buddhists, 249
      Hindus, 249
      Jews, 248
      Moslems, 249
      Sikhs, 249
    & patient with hepatitis B, procedure for, 247
    unexpected, procedures for, 247
decerebrate posturing, 297
decompression sickness & hyperbaric oxygen therapy,
  312
decorticate posturing, 297
defibrillation in treatment of cardiac arrest 86
dehydration
  & constipation, 51
  & nasogastric feeding, 286, 293, 295
  problems of, 4
dentures, 279, 280, 281
deodorants for stoma patients, 392
depression & constipation, 51
dextrose in osmosis, 318
diabetes
  & abnormal changes to the retina, 163
  maturity onset, bowel functioning & bran, 54
  mellitus & pressure sores, 340
  mellitus patient in peritoneal dialysis, 327

diabetic ketoacidosis & hyperventilation, 363
dialysis 318, 319
dialysis fluid
  preparation of, 321, 322
  temperature of 320, 321, 326
dialysing membrane, peritoneum used as, 317
diamorphine solution, prone to deteriorate, 138
diaphragm, 192, 194, 258,
  356, 358, 361
diarrhoea, due to previous radiotherapy, 76
diarrhoea, management of, 49
diastolic pressure, 36, 38, 39, 41
diathermy burns, 333
diet & exercise, key factors in bowel evacuation, 52
diet & pressure sores, 340
diffusion in exchange across peritoneal membrane, 318
dilator pupillae, 168
disinfection of an instrument, emergency, 8
diverticular disease, 383
dizziness & systemic effects of handling cytotoxic drugs,
  112
Dobbie applicator & irradiation of the whole vagina, 76
dorsal nerve root, 271
Doxorubicin, 367
drain, intra pleural, 198, 200, 201, 202, 204
drain, types of chest, 193, 194, 195
drainage, bag
  leg, 448, 449
  for stoma patients, 389
  drainage, changing tubing bottles for, 199, 200
drainage, guidelines for the management of underwater
  seal, 196, 197, 198, 199
drainage, intrapleural, 202, 203, 204
dressing trolley & aseptic techniques 8
dressings, drains & packs, changing &
  use of Entonox, 157
droplet dispersion, masks & aseptic techniques, 8
drowning & cardiac arrest, 84
drug administration, 128-155
  correct form of prescription, 130
  ear drops, guidelines for, 155
  eye medication, guidelines for, 155
  inhalations, guidelines for, 154, 155
  marking of bottles, 130
  & Misuse of Drugs Act, 1971, 128-131
  nasal drops, guidelines for, 155
  oral guidelines for, 142-145
  rectal preparation, guidelines for, 153
  safe custody of controlled, 130
  supplies of controlled, 129
  topical applications, guidelines for, 154
  vaginal preparation, guidelines for, 154
drug overdose, 176, 177
drug registers 130
drugs, controlled, 128, 129
drugs prior to deterioration, 138
drugs in treatment of cardiac arrest, 84
duodenum, 2
dural sac, 266
dysmotility & constipation, 51
dyspnoea, 108, 109, 263
  & pleural effusion, 114

Ear swab, 377
Ebola fever, & formaldehyde for terminal disinfection,
  15
elastic recoil of the arteries & factors affecting
  blood pressure, 37
electrocution & cardiac arrest, 84
electrolyte balance, correcting, stage in treatment of
  cardiac arrest, 84, 90

electrolyte maintenance & central venous
catheterization, 92
electrolytes absorbed by the colon, 49
electrolytes, exchange of imbalance in, 2, 4, 26, 54, 60,
61, 286
embolisms air, 94, 103, 104, 108
228
acute gas & hyperbaric oxygen therapy, 312
particle, 228
emesis, induced vs gastric lavage, 177
emphysema, subcutaneous, 203
empyema, draining of intra-abdominal, 401
encephalitis & monocytes, 267
endocrinal causes of unconsciousness, 439
endoscopy, enema used to clean lower bowel prior to, 54
endothelium, capillary, 318
enema
administration of, procedures for, 62, 63, 64
dangers of green soap, 56
dioctyl sulphosuccinate & stool softening, 55
evacuant, 55, 56
phosphate, prior to X-ray examination & surgery, 55
reasons prescribed, 54,55
retention, 56
& short term management of severe constipation, 50,
54, 55, 56
tap-water & danger of circulatory overload,
55, 56
types of, 55, 56
Entonox
administration, 156-161
composition of, 156
contraindications for, 157
vs opiates, 158
indicated prior to painful procedures, 157
epidural space, 66
epiphora, 168
equilibrium in osmosis, 318
equipment as a source of infection, 13
ergometrine solution, prone to deteriorate, 138
erythema 225
Escherichia coli, 21
ethambutol & damage to the optic nerve, 169
excoriation, 49
eye
care 162-175
anatomy & physiology, 162, 163, 164
of an insensitive, 166
& risk of infection, 162
drops
anaesthetic, 165, 167
antibiotic, 168
as artificial tears, 168
instillation of, 165, 166
oil based, 165
'one-drop' rule with, 165
dry, 169
irrigation, 166
guidelines for, 173, 174, 175
medications, 166, 167,168
ointment, 172, 173
swab, 374, 375
toxic effect of common systemic drugs on, 168, 169
swabbing, 169-171
eyes, drugs having same effect on healthy & diseased,
166, 167, 168

facial & jaw injuries & nasogastric feeding, 283
faeces
composition of, 49
investigation of, 378, 379

fasting, preoperative, 330, 331, 332
fat emulsion administered intravenously, 209
femoral pulse site, 351, 352
fibrin formation, 192, 224, 321
fibrinogen, 259
film badges for radiological protection, 230, 242
fire, emergency procedures for iodine [131] patient in a,
238
firearms, threat with & management of violence, 480
fistulae, internal
& gastronasal feeding, 283
rectal lavage contraindicated in, 59
5 - fluorouracil (5-FU), 169
fixed traction, 430, 431
Fletcher applicator for carcinoma of the corpus or
cervix, 74, 75
flora normal to the human body, 13
flora, pathogens in, 13
fluid balance chart, patient's, 4
foam sticks, 276, 278, 279, 280
food, bacterial contamination in, reduced by microwave,
15
fovea centralis, 162, 163
Fowler's position, 3, 337
Framycetin, 168
Frusemide & treatment of cardiac arrest, 84
fungal infections in neutropenia, 21, 22
fungal investigations of specimens, 374

gag & swallow reflex, 298, 303
gallbladder, 258
gangrene & soap solution in rectal lavage, 60
gas gangrene & hyperbaric oxygen therapy, 312
gases, exchange of & respiration, 360, 361
gastric lavage 176-181
contraindicated for caustics & corrosives, 177
vs induced emesis, 177
tubes, 177
gastric motility, factors affecting, 331
gaestrointestinal
operations, suppositories contraindicated after, 57
tract neoplasms & malignant pleural effusions, 155
gastrostomy, 282
Gieger counter, 232, 236, 237, 242, 247
gingival tissue, 279
Glasgow Coma Scale, 300, 440
glaucoma, treatment of, 167
Glisson's sling, 432
globulin, 259, 267
globulin levels raised in cerebrospinal fluid, 267
glossopharyngeal nerve, 35
glutethimide, 177
glycerin, as an oral hygiene agent, 275, 279
glyceryl trinitrate tablets, prone to deterioration, 138
gowns & aspetic technique, 8
Gram-negative organisms, 13, 21, 23, 275
Gram-positive organisms 14, 26, 275
granulocytes, 21, 23
green soap enema, dangers of, 56
gynaecological applicators of caesium [137] 74, 75, 78
& preparation of the patient for, 76
removal of, guidelines for, 79, 80, 81, 82
gynaecological operations, suppositories contraindicated,
57
gynaecological radioactive sources, care of patients with,
79

haematoma, prevention of formation of, 47, 48, 152,
208, 459, 469
haematopesis, evaluation of through bone marrow
aspiration, 44

haematuria
    bladder erosion & chlorhexidine gluconate, 26
    intravesical administration of cytotoxic drugs, 126
haemodialysis vs peritoneal dialysis, 317
haemoglobin, 286
    liver reprocesses, 259
haemorrhage
    & hazards of catheter insertion, 94
    & liver biopsy, 260, 262, 263
    local, enema used to stop, 55
    postoperative, 203
    primary postoperative, 335
    severe & green soap enema, 56
    subarachnoidal, 267
haemorrhoids
    prolapsed, rectal lavage contraindicated, 59
    treatment of with suppositories, 56
haemopneumothorax, 90
haemothorax,
    & cardiac arrest, 84
    & hazards of catheter insertion, 94, 108
Hair-loss
    distress to patients of, 367, 370
    methods of prevention, 367
    psychological trauma of, 367
    & scalp cooling, 367-370
halitosis, 275
hallucinogenic drugs, 129
Hamilton-Russell traction, 431
hand washing & aspetic technique, 7, 14, 23
headache & systemic effect of handling cytotoxic drugs,
    112
heparin 97, 109, 110, 208, 216, 218, 219, 220, 321
    lock & intravenous drug administration, 212, 219, 222
solution prone to deteriorate, 138
hepatic
    blood vessel, intra- or extra-, 260
    coma & hyperventilation, 362,
Hepatitis B, 82-188
    antigen carriers, 183,
    clinical responses to, 182
    core antigen, 183
    epdiemiology, 182
    guidelines for, 184-188, 373, 470
guidelines in case of accidental innoculation, 186
    immunoglobulin, 186
    precautions if bleeding is present, 186, 187, 188
    procedures on death of a patient with, 188, 247
    serological markers for diagnosis of, 183
    surface antigen, 183
Hepsal, 97, 105
    herniation & lumbar pressure, 266, 270, 271, 272
herpes simplex virus, 22
herpes zoster virus, 22
herpetic lesions, consequences of, 22
Heyman's capsules & treatment of carcinoma of the
    corpus, 76
Hibiscrub: 7, 9, 10, 14, 17, 19, 29, 31, 104
    & possibility of skin reaction, 7
Hibisol, 7, 9, 11, 20, 28, 29, 31, 102, 103, 199, 395,
    423, 424, 426, 449, 450, 452
Hibispray, 9
Hibitane, 103, 105
Hindus, religious requirements for on death, 249
Hirschsprung's disease 51, 56
    & constipation 51, 56
    death in & potassium based green soap, 56
humidification
    guidelines for immediate postoperative, 191
    indicated, 189, 191, 311, 312, 315, 316
humidifiers, types of, 189, 190

hydration, systemic oral, 273, 280
hydrogen peroxide as an oral hygiene agent, 274, 275,
    281
hydrothorax & hazards of catheter insertion, 94, 108
hyperaemia & soap solution in rectal lavage, 60
hyperbaric therapy, 312
hypercalcaemia & constipation, 51
hypercatabolic states & nasogastric feeding, 283
hyperglycaemia & peritoneal dialysis, 327
hyperkalaemia & cardiac arrest, 84
hyperkalaemia & green soap enema, 56
hypernatraemia, 286
hypernoea, 36, 72
hypertension, 36, 42, 299, 305
    & abnormal changes to the retina, 163
hyperventilation 161, 362
    hypervolaemia, postoperative, 337
hypoglycaemics & bran as a laxative, 54
hypokalaemia, 1
    & cardiac arrest, 84
hyponatraemia, 1
hypoproteinaemia, 340, 349
hypotension 36, 42
    & cardiac arrest, 84
    as first sign of septicaemia in neutropenia, 23
    in peritoneal dialysis & fluid loss, 322
    postoperative, 336
hypotensives & constipation, 51
hypothalmus, damage to & temperature fluctuation, 299
hypothermia & cardiac arrest, 84
hypoventilation, 307, 362
hypovolaemia, 1
    postoperative, 337
hypoxia, 89, 307, 308, 333
Hypromellose, 168
hysterectomy, 399

idiopathic slow bowel & constipation, 51
Idoxuridine solution, prone to deterioration, 138
ileal
    conduit, 382
    loop, 382, 387
ileocaecal sphincter, 49
ileostomy, 382-387
    & diet, 384
iliac crest, 44, 45
immunosuppressed patient & need of barrier nursing, 21
immunosuppression
    & oral hygiene, 281
    & pressure sores, 340
inanition & pleural effusion, 114
incontinence
    in iodine[131] patient, emegency procedures for, 237
    intractable & stoma, 383
    & pressure sores, 340
Indomethacin, 169
infection
    control measures for hepatitis B, 184
    local or systemic in abdominal paracentesis, 5
    risk of in recatheterization, 26
    sources ofcross infection, 13, 30
        in hand washing, 7
        self-infection, 13
infections
    causing unconsciousness, 439
    common in neutropenia, 21, 22
infectious diseases & barrier nursing, 12
information & patient's well-being, 330
infusion, guidelines for drug administration by
    continous, 210, 213, 214, 215
    intermittent, 210, 211, 215, 216, 217, 218, 219

injections
  guidelines for the administration of, 145-152
  guidelines for drug administration by
    bolus, 219, 220, 221, 222
    direct, 219, 220, 221, 222
  intra-arterial, 133, 137, 138, 141
  intra-articular, 133, 137, 138
  intracardiac, 137, 138
  intradermal, 133, 137, 138
  intralesional, 137, 138
  intramuscular, 137, 138, 150
    sites for, 138, 139
  intrathecal, 133, 137, 138
  intravenous, 133, 137, 141
  multidose vial, 147, 148, 149, 150, 151
  push, 219, 220, 221, 222
  single dose ampoule, 146, 147
  site & needle size, 140, 141
  sites of, 138, 139
  skin preparation for, 139, 140
  subconjunctival, 134
  subcutaneous, 133, 137, 138, 151, 152
  Z-track, 138, 139
inspiratory capacity, 359
Inspiron system nebulizer, 189, 191
instruments, cleaning & aseptic technique, 7, 8
insulin solution, prone to deterioration, 138
intercostal muscles, 258, 259, 356, 361, 363
intercostal vessels, 258
intercranial pressure, raised & herniation, 264, 272, 305
interstitial therapy with iridium[192], 239
intoxicated patient, Entonox contraindicated for,
intra-abdominal pressure, 251, 254
intra-oral iridium[192] implants, 240, 241
intraperitoneal pressure & central venous pressure, 96
intrapleural
  drain, removal of an, 200, 201, 202
  drainage, 192-204, 263
  drugs, guidelines for administration of, 122, 123
  instillation of cytotoxic drugs, 114
intrathoracic
  pressure & central venous pressure, 96
  surgery, 193
intravenous
  administration of cytotoxic drugs, 120, 121
  drug administration, 205-228
    dangers of contamination in, 208, 209
    diagnostic, 208
    1976 DHSS guidelines for, 205, 206, 207
    responsibility for procedures in, 205, 206
    a risk of infection, 206, 207, 208
    safety & drug addition, 209
  methods of administering
    direct intermittent injection, 211, 212
    continous infusion, 210
    intermittent infusion, 210, 211
intravenous infusion
  in cardiopulmonary resuscitation, 90
  & intubation in treatment of cardiac arrest, 86, 89, 90
intravesical installation of cytotoxic drugs, 123, 124, 125
intubation, endotracheal, 86
iodine concentrating organs, 229
iodine[131], contamination of bare hands, emergency
  procedure, 237
iodine[131], patient, emergency procedure for: cardiac
  arrest, 238
  death of, 237, 238, 247
  in case of fire, 238
  protocols for, 229-238
iodine [131] therapy room, preparation of & cleaning of,
  232

iodine [131] treatment: discharge of patients, 233
  emergency procedures in, 237, 238
  nursing patient before, 234
  nursing patient after, 234, 235, 236, 237
  preparation of patient, 233
ipecacuanha, 177
iridium[192] implants, 239-243
  removal of, 241
interstital treatment with, 239
  patient discharge of, 241
& post-treatment local reaction, 241
    reasons indicated, 239
iris, 162, 163, 167
isolation
  accommodation, design & construction of,
    13-14
  of the patient in barrier nursing, criteria, 15
  room in barrier nursing, entering & leaving, 18, 20
  room, preparation of, 17, 18, 23
isoprenaline in treatment for cardiac arrest, 84
isoprenaline tablets & solution, prone to deterioration,
    138

Jaques stomach tube, 30 gauge, 177
jaundice, 182, 257
jejunostomy, 282
Jews, religious requirements on death of, 248
jugular pulse site, 351, 352
jugular vein, internal, external as catheterization site,
    92, 93

klebsiella, 21, 23
Korotkoff's sound, 37, 38, 39
Kussmaul's respiration, 363

lacrimal
  canaliculi, 164
  gland, 164
  puncti, 164, 170
lactose intolerance, 293
laparotomy, 263
laryngectomy, Entonox contraindicated for, 157
Lassa fever & formaldehyde for terminal disinfection of,
    15
last offices, 244-249
lateral rectus, 162
laxative abuse, 52
laxatives
  dependence upon, 53
  illicit use of & constipation, 51
  & short term management of constipation, 50, 53, 54
  types of, 53
lemon juice as an oral hygiene agent, 274
lens, 162, 164
lesions
  cerebral & abnormal respiration patterns, 300
  small primary, iridium[192] treatment for, 239
  upper motor neurone, test for, 303
lethargy & levels of consciousness, 296, 297
leucopoenia, danger of, Entonox contraindicated when,
    157
leukaemia, 44, 367
  & chemotherapy via lumbar puncture, 267
lifting, 250-256
  guidelines for, 255, 256
  mechanical aids to, 254
  potential hazards of, 250
technique
  the orthodox lift, 254
  the shoulder lift, 252, 254
  the through arm lift, 254

techniques compared, 254
ligament
    interspinous, 266
    supraspinous, 266
lightheadedness & systemic effects of handling cytotoxic
    drugs, 112
lignocaine & treatment of cardiac arrest, 84
Listerine as an oral hygiene agent, 276
liver, 2, 258
    functions of , 258, 259
    function, diagnosis & intravenous drug administration,
       208
    needle biopsy 257-263
       complications in, 260
       contraindications for, 257
       guidelines for, 260, 261, 262, 263
       investigations prior to, 259
       vs needle, 257
    tear, risk of, 262, 263
locus of control & postoperative patient recovery, 330
lubricating laxatives, 53
lumbar
    puncture, 264-272
       contraindications to, 264
       guidelines for, 268, 269, 270, 271
       & instillation of chemotherapy, 267
    subarachnoid space, 264, 265, 268, 269
lung
    anatomy, normal altered by pleural effusion, 115
    capacity, total, 358
    defence mechanisms, 362
    neoplasm causing malignant pleural effusions, 115
lungs, 192, 194
lymph nodes, deposits in local, 230
lymphocytes & cerebrospinal fluid, 267
lymphoma, 367
    neoplasms causing malignant pleural effusions, 115
lysozyme, 164

macula lutea 163
malignancies, gynaecological treated by radioactive
    applicators 74, 75, 76
managing violence 473
mannitol solutions administered intravenously, 209
manual traction, 430
Manusept, 9
Marburg disease & formaldehyde for terminal
    disinfection 15
masks & aseptic techniques 8
maxillofacial injuries, & Entonox contraindicated for,
    157
MC masks & oxygen therapy, 310, 314
mechanical ventilation & oxygen therapy, 311
mediastinal shift, 203
mediastinum 192
medicinal preparations
    inhalations, 134
    injections, 133, 134
    lipsomes, 135
    oral, 132, 133
    rectal & vaginal 133
    solutions, 134
    topical applications, 134
medicines, 128
Medicines Act 1968, 131-135
medicines, storage of, 135, 136
medulla oblongata 35, 361
Meibornian glands, 168
melanosis coli from chemical stimulants as laxatives 54
meninges
    arachnoid, 265

dura, 265
    pia mater, 265
meningitis
    & lumbar puncture, 264, 267
    tubercular & monocytes, 267
    viral & monocytes in, 267
mesenteries, functions of, 2
mesothelium, 318
metabolic abnormalities of gastrointestinal tract, 283
metabolic causes of unconsciousness, 439
metastases, 229, 230
metastatic carcinoma, 44
metastatic disease & liver:
    severe hair loss, 367
methanol poisoning, 177
methotrexate, & related antimetabolites, effects on the
    eye, 168
methyl cellulose, 168
microbicides, wide-spectrum 9
micrococcus, 13
mid-axilla & reading central venous pressure 96, 98, 109
miliary tuberculosis, liver biopsy indicated for, 257
Milton 291, 292
    as an oral hygiene agent, 276
miotics, 167
Misuse of Drugs Act 1971, 128, 129, 130, 131
mortuary, 245, 246, 247, 248
Moslems, religious requirements on death, 249
Motor function, 296, 298, 299
mouth care 273-281
    guidelines for, 278, 279
    instruments used in, 276, 277
    reasons for indication of, 273
mouth, dry, 273, 275, 276, 277
mucosa buccal, 274, 275, 276, 277
mucosal damage & green soap enema, 56
mucus
    produced by the colon, 49
    removal of hardened oral, 274, 275
multiple sclerosis
    & constipation, 51
    & raised globulin in cerebrospinal fluid, 267
mustine, blistering associated with, 112
mutagenesis vs carcinogenesis, 113
mutagenic effects of cytotoxic drugs at therapeutic
    levels, 112
myasthenia gravis, diagnosis of & intravenous drug
    administration, 208
mydriatics, 166, 167, 169
myelitis & raised protein levels in cerebrospinal fluid,
    267
myeloma, 44
myelosuppresion, 124
myocardial infarction & Entonox, 157
myocardial stress, 308
mysenteric plexi, from chemical stimulants as laxatives,
    54
myxoedema & pulse, 355

Narcotics, 128
Nasal cannulae & oxygen therapy, 310, 311, 315
nasogastric feeding, 282-295
    administration of, 285, 286, 291, 292
    assessment of patient prior to, 283, 284
    contraindicated in patients, 282, 283
    frequency of, 286
    & patient monitoring, 286, 294, 295
    temperature of feed, 285
nasogastric intubation, 289-291
    with Clinifeed tubes, 287-289
nasolacrimal duct, 164, ,165

nausea & systemic effects of handling cytotoxic, drugs 112
necrosis
    danger of & intra-arterial drug administration, 141
    & green soap enema,56
Neomycin, 168
neoplasms causing malignant pleural effusions,115
Neostigimine, 326
neurogenic factors & factors affecting blood pressure, 37
neurological
    damage & stoma, 383
    observations, 296-305
        guidelines for 301-305
neurosyphilis & raised globulin in cerebrospinal fluid, 267
neutropenia 6, 21
    barrier nursing for, 21-24
    infections common in, 21, 22
    infections occurring in, 21, 22
    & oral hygiene, 281
neutrophil count 21, 42
nitrogen mustard, 116
nitrogenic balance, 286, 295
nitrous oxide, 156, 157, 160, 161
Norton scores, 342, 343, 349
nose swab, 375
Norton Morgan drainage system, 408, 409, 410, 411
noxythiolin (Noxyflex) 26, 28
nursing staff, guidelines for the protection of when handling cytotoxic drugs, 116-119
Nutricath, 93
Nystatin, prone to deteriorate, 138

oblique, external 258, 259
obtundation & levels of consciousness, 297
occipital cortex, 163
ocular pemphigus, 169
occulocephalic reflex, 298
oedema, 109
    local, 226
oesophageal surgery, 283
oesophagus, 177, 192
    fungal infection of in the neutropenia, 22
Ohio nebulizer, 189, 190, 191
omentum, 321
operative care, pre & post, 329-338
opiates, 129
    vs Entonox, 158
OpSite, 102
optic chiasma, 163
optic discs,162
optic nerve, 162, 163
optic neuritis, 169
oral
    administration of cytotoxic drugs, 121, 122
    contraceptives, 169
oral hygiene, 273
    agents for, 273, 274, 275, 276
oral mucosa, 274-277
    stressors to, 277, 280
oral ulcers, 274, 275, 279
Oraldene, as an hygiene agent, 275
orthopaedic traction, application of & entonox, 157
osmosis across peritoneal membrane, 318
osmotic
    agents as laxatives, 53, 54
    pressure, 318
osteodiponecrosis & hyperbaric oxygen therapy, 312
osteomyelitis & hyperbaric oxygen therapy, 312
ostomist
    & fear of maladour, 348, 385, 397

& sex, 385
ovary neoplasms causing malignant pleural effusions, 115
overdoses of depressant drugs & cardiac arrest, 84
overhydration in peritoneal dialysis & pulse, 322
oxygen
    care need with, 307, 308
    giving sets, types of, 308-312
    tent
        therapy, 263, 306-316
            continous, 277, 289
            humidification indicated in, 189, 191
oxyhaemoglobin dissociation curve, 307
oxyphenabutazone, 167
oxytocin, prone to deteriorate, 138

pads, heel & elbow pressure relief, 342
pain
    of bone marrow aspiration, 45, 47, 48
    incisional, 203
    & injections, 141
    postoperative & patient education, 320
painful procedures, indication of Entonox, 157
pancreas, 2
pancreatitis, 283
paraffin, repeayted use of liquid, dangers of, 53
paraldehyde, prone to deteriorate, 138
paracentesis, 166
paralytic ileus, suppositories contraindicated in, 57
paraplegia & constipation, 51
parenteral nutrition & central venous catheterization, 92, 95
parietal peritoneum, 2, 317
parietal pleura, 115, 192, 194, 258, 358
paroleine, 165, 166
Paul's tubing system, 408, 409, 410, 411
pedal pulse site, 351, 352
pelvic
    abcess, 82
    cellulitis, 82
    traction, 432
penile swab, 378
Penrose drainage system, 408, 409, 410, 411
perforation of bladder or bowel & peritoneal dialysis, 325
pericardial tamponade, 84
pericarditis, purulent, drainage of, 401
periorbital oedema, 168
periosteum, 45,47
peritoneal cavity, 2, 3, 318, 319, 320, 321, 322
peritoneal dialysis, 317-328
    checklist for, 323
    continous ambulatory, 319
    guidelines for, 320-324
    intermittent, 319
    reasons indicated, 317
peritoneal fluid, removal of & abdominal paracentesis,dangers of, 1, 3,
peritoneal membrane, osmosis & diffusion across, 318
peritoneum
    anatomy & physiology of, 1, 2, 259, 317, 318
    functions of, 2, 318
    pelvic, 2
peritonitis
    due to perforation of the uterus, 82
    & liver biopsy, 260, 263
pernasal swab, 375, 376
perperitoneal cavity, insertions to, 1
personal attack & management of violence, 475, 476
personal contact as source of infection, 13
peristaltic action, 50, 53, 54

Phenylephrine solution, prone to deteriorate, 138
phlebitis
    chemical, 209, 225
    septic, 209
photophobia, 168
physics department, role of & radiological protection,
    230, 231, 232, 233, 236, 237, 238
plantar reflex, 298, 303
plaque, 275, 279, 280
plasma administered intravenously, 209
plasma proteins, liver's production of, 257
platelet concentrate administered intravenously, 209
platelet count, 48, 124
pleura, 192
    diaphragmatic, 258
    parietal, 115, 192, 194, 258, 358
    visceral, 115, 356, 358
pleural effusion, effects of, 114
pleural effusions, methods of treatment for malignant,
    115
pleural space, 192, 193
    in healthy subject, 192
    pressures in, 192, 19, 198
pleuritis, right lower lobe, 257
pneumonia, 22, 362
    aspiration, 276
    humidification indicated in, 189
    lipoid, 53
    right lower lobe, 257
pneumothorax, 192, 198
    & cardiac arrest,
    Entonox contraindicated for, 157
    & hazards of catheter insertion, 94, 108
    & liver biopsy, 260, 262, 263
    tension, 201, 203
poisons
    liver detoxification of,259
Poisons Act, 1972, 131
poisons & drugs as causes of unconsciousness, 439
polymorphonuclear leucocytes & cerebrospinal fluid, 267
popliteal pulse site, 351, 352
porphyria, acute & constipation, 51
positioning, correct & pressure sores, 341
postmortem, 244, 245, 247, 249
postoperative care
    guidelines for, 334-335
    physical, 329
    psychological, 329
posture, 298
pregnancy & constipation, 51
pregnant client & blood pressure, 42
preoperative care
    guidelines for, 332, 333
    physical, 329
    psychological, 329
pressure
    in pleural space & thoracic cavity, 192, 193, 198
    sores, 339-350
        dressing for treatment of, 346, 347
        & hygiene, 344
        mechanical methods for relief, 342, 343
        patients at risk of, 340, 341
        prevention of, guidelines for, 349
        treatment of, 341, 342, 343, 344, 345, 349,   350
prevention & the management of violence, 473
proctitis, postradiation, rectal lavage contraindicated, 59
prostate neoplasms causing malignant pleural effusions,
    115
prostatic surgery, bladder irrigation & blood clots, 25
protein & cerebrospinal fluid, 267
proteins, depletion of in abdominal paracentesis, 1

proximal arterial tree, 35
proximal vascular system, 55
pruritis, 168
    & systemic effects of handling cytotoxic drugs, 112
pseudomonas, 21
psychological preparation of patients for surgery, 329
psychoses, chronic & constipation, 51
pulmonary
    disease, chronic obstructive, 306
    embolism, 203, 225, 337
        & cardiac arrest, 84
        & catheterization, 110
    oedema, 306
        reduction of aminophylline, 84
    tumours, risk of & inhalation of liquid paraffin, 53
pulp traction, 432
pulse, 351-353
    amplitude, 351, 353
    elasticity, 351, 353
    guidelines for, 354
    quality, 351, 353
    rate, 351, 352
        raised, 109
    rhythm, 351, 352, 353
    sites of, 351, 352
pupil, 167
pupillary activity, 296, 297
Purpura, severe, 257
pus, draining of intra-abdominal, 401
pyrazole derivatives, 167
pyrexia, 42, 82, 94, 116, 209, 227, 413, 416

Queckenstedt's manoeuvre, 266, 270

radial pulse site, 351, 352, 353
radiation
    beta, 229, 239
    gamma, 229, 239
    enteritis, 283
radioactive
    implants & applicators, 72-82, 229-238,
        239-243
    interactivity gynaecological applicators & Entonox,
        157
    patient's body fluids after iodine[131], 231
    phosphorus as sclerosing agent in pleural space, 116
    sources
        care of patients with gynaecological, 79
        care of patients with intraoral, 78, 79, 241, 243
        patient with in cardiac arrest, 91, 238
        sealed & care of patients, 77, 78, 241, 242
radiological
    examination & lumbar puncture, 264
    protection policy & procedures, 230-233
    protection & role of physics department, 230, 231,
        232, 233, 236, 237, 238
radiotherapy, 72-82, 115, 229-238, 239-243
    & dry mouth, 273, 275, 280
rectal
    examination for degree of constipation, 52
    lavage
        administration of, equipment for, 67
        choice of catheters for, 61
        contraindications for, 59
        hypertonic solutions for, 60
        isotonic saline for, 61
        reasons for use of, 58, 59
        soap solutions for, 59, 60
        tap water for, 60
    swab
rectum

need to avoid manual evacuation of, 52
sensitive to pain, 50
Redivac & closed drainage systems, 406, 407, 408
reflex
arcs & maintenance of normal blood pressure, 35
tachycardia, 35
vagal slowing of the heart, 35
reflexes, 298, 302
relatives & death of a patient, procedures for, 248
religious requirements on death for
Buddhists, 249
Hindus, 249
Jews, 248
Moslems, 249
Sikhs, 249
renal
dysfunction
& bladder lavage & irrigation, 25, 32
postoperative, 337
failure, 363
magnesium salts contraindicated, 54
& peritoneal dialysis for chronic, 317
flow, fall in, consequences of, 35
function, impaired & rectal lavage contraindicated, 59
insufficiency & bocasan as an oral hygiene agent, 275
insufficiency & thymbol as an oral hygiene agent, 276
underperfusion, postoperative, 336
units & hepatitis B, need for screening for, 183
respiration, 356-366
& anatomy of the pleural space, 192
guidelines for, 363, 364
interference to & abdominal paracentesois, 1
patterns, abnormal, 300, 304
& vital signs, 299
respiratory
alkalosis, 363
centre, 361
chemical control of, 361
depression of & cardiac arrest, 83, 84
neural control of, 361
dysfunction & postoperative care, 335
infections, lower, 306
insufficiency & pleural effusion, 114
reticular activating mechanism & levels of consciousness,
297
retina, 162, 163
retinal
lesions, 169
pigmentary toxicity, 169
vessels, 162
reverse barrier nursing & protective isolation, 13, 21
rhinitis, humidification indicated in, 189
rib cage, 192, 194
rickettsial vaccines, storage conditions for, 136
rigor mortis, 245
Robert's suction pump, 196, 197
Roger's spray & humidification for tracheostomy, 190,
191
rotation of patient & administration of intrapleural
drugs, 122, 123

salicylate
overdose & hyperventilation, 363
poisoning & gastric lavage, 176, 177
saline, normal, 344
as a bladder washout, 26
for eye irrigation, 166
as an oral hygiene agent, 274, 280, 281
saliva
production of sufficient, 273
synthetic as an oral hygiene agent, 275, 280

sarcoma neoplasms causing malignant pleural effusions,
115
Savlodil, 28, 29, 31, 80, 287, 344, 395, 396, 499, 450
scalp cooling, 367-370
guidelines for, 368, 369
ice phobia following, 368, 370
inadequate, 367
scalp tourniquet, 367
scapulae, 44
sciatic nerve & intramuscular injections, 138
sclera, 162, 163
sclerosing agents in pleural space, 115, 116
scopalamine, 169
scrub, preoperative, 9
scrub, surgical, 9
seborrhoeic blepharitis, 168
sedated patients, heavily, & Entonox contraindicated,
157
sediment from infection, removal & bladder lavage, 25
seizures causing unconsciousness, 439
self-poisoning & gastric lavage, 176, 177
sensory functions, 296, 299
sepsis as hazard of catheter insertion, 94
septicaemia 22, 23, 42, 209, 225, 227
& postoperative care, 338
serology for syphilis, 267
shaving, preoperative, 330, 332
shearing & pressure sores, 340
shock
& central venous catheterization, 92
in peritoneal dialysis & pulse change, 322
speed, & intravenous drug administration, 208, 228
syndrome, 4, 42
short bowel syndrome, 283
sigmoidoscopy & Entonox, 157
Sikhs, religious requirements for on death, 249
sinus arrhythmia, 353
Sjörgen's system, 169
skeletal traction, 432, 433, 435, 436
skin
barriers for stoma patients, 390, 391
flora, resident, 7
preparation for venepuncture, 462
traction, 432, 434, 435
skull
traction, 432
sliding traction, 431
smallpox & formaldehyde for terminal disinfection, 15
soap & water in handwashing, drawbacks of, 7, 14
sodium bicarbonate
& correction of acidosis in cardiac arrest, 84
as an oral hygiene agent, 274, 280
solution administered intravenously, 209
solvent drag effect, 318
specimen collection 371-380
documentation for, 372
guidelines for, 374-380
specimens
of fluid for analysis & abdominal paracentesis, 1
necessary quantities, 371
transportation of, 372, 373
sphygomanometer, 37, 38, 40, 42, 43
spinal
canal, 265, 266
cord, 264, 265, 266
degenerative & globulin level in cerebrospinal fluid,
267
suspected compression, 264
joint disease, degenerative, 264
stress during lifting, 251, 252, 254, 255, 256
spinous processes, 265, 269

spleen, 2
sputum, 376
staphylococcus aureus, 7, 13, 22, 23
staphylococcus epidermis, 21
sterile supplies department, central, 7
sterile water, as a bladder washout, 26
sternal angle & reading central venous pressure, 96, 98, 109
sternum, 44, 45
steroids, 167, 243
stimulus to defaecate, 50
Stockholm applicator & treatment of carcinoma of the body of the uterus & the cervix, 74
stoma, 190, 191
  ability to manage a, 385, 386
  appliances & accessories, 388, 389, 390, 391, 392
  care, 381-398
    guidelines for, 393, 394, 395, 396, 397, 398
  patient, postoperative period for, 387, 388
  in tracheostomy, 419
  surgery, preoperative preparation for, 383, 384
stomach, 2
stomatitis, help prevent & mouth care, 273, 274, 275, 280, 281
stool softening
& dioctyl sulphosuccinate enema, 55
  laxatives, 53
stretch receptors, 35
strychnine, 177
stupor & levels of consciousness, 297
subclavian vein as catheterization site, 92, 93
suction pump, Robert's, 1976, 197
sulphaecetamide, 168
  solution prone to deterioration, 138
suppositories
  administration of, equipment for, 65
  contraindications, 56,57
  procedure for administration of, 66, 67
  & short-term management of constipation, 50
  uses of, 56
suprarenal glands, stimulation of & salt & water retention, 35
surgery
  enema used to clean lower bowel prior to, 54
  major & central venous catheterization, 92
  phosphate enema prior to, 55
surgical
  ablation of the pleural space, 115
  drain
    dressing, 406, 407, 408, 409
    removal of, 407, 408, 411
    shortening, 409, 410
    types of, 402
  incision, recent & aseptic technique, 6
  wounds & drains, 399-411
suspensory ligament of the lens, 162
sutures, removal of from sensitive areas & entonox, 157
suxamethonium solution, prone to deterioration, 138
swabbing, 276, 280
Swedish nose, laryngectomy & humidification, 190
syphilis, serology for, 267
systemic drugs, common toxic effects of on the eye, 168, 169
systolic pressure, 36, 38, 39, 41, 43

tachycardia, causes of, 227, 352
tachypnoea, 362
  & catheter insertion, 108
talc powderage as sclerosing agent in pleural space, 116
tamoxifen, 169
temperature

body, 412-418
  enema used to decrease, 55
  guidelines for recording, 415, 416
  liver & maintenance of, 259
  recording sites
    axilla, 41
    oral, 412
    rectal, 412, 413
  & vital signs, 299
temporal pulse site, 351, 352
tension pneumothorax, 201, 203
terminal disinfection in barrier nursing, 15
tetracyclin as sclerosing agent in pleural space, 116
tetraiodothyronine, 233
therapy room for iodine [131], 232, 233
thermometer
  electronic, 413, 141
  mercury in glass, 413, 414
thiotepa, 116
Thomas's splint, 431
thoracentesis, repeated, 115
thoracic
  cavity, 192
    pressure in, 192, 193, 198, 356
  duct trauma as hazard of catheter insertion, 94
  wall,192
throat swab, 376, 377
thrombocytopenia,
thrombosis
  as a hazard of catheter insertion, 94
  prevention of & intrenous drug administration, 208
  risk of deep vein & postoperative care, 337
thyroid
  cancers, 229
    follicular, 229
    papillary, 229
  gland, 229
  stimulating hormone, injections of, 233
  treatment programme for carcinoma of, 229, 230
thyrotoxicosis, 229, 355
thyroxine, 233
tibial pulse site, 351, 352
tidal volume of air breathed, 358, 359
tissue death in pressure sores from anoxia, 339
tongue lesions, iridium [192], treatment for, 239
toothbrushes, 276, 277, 278, 279, 281
toxic effects of common systemic drugs on the eye, 168, 169
toxins storage conditions for, 136
toxoids, storage conditions for, 136
trachea, 192, 419
tracheostomy
  care, 419-429
  dressing, changing, 423, 424
  emergency, 420
  humidification indicated after, 189
  mask & Ohio nebulizer, 189
  patients & suction, 424, 425
  permanent, 419, 420
    tubes for, 421, 422, 423
  reasons indicated, 419
  Roger's spray & humidification, 190, 191, 424
  temporary, 420
    tubes for, 421
  tube
    & blower humidifier, 189
    changing, 426, 427
    tubes for, 420, 421, 422, 423
traction, 430-437
  patient care, principles of, 433, 434
  reasons indicated, 430

transplant units & hepititis B, need for screening for, 183
transudate fluid, 115
transversus abdominis, 258
trauma
  & cardiac arrest, 84
  humidification indicated in, 189
Trendelenburg position, 93, 94, 108
Triclosan, 9
triiodothyronine, 233
trocar puncture to peritoneum, 320, 321, 323
tube thoracostomy, 115, 123
tumours
  of central nervous system & cells in cerebrospinal fluid, 267, 270
  & constipation, 51
  large, in rectum of sigmoid colon, & rectal lavage contraindicated, 59
  oral & caesium¹³⁷ implantation, 72
ulcerative colitis & stoma, 383
ulnar pulse site, 351, 352
unconscious patient 438-445
  guidelines for care of, 440, 441, 442, 443, 444, 445
unconsciousness
  causes of, 439
  indications of, 438
undertakers, 247
uraemia, 286
uraemic toxins, 317, ,318
ureterostomy, 382
urinary
  bladder, removal of contaminated material from, 25
  infection, 82
    bladder lavage & prevention of spread, 25,
urine
  catheter specimen of, 380,454, 455
  ilieal conduit, specimen from, 380, 395, 396
  midstream specimen
    female, 80
    male, 379
  solute concentration, monitoring patient's, 286
  specimens of, 379, 380
urostomy, 382
  a diet, 284
  specimen, 397, 398
uterus, anterior & posterior surfaces of, 2

Vagina
  fungal infection of in neutropenia, 22
  irradiation of whole & Dobbie applicator, 76
vaginal swab, 378
vagus nerve, 35, 361
Valsalva manoeuvre, 93, 94, 103, 109
vascular
  causes of inconsciousness, 439
  factors & pressure sores, 340
  irritation, 209
  pressure, 35
  space, movement of fluid from, 1,4
Vaseline as an oral hygiene agent, 276, 279, 280
vasoconstrictor tone in the peripheral blood vessels, release of, 35
vasodilatation, 4
vasometer centre in the medulla oblongata, 35
vena cava, superior & inferior, 92, 95, 259
venepuncture, 374, 459-470
  choice of device for, 462, 463
  criteria for choosing site for, 460, 461, 462
  guidelines for, 464, 465, 466, 467, 468, 469, 470
venous tone & central venous pressure, 96
Ventimask & oxygen therapy, 308, 309, 313

ventilation, 356, 358
ventricular fibrillation, left, reduction of & aminophylline, 84
vertebra, sacral, 265
vertebrae, 44, 265
vertebral venous plexus, 266
violence
  & its causes, 471, 472
  follow-up after incidents of, 473
  & management of personnel involved, 480, 481
  & its management, 471-481
violent
  patients, care of, 472, 473, 474
  behaviour, predisposition to, 472
viral
  illnesses, prodromal phase of, 373
  investigations of specimens, 373
  vaccines, storage conditions for, 136
visceral
  peritoneum, 2, 317
  pleura, 192, 194, 356
visitors & barrier nursing, 15, 16, 24
vital
  capacity, 359
  signs, 296, 299
vitamins
  B & K synthesized in colon by bacterial flora, 49
  C levels, low, & pressure sores, 340, 349
  fat soluble & repetitive use of liquid paraffin, 53
  storage & liver, 259
vitreous humour, 162, 164
vomiting in iodine¹³¹ patients, emergency procedures for, 237

ward, organization of & management of violence, 473
warfarin, 111
waster handling in barrier nursing, 15
water
  in flower vases, a source of infection, 9, 13
  intoxication, 60
weight & pulleys for traction, 431
white blood cell count, 124
whole gut irrigation vs suppositories, 57
whooping cough, specimen collection for, 376
wound
  healing, delaying factors of, 345
  infection, 6
  swab, 378
wounds
  clean, 399
  clean contaminated, 399
  clean & with exudate, 403
  clean & without exudate, 402, 403
  complex, 399
  contaminated, 400
  dehiscent & with copious exudate, 405, 406
  dehiscent & with minimal exudate, 404
  dirty, 400
  order for dressing clean & contaminated, 9, 11
  repair, Westaby's stages of, 400, 401
  simple, 399

X-ray examination
  with contrasting medium of bowel, enema prior to, 54
  phosphate enema prior to, 55
  of bowel using braium & constipation, 51
X-ray therapy to pelvis, deep, rectal lavage contraindicated with previous, 59

Zinc deficiencies & pressures sores, 340